To Dr. Phil Routledge

With grateful thanks for all your —

John W. Thompson.

Robin Seymour

John Walton

OXFORD MEDICAL PUBLICATIONS

TEXTBOOK OF
DENTAL PHARMACOLOGY AND THERAPEUTICS

TEXTBOOK OF
DENTAL PHARMACOLOGY
AND THERAPEUTICS

•

JOHN G. WALTON
JOHN W. THOMPSON
AND
ROBIN A. SEYMOUR

Oxford   New York   Tokyo
OXFORD UNIVERSITY PRESS
1989

Oxford University Press, Walton Street, Oxford OX2 6DP

Oxford New York Toronto
Delhi Bombay Calcutta Madras Karachi
Petaling Jaya Singapore Hong Kong Tokyo
Nairobi Dar es Salaam Cape Town
Melbourne Auckland

and associated companies in
Berlin Ibadan

Oxford is a trade mark of Oxford University Press

Published in the United States
by Oxford University Press, New York

British Library Cataloguing in Publication Data
Walton, J.G.
Textbook of dental pharmacology and
therapeutics
1. Dentistry
I. Title.   II. Thompson, John W.
III. Seymour, Robin A.
617.6
ISBN 0-19-261823-7
ISBN 0-19-261235-2 (Pbk)

Library of Congress Cataloging in Publication Data
Walton, J. G.
Textbook of dental pharmacology and therapeutics/J.G. Walton,
John W. Thompson, and Robin A. Seymour.
(Oxford medical publications)
Includes bibliographies and index.
1. Pharmacology.   2. Dentistry.   I. Thompson, John W. (John Warburton)
II. Seymour, R. A.   III. Title.   IV. Series.
[DNLM: 1. Dentistry.   2. Pharmacology.   QV 50 W239t]
RM300.W36   1989   615'.1—dc19   88-28909 CIP
ISBN 0-19-261823-7
ISBN-0-19-261235-2 (pbk.)

Typeset by Cotswold Typesetting Ltd, Gloucester
Printed in Great Britain
at the University Printing House, Oxford
by David Stanford
Printer to the University

FOREWORD

ROY STORER

Dean of Dentistry, University of Newcastle upon Tyne

THOSE conversant with the publications on Dental Pharmacology will recall the highly successful British Dental Journal booklet entitled *Pharmacology for the Dental Practitioner* by Mr John Walton and Professor John Thompson. They have been joined by Dr Robin Seymour in this textbook which is an expansion of that earlier publication. John Walton has been lecturing to dental students on pharmacology since 1960 and John Thompson began his academic career in medical pharmacology by presenting a course to dental students. Robin Seymour is a more recent addition to the Newcastle team and he has developed a particular interest in analgesics. The three authors have encouraged others in the Sub-Faculty of Dentistry at Newcastle to participate in research in the pharmacological field and the projects will be a valuable contribution to pharmacology in relation to dentistry, which is emerging as a specialist subject within the dental curriculum.

In this book, the authors have not only dealt with, in appropriate detail, those drugs used by the dentist but also those the dentist is likely to encounter in patients who are receiving medication from their medical practitioners.

As an increasing proportion of the population move into the elderly category, it is likely that more of those who seek dental health care will be on long-term medication. Therefore it is very important that the dental practitioner should have 'a thorough understanding of the principles of pharmacology so that he can anticipate drug interactions, allergies, incompatibilities, side effects, and other dangers.' (An Inquiry into Dental Education—A Report to the Nuffield Foundation, 1980, The Nuffield Foundation, London).

The chapter on Emergencies in Dental Practice is based on the authors' annual postgraduate course for dental practitioners in the Northern Region, which must be one of the most successful of its kind.

This book will be appreciated by undergraduates, by those studying for higher diplomas, and, not least, by general dental practitioners who, in the provision of whole mouth care for their patients, will be better able to deal with those who are on complex medication.

March 1988

PREFACE

OVER the past 30 years or so the subject of pharmacology has developed explosively with the result that there are now many groups of potent drugs used for the treatment of disease. This has had two important consequences for dentistry. First, a number of the newer drugs have found important roles in dental treatment. Second, many patients who attend for dental treatment are taking drugs for the treatment of medical conditions and it is therefore important for the dentist to be aware of this fact and to be fully conversant with the pharmacology and rationale behind the use of these drugs. Furthermore, it is obviously important for the dentist to be aware of the unwanted effects that may be produced by the drugs prescribed, some directly concerned with the mouth. Of equal importance is the need to know about possible interactions that might occur (and must therefore be avoided) in the event that the dental practitioner prescribes one or more drugs for dental treatment that have the potential to interact with those already being taken by the patient for medical reasons. Thus the need for the present-day dental student and dental practitioner to have a sound working knowledge of pharmacology and therapeutics is a pressing one, and this book has been written to meet these needs.

The book is divided into two sections. The first deals with general pharmacological principles together with those drugs that are part of the day-to-day pharmacological armamentarium of the dental practitioner. The second part deals with the pharmacology and therapeutics related to drugs which, although unlikely to be prescribed by the dental practitioner, are nevertheless of considerable importance for reasons already given.

This book is based on an earlier and much shorter book entitled *Pharmacology for the Dental Practitioner*, which was written by two of the authors of the present book (J.G.W. and J.W.T.). That original book has now been expanded into a comprehensive textbook for dental students and dental practitioners and, in tackling this difficult and lengthy task, the original authors have had the good fortune to acquire the invaluable help of Dr Robin Seymour, who has for some time assisted his colleagues in the teaching of pharmacology to dental students.

The authors are grateful to many colleagues and others who have willingly helped in various ways, and the names of these individuals are listed in the Acknowledgements. However, the authors alone are responsible for any errors of omission or commission that are to be found in this book. Furthermore, they would be most grateful to any reader who takes the trouble to point out mistakes or to make suggestions for a further edition.

Newcastle upon Tyne
February 1988

J.G.W.
J.W.T.
R.A.S.

ACKNOWLEDGEMENTS

The authors gratefully acknowledge the generous help and assistance they have had from colleagues in the preparation of this book. Those who have kindly read, and constructively criticized various chapters or sections of the text include Dr Heather Ashton, Professor R. W. F. Campbell, Dr T. S. J. Elliott, Professor B. T. Golding, Professor C. J. Hull, Professor M. D. Rawlins, Dr P. A. Routledge, and Mr A. K. Watson (Astra Laboratories). They also wish to acknowledge the valuable help given by the Audio Visual Centre and the Medical and Dental Library of the University of Newcastle upon Tyne. They are deeply indebted to Mrs Margaret Cheek for her tireless work in typing the seemingly endless drafts and also for her conscientious and painstaking labours concerned with the bibliography of this book. The help and forbearance of the staff of Oxford University Press is gratefully acknowledged. Finally, the authors wish to thank Mrs Judith Thompson for her help in preparing the index.

FIGURE AND TABLE ACKNOWLEDGEMENTS

The authors of this book wish to thank the following authors, editors, and publishers for kindly granting permission to reproduce published material as indicated.

Fig. 1.1: Adapted from Fig. 1.1 on p. 5, Grahame-Smith, D. G. and Aronson, J. K. (1984). *Oxford Textbook of Clinical Pharmacology and Drug Therapy*. Oxford University Press, Oxford. **Fig. 1.4**: Redrawn from Fig. 1, p. 201, Brodie, B. B. (1964). *Absorption and Distribution of Drugs*, (ed. T. B. Binns). Livingstone, Edinburgh. **Figs. 1.5 and 1.6**: Based partly on Fig. 2, p. 37, Gillette, J. R. (1967). In, *Drug Responses in Man*. (eds. G. Wolstenholme and R. Porter). Churchill, London. Based partly on Fig. 1, p. 17, Brodie, B. B. (1964). *Absorption and Distribution of Drugs*, (ed. T. B. Binns). Livingstone, Edinburgh. **Fig. 1.7(b)**: Fig. 1, p. 995, Drew, G. C., Colquhoun, W. P., and Long, H. A. (1958). Effects of small doses of alcohol on skill resembling driving. *British Medical Journal*, **2**, 993–9. **Fig. 1.9**: Fig. 2.2, p. 22, Creasey, W. A. (1979). *Drug Disposition in Humans*. Oxford University Press, Oxford. **Fig. 1.10(a and b)**: Fig. 13.8, p. 189, Rowland, M. and Tozer, T. N. (1980). *Clinical Pharmacokinetics: Concepts and Applications*. Lea and Febiger, Philadelphia. **Fig. 1.12**: Fig. 3–10, p. 27, Schild, H. O. (1980). *Applied Pharmacology*. Churchill Livingstone, Edinburgh. **Tables 1.3 and 1.4**: Adapted from Table I, p. 453. Lefkowitz, R. J. (1979). Direct binding studies of adrenergic receptors: biochemical, physiologic and clinical implications. *Annals of Internal Medicine*, **91**, 450–8. Table II, pp. 68 and 88. Lefkowitz, R. J. and Hofman, R. J. (1981). New directions in adrenergic receptor research. Parts I and II. In, *Towards Understanding Receptors*, (ed. J. W. Lamble). Elsevier/North Holland, Amsterdam. **Table 1.5**: Adapted from Fig. 1, p. 228, Koch-Weser, J. (1972). Serum drug concentrations as therapeutic guides. *New England Journal of Medicine*, **287**, 227–31. **Fig. 6.1**: Thompson, J. W. (1984). Pain: mechanisms and principles of management. In, *Advanced Geriatric Medicine 4* (ed. J. Grimley Evans). Pitman, London. **Fig. 13.1**: Adapted from Fig. 8–16, p. 25, Schmidt, R. F. (ed.) (1978). *Neurophysiology*. Springer-Verlag, New York, Heidelberg, Berlin. **Fig. 13.3**: Wilson, A. and Schild, H. O. (1968) *Applied*

Pharmacology, (10th edn), p. 77. Churchill, London. **Fig. 13.5**: After Axelrod, J. (1960). *Proceedings of the 2nd International Pharmacology Meeting*. Churchill Livingstone, Edinburgh. **Figs. 15.1 and 15.2**: Adapted from Fig. 11.1, p. 141. Noble, D. (1975). *The initiation of the heart beat*. Oxford University Press, Oxford. **Fig. 21.3**: Drawn from data of Kalow, W. and Gunn, D. R. (1957). *Journal of Pharmacology*, **120**, 203.

CONTENTS

PART II · GENERAL DRUGS

1

General principles of drug action

THE word 'pharmacology' means nothing more nor less than the study of the effects of chemical substances upon living tissues; it is derived from two Greek words; *pharmakon*, drug; *logos*, study. Living cells, tissues, and organs consist of biological systems and a chemical substance that is capable of modifying a biological system in a relatively selective way is known as a drug. Whilst many chemical substances could be said to fall into this category, only a small proportion of them are sufficiently selective and safe to use for the prevention or treatment of disease or, in other words, as therapeutic agents. For example, phenol and many other chemical substances when applied to nerves can block impulse transmission but cannot be used for this purpose routinely because they cause irreversible damage to nerve tissue. The actual number of clinically acceptable local anaesthetics used by the average dental practitioner can be counted on the fingers of one hand.

The rapid increase in the number of new drugs during the past quarter century has been aptly described as the 'drug explosion'. Prior to this, the number of drugs of real value was very small; there were many virtually useless preparations but they did not do much harm even if they did not do much good! Today, the situation is vastly different; a bewildering and ever-increasing number of new and powerful drugs is available for therapeutic use. The subject of pharmacology has developed at a phenomenal pace, particularly when one considers that it was only in the 1930s that it crystallized out as a separate subject from related disciplines such as physiology and chemistry (Paton 1963). Pharmacology has received its greatest impetus from progress made in the field of synthetic organic chemistry and the momentum has been maintained by the ever-present need for chemical substances that can be used to prevent or control disease.

The dental practitioner, in the same way as the medical practitioner, is faced with the problem of keeping abreast of developments in pharmacology and therapeutics. In order to use drugs rationally, it is important to understand the basic principles of drug action. The clarification of old ideas of drug action coupled with the discovery of new mechanisms have made it possible to begin to interpret the effects of drugs in terms of molecular events governed by physico-chemical laws. The stage has therefore been reached when it is now possible to enumerate the different processes involved in the absorption, distribution, mechanism of action, fate, and excretion of drugs. Furthermore, it is in the study of the mechanism of drug action that major progress has been achieved. Sufficient knowledge is now available to make it possible, in many instances, to present a coherent account of the action of a drug. It is the authors' fervent belief that the administration of any drug, irrespective of type and route, should always be carried out with these principles constantly in mind. Drugs will come and drugs will go; but basic principles will always remain even though these may be modified and extended as new knowledge becomes available.

The dental practitioner most commonly applies drugs locally; much less often is he or she concerned with their systemic administration, with the exception of analgesics, antibiotics, and drugs used for sedation. Nevertheless, many of the same pharmacological principles apply whether the drugs are used systemically or locally. When a drug is given locally, some proportion of the total dose will be absorbed into the general circulation, the amount depending upon the drug, the dose, and the area to which it is applied. It is possible therefore that under certain conditions, local application of a drug may be followed by undesirable systemic effects. Today, many patients who come to the dental surgery are already taking drugs prescribed by their medical practitioners or even by themselves. The dental surgeon should always be aware of the risk of a drug interaction between the drug(s) to be prescribed and those the patient is already taking. Thus, the problem of drug interaction is another reason why the dental practitioner needs to be conversant with the general principles of drug action. This is also an appropriate moment to remind ourselves of a particularly important point, namely, that to the layman the word 'drug' usually means something different from that understood by the prescriber. Furthermore, in the mind of the average patient, there is often a vast difference between the meanings of the words 'drug', 'pill', 'tablet', 'medicine', and 'mixture'. If this is not appreciated by the practitioner the fact that a particular patient is under the influence of a powerful drug may be missed to their possible detriment.

SOURCE OF DRUGS

In the past, drugs were obtained from natural sources and some of the most important drugs are still derived in this way. For example, insulin is obtained from the pancreas of cattle or pigs; digitalis from certain species of the foxglove plant; and iron, commonly used in the form of ferrous sulphate, is derived from mineral sources. Nevertheless, today, the majority of drugs are synthesized by chemists and every year many thousands of new compounds are made and screened for possible use as drugs. Table 1.1 indicates the stages involved in the development of a drug (Thompson 1967; Goldberg and Griffin 1984; M. D. Rawlins, personal communication). It also shows the points at which the Committee on Safety of Medicines operate in order to weigh the evidence about new drugs submitted to it by the pharmaceutical industry and by the dental and medical professions, so that

Table 1.1. Development of a drug

Principal individual(s) concerned	Stages in the development of a drug	Regulatory involvement
Various	Ideas	
Chemist	Natural or synthetic chemical compounds	
Pharmacologist Biochemist	Pharmacological tests including: pharmacodynamics $\Big\}$ in animals pharmacokinetics	
Toxicologist	Acute toxicity (e.g. LD_{50}) Chronic toxicity tests including: studies on two species of animals, one rodent and the other non-rodent Reproduction toxicity (fertility and reproduction teratogenesis, fetal and embryological toxicology) Mutagenicity Carcinogenicity	
Pharmacist	Pharmaceutical formulation Clinical trials	
Clinical pharmacologist Normal volunteers	Phase 1: a pilot investigation made in a small number of normal volunteers	
Dentist/Doctor Clinical pharmacologist Nurse Patients Statistician	Phase 2: an 'open' clinical trial carried out in a small number of patients Phase 3: large-scale clinical trial (double blind)	Clinical trial certificate (or clinical trial exemption) required
Practising dentists/doctors and their patients	Phase 4: monitored release and post-marketing surveillance of new drug	Product licence required Post-marketing surveillance
	Accepted drug	For unforeseen reasons, usually toxicological, it may prove necessary to withdraw a drug at any time

it can act as an independent assessor. As can be seen from Table 1.1, the development of a drug is a long and complicated process involving many stages and many individuals.

CLASSIFICATION OF DRUGS

The most logical way to classify drugs would be according to their mechanism of action, but this is not yet feasible because for many drugs this information is still incomplete. One of the largest areas where knowledge is lacking concerns drugs which act on the central nervous system, a situation which is slowly improving as new knowledge becomes available about the biochemistry and pharmacology of the brain.

At present, the most practical way to classify drugs is according to their main site(s) of action and this is the method adopted by (see Chapter 3) the *British National Formulary* and also by the *Dental Practitioner's Formulary* (a joint publication of the British Dental Association, the British Medical Association, and The Pharmaceutical Society of Great Britain).

MODE OF ACTION OF DRUGS

The subject of pharmacology exists because a large number of substances exert a selective action, so modifying the behaviour of some cells or tissues more than others. Indeed, were it not for selective action, it would be impossible to use chemical substances therapeutically. Unfortunately, with many of the drugs at present available, the degree of selective action is less than is desirable, so that in order to produce the required effect it may be necessary to use a dose that also gives rise to certain unwanted actions. In some instances these are of trivial inconvenience to the patient but in others, unwanted effects of a more serious nature may occur. Pharmacologists, particularly those in the pharmaceutical industry, are constantly striving to produce drugs that exert a higher degree of selective action than existing drugs of the same type. However, it is likely to be a long time before the majority of drugs available exert such a high degree of selective action that they are incapable of producing any unwanted effects.

THE PROCESSES OF DRUG THERAPY

Four main processes are involved in drug therapy:

(1) the pharmaceutical process;
(2) the pharmacokinetic process;
(3) the pharmacodynamic process;
(4) the therapeutic process.

As has been pointed out by Grahame-Smith and Aronson (1984), each of these four processes can be formulated as a simple question:

(1) Is the drug getting into the patient?
(2) Is the drug getting to its site of action?
(3) Is the drug producing the required pharmacological effect?
(4) Is the pharmacological effect being translated into a therapeutic effect?

These closely interrelated processes will now be discussed in detail and Fig. 1.1 illustrates them diagrammatically.

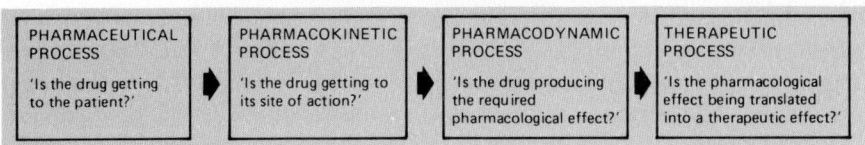

Fig. 1.1. Processes involved in drug therapy. (Grahame-Smith and Aronson 1984.)

THE PHARMACEUTICAL PROCESS:
IS THE DRUG GETTING INTO THE PATIENT?

The fundamental importance of the pharmaceutical formulation and presentation of a drug is often insufficiently appreciated. Thus, an oral preparation of the most powerful drug would be useless if, through a faulty formulation, it failed to disintegrate on contact with the gastro-intestinal contents and therefore was not absorbed. Likewise, the injection of a preparation of local anaesthetic would be not only fruitless but positively dangerous if it had been formulated in an insoluble form. Scant attention and thought is given to the enormous amount of time and effort taken to produce a formulation and presentation that meets, as far as possible, the needs of the patient and of the clinician. Although the pharmaceutical process is mainly the concern of the pharmaceutical chemist and the pharmacist, the dental practitioner should take an intelligent interest in the subject for the good of the patient. Occasionally, therapeutic problems arise with respect to a particular drug or patient and these may be due to a formulation problem concerned with the particle size, excipients, and coating materials used in the preparation of a drug. The outbreaks of toxicity from digoxin and phenytoin in the late 1960s and early 1970s are striking and important examples of this type of problem (for further details see Tyrer *et al.* 1970; Smith and Dodd 1982).

Drug compliance

It should be remembered that the simplest cause of an apparent therapeutic failure is because the patient has failed to take an adequate quantity of the drug! This may be unintentional, for example, where they have misunderstood the directions; or it may be due to a wilful determination on their part not to take the drug. It should also be noted that for a given patient the greater the number of drugs prescribed the less likely are these to be taken correctly.

THE PHARMACOKINETIC PROCESS:
IS THE DRUG GETTING TO ITS SITE OF ACTION?

Pharmacokinetics is concerned with the absorption, distribution, and elimination (by means of metabolism and excretion) of drugs. The term 'pharmacokinetics' was introduced by Dost (1953) and is concerned with the mathematical analysis of the time course of drug absorption, distribution, metabolism, and excretion. After oral administration of a drug, a given fraction is absorbed and the amount of drug in the body at any moment depends upon the balance between the rate of absorption and the rate of elimination.

Factors governing the fate of a drug in the body

Whether a drug is applied locally or is administered systemically, there are four main factors that determine its subsequent fate in the body:

(1) molecular weight;

(2) chemical stability;

(3) lipid solubility;

(4) degree of ionization.

Each drug has its own characteristic profile of these factors, which may be conveniently termed its physico-chemical profile. This topic will now be discussed in more detail.

Molecular weight (MW)

Substances with a high molecular weight are not usually absorbed intact except in minute quantities. Moreover, they may be altered by enzymatic action so that following oral administration, proteins, for example, will be broken down to their constituent amino acids. Thus insulin, which is a protein, undergoes enzymatic breakdown in the gastro-intestinal tract and is, for practical purposes, not absorbed.

Chemical stability

Unstable drugs may be inactivated in the gastro-intestinal tract. Benzylpenicillin is unstable in an acid medium and therefore cannot be relied upon to produce satisfactory results if given by mouth because a high proportion of the original dose is rendered inactive by the acid contents of the stomach. Phenoxymethyl-penicillin is more stable in an acid medium than benzylpenicillin so that adequate doses given by mouth are therapeutically effective.

Lipid solubility

If a drug is to be absorbed from any part of the gastro-intestinal tract, including the mouth, it is necessary for it to pass through cell membranes. Thus, it must first pass through the cells of the mucous membrane of the gastro-intestinal tract and thence into the circulation either directly via the capillary walls or indirectly via the lymphatic drainage of the area. As cell membranes are lipid in nature, the degree and rate of penetration of them by a drug is dependent to a large extent on its lipid solubility (for a more detailed discussion on this topic see below and Chapter 7).

Degree of ionization

Under physiological conditions some substances, such as ethanol (ethyl alcohol), are un-ionized whilst others, for example acetylcholine, are highly ionized. The important fact is that the majority of drugs are weak bases or weak acids so that at a physiological pH (7.4) they exist partly in the un-ionized form and partly in the ionized form, the proportion of each form varying with the environmental pH. At a particular pH, the proportion of un-ionized to ionized molecules of a drug depends upon its dissociation constant (K_a; $-\log K_a = pK_a$). The pH, pK_a, and ratio of un-ionized to ionized molecules are related by the Henderson–Hasselbach equation as follows:

$$\text{For acids, pH} = pK_a - \log_{10} \frac{\text{un-ionized acid}}{\text{ionized acid}}$$

$$= pK_a - \log_{10} \frac{[AH]}{[A^-]}.$$

$$\text{For bases, pH} = pK_a - \log_{10} \frac{\text{ionized base}}{\text{un-ionized base}}$$

$$= pK_a - \log_{10} \frac{[BH^+]}{[B]}.$$

Where pK_a is the dissociation constant expressed as its negative logarithm to base 10; pH, the concentration of hydrogen ions in the solution expressed as the negative logarithm to base 10; [AH], concentration of un-ionized acid; [A$^-$], concentration of ionized acid; [BH$^+$] concentration of ionized base; [B] concentration of un-ionized base.

The fundamental and important relationship between the degree of drug ionization and drug absorption is that the un-ionized portion of a drug is lipid soluble and so readily absorbed (see later under Cell membranes) whereas the ionized portion is lipid insoluble and so very poorly absorbed.

The physico-chemical profile of a drug (i.e. the molecular weight (MW), chemical stability, lipid solubility, and degree of ionization) principally governs its fate in the body. We must now consider the processes involved in the absorption of drugs. This can be put in the form of a question: how do drugs cross the cell membrane? In order to answer this question the structure of cell membrane itself must first be examined.

The cell membrane

Various studies have shown that the plasma membrane of mammalian cells consists of three principal organic components, which are arranged as shown in Fig. 1.2. The major part of the plasma membrane consists of a double-layer of lipid

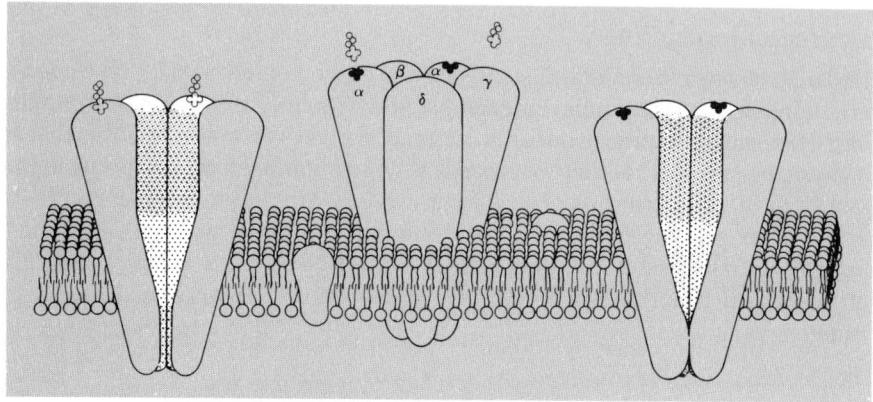

Fig. 1.2. Model of cell membrane with acetylcholine receptor (nicotinic type). Note the following: (i) The cell membrane consists of a double layer of lipid molecules orientated with hydrophilic groups situated at inner and outer surfaces, and hydrophobic portions occupying the inner and central part. (ii) Integral protein occupies the full width of the membrane. (iii) Middle of figure shows reconstruction of acetylcholine receptor and associated ion channel consisting of five protein subunits: alpha (α) (two), beta (β), gamma (γ), and delta (δ), which surround a central pore. Acetylcholine binds to the α subunits and two molecules of acetylcholine must bind in order to open the channel. *Right channel:* closed because two molecules of acetylcholine have not yet occupied the receptors. *Left channel:* open in response to occupation of both receptors by molecules of acetylcholine.

molecules orientated so that their hydrophilic groups are situated at the inner and outer surfaces of the membrane, whilst their hydrophobic portions, which consist of hydrocarbon chains, occupy the inner and central part.

Proteins also form an important component of the plasma membrane and are present in two forms:

(1) integral protein, which occupies the full width of the cell membrane;

(2) peripheral protein, which is attached either to the integral protein on the inner aspect of the membrane or attached to the hydrophilic ends of the lipids at the external or internal surfaces.

In addition, several varieties of glycoproteins or glycolipids may be attached to the integral protein or hydrophilic lipid, respectively, on the external surface of the plasma membrane.

It is important to note that the cell plasma membrane is not a fixed structure but a dynamic one in which the various components are mobile. The membrane contains membrane-bound water that interacts with ionized groups and thus forms a barrier to the diffusion of water-soluble agents. The membrane is asymmetrical both structurally and electrically; it also contains pores formed both within the membrane of an individual cell and between the membranes of adjacent cells. As a consequence, substances (including drugs) with a molecular weight not exceeding 100 daltons are able to diffuse freely across the membrane (see next section). The external surface of the membrane also contains pharmacological receptors (described later). These are linked with intracellular mechanisms that can thus be switched on or off by the interaction of appropriate drug molecules with the membrane receptors. For general references on the structure of the cell membrane see Houslay and Stanley (1982).

The principal mechanisms involved in the passage of drugs across cell membranes

A drug is unlikely to be absorbed unless it is able to go into solution. For example, barium ions are very poisonous but barium sulphate can be used safely in radiology as a contrast agent because it is highly *insoluble*.

Pharmaceutical formulations of a drug can greatly influence the amount and rate at which it is absorbed. The rate at which acetylsalicylic acid (aspirin) is absorbed and the maximum plasma concentration attained varies widely according to the formulation used. In one study (Leonards 1963), effervescent aspirin (0.6 g) caused more than double the plasma level produced by an equivalent dose of ordinary aspirin (both measured after 30 minutes). However, when the same dose of ordinary aspirin was given in hot water it resulted in a plasma concentration almost as high as that attained with the effervescent preparation. Sometimes tablets or capsules may fail to disintegrate so that absorption cannot take place. Under these circumstances, the absence of a therapeutic effect may be wrongly attributed to other factors such as too small a dose or failure of the patient to take the medicine.

Lipid diffusion

Figure 1.3 illustrates diagrammatically the principal mechahisms involved in absorption of drugs, for example from the gastro-intestinal tract (Brodie 1964; Smyth 1964; Gilette 1967). The majority of drugs cross membranes by lipid diffusion (simple diffusion) at a rate related to their lipid solubility or, to be more exact, to their lipid/water partition coefficient. The rate can be expressed by Fick's law, which states that:

$$m = \frac{PA(C_o - C_i)t}{W}.$$

Where m = amount of unchanged molecule diffusing passively through an area; A = area of cell membrane over which diffusion is under consideration; t = time over which diffusion takes place; C_o = concentration of solute on outer side of membrane; C_i = concentration of solute on inner side of membrane; P = permeability constant; W = thickness of cell membrane.

A lipid-soluble non-electrolyte is readily absorbed whilst a lipid-insoluble non-electrolyte will only be absorbed exceedingly slowly. As noted earlier, the

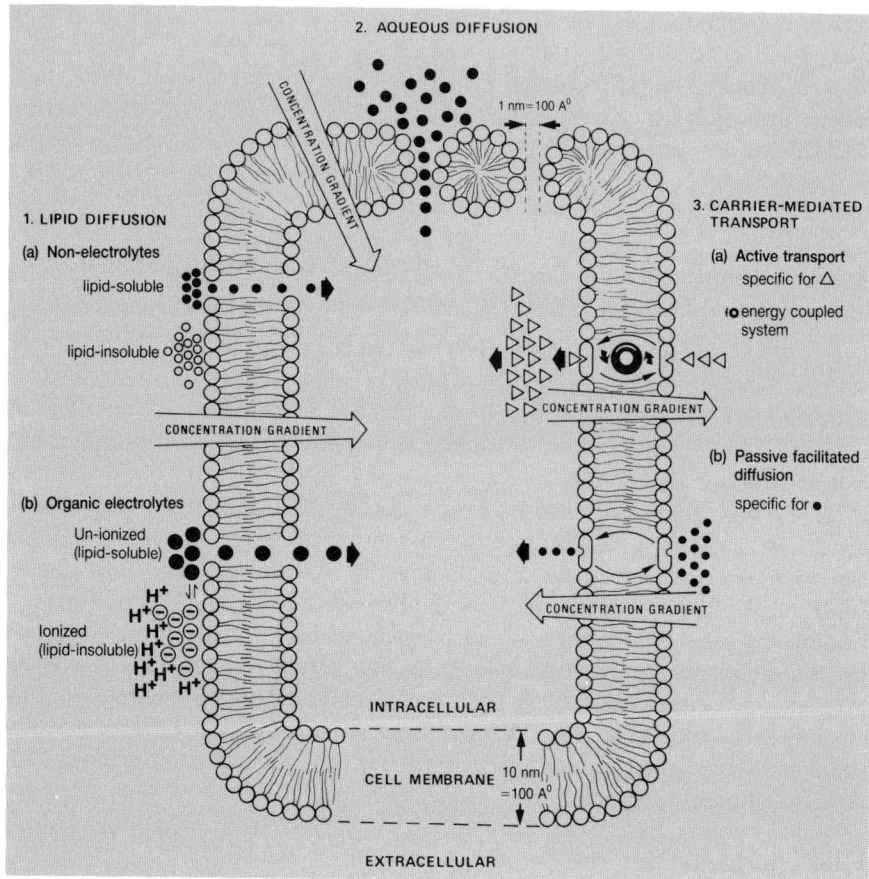

Fig. 1.3. Illustration of the principal mechanisms of (1) lipid diffusion, (2) aqueous diffusion, and (3) carrier-mediated transport ((a) active transport and (b) passive facilitated diffusion) by which drugs and other substances cross cell membranes. Note that the direction of molecular movement is down the concentration gradient with the exception of active transport, where it is distinguished by molecular movement *against* the concentration gradient. See text for further details.

majority of drugs are weak organic electrolytes that exist partly un-ionized and party ionized, the proportion of each depending on the dissociation constant (pK_a) of the particular drug and the pH of its environment. The un-ionized form is lipid-soluble, whereas the ionized form is not (see Fig. 1.3), so any factors which tend to increase the un-ionized fraction will also increase the rate of absorption; the converse is also true.

Diffusion can take place either:

(1) directly via the lipoprotein membrane or;

(2) through the paracellular spaces (as indicated earlier).

Lipid diffusion is the most common mechanism by which drugs cross cell membranes to enter the body, and also the mechanism by which they are subsequently distributed around it and ultimately excreted.

Aqueous diffusion (filtration through pores)

Water-soluble (lipid-insoluble) drugs of sufficiently small molecular size (MW less than 100 daltons) are able to cross cell membranes by passing through the polar pores or spaces between membranes of adjacent cells (see Fig. 1.3). Ethanol (MW = 46) and urea (MW = 60) are believed to pass through membranes by this means. The size of the drug molecule relative to the size of the pore is of considerable importance in determining the ease or difficulty with which the drug can pass through pores (see Fig. 1.3). Moreover, pore size differs in the cell membranes of different tissues (Lindemann and Solomon 1962). Pores found in the capillaries and the renal glomeruli are probably the largest (50–100 nm diameter) and offer greater ease of passage than those available in other tissues.

Active transport (specific carrier-mediated transport systems)

A number of substances essential to the body but too lipid-insoluble to dissolve in the cell membrane (lipid diffusion) and too large to flow through pores (aqueous diffusion) are nevertheless readily transported across cell membranes. Important examples are sodium, potassium, calcium, and chloride ions; others are iron, amino acids, and glucose; for each of these substances, there are highly specific carrier-mediated transport systems (see Fig. 1.3). Three features distinguish these active transport systems from the other mechanisms involved in passage of drugs across cell membranes. These are:

(1) Ability to work against concentration, osmotic, electrical, or hydrostatic gradients.

(2) Specificity, such that these systems have the ability to concentrate a selected substance on one side of the cell membrane.

(3) Each system requires an energy source, usually adenosine triphosphate (ATP), to which it is directly coupled.

The actual transport is carried out by large proteins that lie within the substance of the membrane and act as a two-state gated pore passing the specific substrate in one direction only. This is a saturable system but only at high substrate concentrations. Although active transport systems possess high specificity they will often transport substances that are closely related chemically to their natural substrates. For example, the system for aromatic amino acids in the gut wall will also transport the chemically related drugs, L-dopa and α-methyl dopa.

The kidney also has at least three special transport mechanisms. The proximal renal tubule contains a mechanism for the transport of acids and another for the

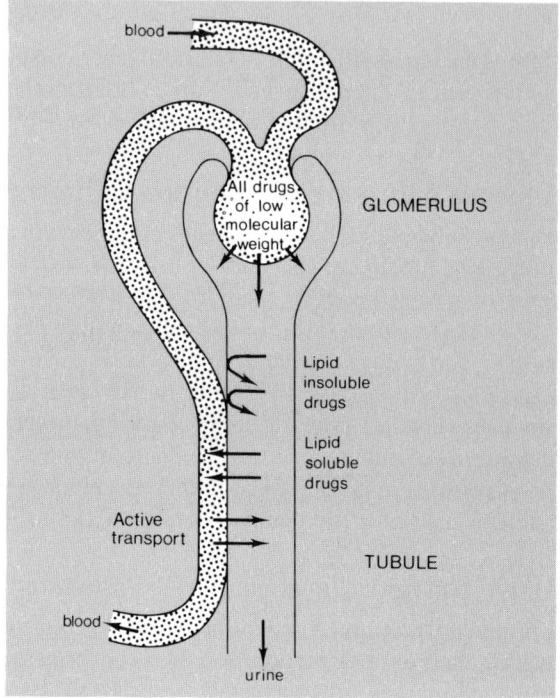

Fig. 1.4. The excretion of drugs by the kidneys. (After Brodie 1964.) (See text for details.)

transport of bases. The third is located in the distal tubule, which actively transports the cardiac drug, digoxin. Benzylpenicillin is actively transported into the renal tubules through the acidic transport system (see Fig. 1.4) and, as it also passes into the glomerular filtrate, this dual channel of excretion accounts for the rapid removal of this drug from the body. The half-life of benzylpenicillin is less than an hour (the half-life is the time taken for the original amount of drug in the body to be reduced by half; see later sections of this chapter).

Facilitated diffusion

This is a passive process whereby drugs can move across membranes more rapidly than by simple diffusion; it involves the action of a specific but saturable carrier system. However, it differs from active transport in that it *can only work in the presence of an appropriate concentration gradient* and so, for example, can only move drugs into a cell provided that their extracellular concentration is higher than their intracellular concentration.

Distribution of drugs

The principal factors concerned in the distribution of drugs in the body are indicated in Fig. 1.5 (after Brodie 1964; Gillette 1967). If a drug is taken by

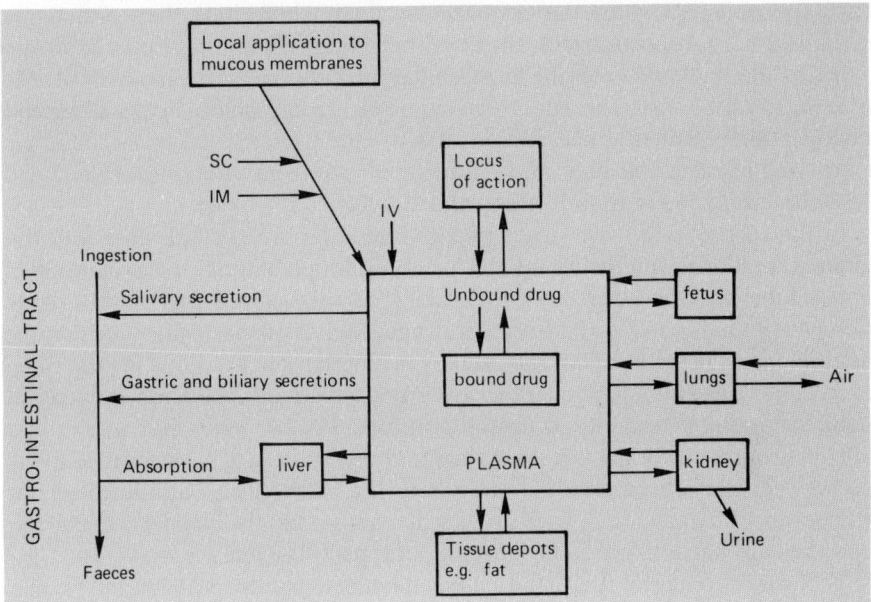

Fig. 1.5. Factors concerned in the distribution of a drug in the body. (Adapted from Brodie 1964, and Gillette 1967.) An arrow represents the direction of movement of the drug in question. Double arrows indicate that a drug and/or its metabolites move in both directions between the points indicated. (SC = subcutaneous; IM = intramuscular; IV = intravenous.)

mouth it will become mixed with the various secretions associated with the gastro-intestinal tract and a varying proportion of the total dose will be absorbed (depending on factors already discussed). The faeces may contain only unabsorbed drug or may also include a certain amount of drug that was originally absorbed and subsequently excreted into the gut either unchanged or partly metabolized. After absorption, the drug passes first into the portal circulation and thence via the liver enters the general circulation. It is important to note that some drugs are extensively metabolized during their first passage through the liver (so-called 'first pass metabolism') such that only a small proportion of the original drug is available to enter the general circulation and thereby produce an effect. Such a drug is referred to as undergoing 'high first pass metabolism', and an example is the β-adrenoceptor antagonist, propranolol (see Chapter 13).

Drugs may be administered parenterally by subcutaneous (SC), intramuscular (IM) or intravenous (IV) injections (Fig. 1.5), or may be applied to mucous membranes, such as in the mouth, where drugs with an appropriate physico-chemical profile may be absorbed with great rapidity.

Once a drug has entered the blood, it is carried to all the vascular tissues in the body. It may be retained within the blood (e.g. heparin) or may pass through the capillary wall and enter the extracellular fluid where it is then principally confined (e.g. D-tubocurarine). On the other hand, it may then pass from the extracellular fluid and enter the intracellular fluid of some or the majority of cells (e.g. thiopentone, ethanol). Thus, the volume of distribution of a drug will depend upon its compartmental distribution; if it is widely distributed throughout the extra- and intracellular fluid compartments, the concentration in the blood will be considerably lower than if it is confined solely to the blood.

In the kidney (Fig. 1.4), drugs of low molecular weight will pass into the glomerular filtrate and thence into the urine, although a significant proportion of lipid-soluble drugs will be reabsorbed by the renal tubules and thus leave the body slowly. As mentioned earlier, certain drugs, such as benzylpenicillin, may be actively transported by the renal tubules, which largely accounts for the rapid excretion of this antibiotic from the body. Thus, once again, the physico-chemical profile of a drug determines its distribution. Drugs of low molecular weight that are lipid-soluble and exist largely in the un-ionized form will be distributed freely across cell membranes and will enter both the extracellular and intracellular compartments. In addition, such drugs will readily cross the blood–brain barrier, and they are liable to cross the placenta and reach the fetus.

There are two special additional factors, binding to plasma proteins and to cells, which must be taken into account when considering the distribution of drugs in the body.

Binding to plasma proteins

Most drugs to varying extents become reversibly bound to various constituents of the tissues and especially to plasma proteins. Thus, acidic drugs (e.g. salicylic acid, warfarin) bind to albumin whereas some basic drugs (e.g. propranolol, diazepam) bind to α_1-acid glycoproteins and also to lipoproteins. As a result, a state of equilibrium becomes established between the bound and unbound portions according to the law of mass action. Figure 1.6 illustrates this effect in relation to the distribution of a drug between plasma and cerebrospinal fluid.

The plasma binding of drugs has several important consequences. First, it is only the unbound portion that is pharmacologically active, and free to leave the

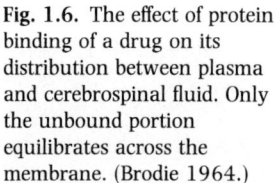

Fig. 1.6. The effect of protein binding of a drug on its distribution between plasma and cerebrospinal fluid. Only the unbound portion equilibrates across the membrane. (Brodie 1964.)

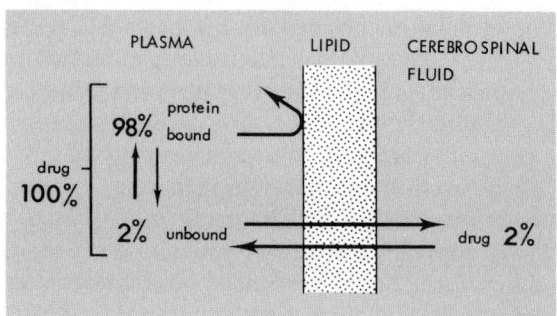

circulation and reach those cells on which it is to act. Second, although the plasma protein–drug complex is pharmacologically inactive, it is a means whereby the total plasma concentration can often exceed the aqueous solubility of the drug and thereby assist in distribution to the tissues. Third, the plasma protein–drug complex forms a reservoir that dissociates to release more free drug as soon as the existing level of free drug falls because of redistribution or elimination, e.g. at the site of action. It thus smooths out any fluctuations in concentration that would otherwise occur. Fourth, acidic drugs compete for binding sites on the plasma albumin such that drugs with a high affinity displace those with a lower affinity. However, when this happens it causes only a transient increase in the concentration of free drug because the effect is followed by an increase in its elimination so that its concentration returns to its previous value. Thus, although it was originally thought that this mechanism might be responsible for the potentiation of, for example, the anticoagulant effect of warfarin by aspirin, it is now clear that this is not so and that aspirin potentiates warfarin by other mechanisms including inhibition of its metabolism (Park and Breckenridge 1981; Routledge 1986; see also Chapters 5 and 22).

Binding in cells

Some drugs become bound onto the surface or inside of cells with the result that a high concentration is slowly built up. For example, the amount of the anti-malarial drug, chloroquine, that becomes bound in the liver, spleen, lung, kidney, and retina may be several hundred times greater than that present in the plasma. If a drug binds reversibly with some intracellular protein, this drug–protein complex will act as a depot from which the drug will be slowly released into the circulation, thus giving rise to a prolonged effect.

Inactivation of drugs: drug metabolism

The statement of Brodie that 'the action of a drug would probably last a lifetime if the body did not have ways of limiting its duration' (Brodie 1956) is certainly not sufficiently appreciated. Moreover, it is rather surprising that when the body is presented, as it increasingly is, with new drugs having chemical structures entirely foreign to any of its constituents, it is apparently able to deal with these compounds in a relatively restricted number of ways. Here again, the physico-chemical profile of any compound plays a major role in determining the eventual outcome. Thus one, or more of two main events may occur namely, excretion in its original form and transformation into one or into several metabolites.

Excretion in the original form

There are very few drugs which are not at least partially metabolized in the body or, in other words, are excreted entirely unchanged. Hexamethonium, a highly ionized ganglion blocker and the first antihypertensive compound, although no longer in clinical use, illustrates certain principles well. As a consequence of being highly ionized it is poorly and erratically absorbed, it is not metabolized to any significant extent, and it is therefore excreted in the urine unchanged. Its variable absorption resulted, not surprisingly, in an unpredictable lowering of the blood pressure in hypertensive patients. It was therefore abandoned as soon as a reliable oral drug had been developed. Most drugs undergo extensive metabolism although a small proportion of the original dose may be excreted unchanged. For example, approximately 15 per cent of a therapeutic dose of acetylsalicylic acid (aspirin) is excreted unchanged whilst the remainder is metabolized in a variety of ways (see Chapter 5).

Transformation to one or more metabolites

Many drugs are metabolized and their metabolites excreted in the urine or bile, or both. The main organ of drug metabolism is the liver, but many other tissues have a limited ability to metabolize drugs and other foreign substances, for example, the gastro-intestinal tract, lung, kidney, skin, and placenta. Biotransformation of drugs has two effects:

1. It alters the pharmacological activity, usually decreasing it but sometimes converting the drug to a compound with similar or greater activity (potency) than the original. Occasionally it converts an inactive compound (a pro-drug) to an active one. A good example is the anticancer drug, cyclophosphamide, which is inactive until it is converted into 4-hydroxycyclophosphamide, and which in turn is converted via two further steps into phosphoramide mustard. Sometimes the metabolism of an active drug will result in a compound with a longer plasma half-life ($T_{0.5}$) than the parent compound. For example, diazepam ($T_{0.5}$ about 30 hours) is converted to desmethyldiazepam ($T_{0.5}$ of 100 hours).

2. It usually results in metabolites that are more water-soluble and less lipid-soluble than the parent compounds and therefore more readily excreted in the urine.

There are two phases of drug metabolism, phase I and phase II.

Phase I metabolism

The drug molecules undergo chemical changes which lead to the exposure or addition of chemically reactive groups. These changes include:

(1) oxidation (requiring NADPH, oxygen, and cytochrome P_{450}), e.g. diazepam, warfarin;

(2) reduction, e.g. nitrazepam, cortisone;

(3) hydrolysis, e.g. suxamethonium, amethocaine.

Phase II reactions

These either replace phase I reactions or form a consecutive step after them. The molecules formed as a result of Phase II conjugation are almost always less pharmacologically active and less lipid-soluble, i.e. more water-soluble, than the molecule before conjugation. Thus the conjugates are more readily excreted especially in the urine.

Phase II reactions involve conjugation to form one or more of the following:

(1) glucuronide, e.g. morphine, paracetamol;

(2) sulphate, e.g. isoprenaline;

(3) acetate, e.g. isoniazid, hydralazine;

(4) glutathione, e.g. paracetamol.

Sites of drug metabolism

The major site of drug metabolism is in the liver although some occurs at other sites such as the kidney (vitamin D), wall of intestine (tyramine), plasma (suxamethonium), lung (5-hydroxytryptamine = serotonin), skin (vitamin D), and placenta (a large range of drugs).

Types of enzymatic reaction

The metabolic changes described above may be due to enzymes located in the endoplasmic reticulum ('microsomes') or at non-microsomal sites.

Factors affecting drug metabolism

It is important to note that the following factors affect drug metabolism and therefore should always be taken into account when prescribing a drug.

Age

The ability to metabolize drugs is reduced at the extremes of age. Thus, children under the age of 6 months and especially premature babies show impaired drug metabolism due to a reduced capacity of hepatic enzyme activity. An example of an unwanted effect of this impairment is the well-documented 'grey syndrome' in which chloramphenicol causes peripheral circulatory collapse when given to young babies. In a similar way, an elderly patient may show intolerance to a normal therapeutic dose of a drug, for example, a tricyclic antidepressant, due to impaired metabolism. Evidence available (Rawlins *et al.* 1987) suggests that this altered response in the elderly is due to a reduced amount of normal enzyme coupled with a reduction in liver blood flow. This problem is easily overcome by ensuring that when a drug is prescribed to an elderly patient the dose chosen is smaller than usual. In practice it is easiest to start off with a dose that is half (or less) than the normal therapeutic one and then to increase it slowly until the desired therapeutic effect is achieved.

Sex

In rodents, drug metabolism appears to be faster in the male than in the female. In humans such an overall difference between the sexes does not seem to occur although several clinical reports suggest that benzodiazepines, salicylates, and oestrogens are metabolized faster in the male than in the female (Katzung 1984). However, in general these differences are not clinically significant and, other things being equal, drugs are prescribed in the same dosage to males and females.

Liver disease

The capacity of the liver to metabolize drugs is very great and as a consequence liver disease needs to be extensive before it is likely to produce a significant effect on the action of normal therapeutic doses of drugs. Thus, for example, chronic alcoholism can greatly reduce hepatic metabolism with obvious consequences. The decreased liver blood flow in heart failure may result in a significant reduction of drug metabolism.

Environmental factors

The presence of other drugs, differences in nutrition, the use of alcohol (see under Liver Disease above), smoking, and exposure to pesticides can all influence drug metabolism. Benzpyrene from heavy cigarette smoking and occupational exposure to chlorinated hydrocarbon insecticides can induce certain drug-metabolizing pathways and thereby modify the response to drugs (Alvares 1978; Jusko 1978). In heavy cigarette smokers the metabolism of theophylline is increased and such patients may therefore need above average doses as compared with non-smokers (Ogilvie 1978). Heavy smokers may also require higher doses of analgesics such dextropropoxyphene. For further details the interested reader should consult Sjöqvist et al. (1980), and Rawlins and Thompson (1985).

Genetic factors (pharmacogenetics)

Pharmacogenetics is concerned with the modification of the responses to drugs by hereditary influences (Kalow 1962). The importance of pharmacogenetics to therapeutics is best illustrated by reference to the antituberculous drug, isoniazid. The major route of metabolism of this drug is under the action of acetylation by the enzyme N-acetyltransferase in the liver. The ability to acetylate isoniazid is inherited as an autosomal recessive trait. When the rate of metabolism of isoniazid is studied in groups of patients it is found that the rate of acetylation may be fast or slow. In Europe and North America approximately half of the population acetylate isoniazid slowly, whereas in other populations the proportion of slow acetylators may be as small as 20 per cent or as high as 90 per cent. This variation is due to a gene which controls the synthesis of hepatic N-acetyltransferase. The abnormal gene controls the synthesis of an *atypical* form of N-acetyltransferase, which acetylates isoniazid more slowly than the typical (normal) enzyme. There are three possible genotypes, namely (i) those with two normal genes (rapid–rapid); (ii) those with one abnormal and one normal gene (slow–rapid or rapid–slow); and (iii) those in whom both genes are of the slow type (slow–slow). As the inheritance is autosomal recessive it was assumed that these three genotypes would give rise to two phenotypes namely rapid acetylators ((i) and (ii)) and slow acetylators (iii). However, more recent and refined work (Lee and Lee 1982) has demonstrated that it is possible to separate the heterozygous rapid phenotype (ii) from the homozygous rapid phenotype (i). Thus, three groups—rapid, intermediate, and slow acetylators—can be identified. The important therapeutic point is that when isoniazid is given in normal doses to a slow acetylator, it is likely to accumulate to toxic levels and thereby produce adverse effects, particularly peripheral neuropathy. The same problem will arise when other drugs that are primarily inactivated by acetylation are given to such patients and these include phenelzine (a monoamine oxidase inhibitor (MAOI)), nitrazepam (a benzodiazepine hypnotic), and sulphasalazine (a complex of a sulphonamide with a salicylic-acid derivative), which is used for the treatment of ulcerative colitis.

The administration of the short-acting neuromuscular blocking drug, suxamethonium, is occasionally followed by prolonged apnoea (see Chapter 8). This effect is likely to be due to an atypical form of the enzyme non-specific cholinesterase (pseudocholinesterase). Here again the abnormality is due to a single gene but with the difference that the type of inheritance involved here is known as autosomal autonomous so that in heterozygotes the trait is partially expressed. Thus, in the population there is a trimodal distribution with one group showing normal enzyme activity, another group with abnormally slow activity of the enzyme, and a third intermediate group. Individuals can be identified by means of the 'dibucaine' test.

Another genetic disorder is the rare condition of malignant hyperthermia (hyperpyrexia), which is due to an abnormality of calcium binding in muscle. As a consequence of this abnormality the general anaesthetic, halothane, and the depolarizing neuromuscular blocking drug, suxamethonium, may, due to depolarization, trigger the intracellular release of calcium which then gives rise to a long, muscle contracture (not contraction) associated with the production of increased heat and lactic acid. Malignant hyperthermia is inherited as an autosomal dominant, as is hereditary porphyria, which is due to an abnormality in haem metabolism. Compounds likely to trigger an attack of acute porphyria (abdominal pain, neuritis, mental changes, and the urinary excretion of porphyrins) are griseofulvin, phenytoin, barbiturates, sulphonamides, and also oral hypoglycaemic drugs.

Excretion of drugs

Drugs are mainly excreted by the kidney, so appearing in the urine. To a lesser extent they are excreted via the bile, skin (sweat), lungs (expired air), saliva, and milk. With the inhalation anaesthetics the expired air is the main route of excretion.

The excretion of a drug by the kidney is best expressed in terms of the renal plasma clearance. This is the volume of plasma effectively cleared of the drug by the kidney in unit time. Thus it is that portion of the apparent volume of distribution (AVD) to be cleared of the drug in unit time (with units of flow i.e. ml/min or litres/h). Therefore, drug clearance (Cl) may be expressed as follows:

$$\text{Clearance (Cl)} = \text{AVD} \times K = \frac{\text{AVD} \times 0.693}{T_{0.5}}.$$

where AVD = apparent volume of distribution; K = elimination rate constant; $0.693 = \log_e 2$; $T_{0.5}$ = half life of drug.

The excretion of a drug by the kidney involves several processes, each of which is now considered.

Glomerular filtration

Under normal conditions the glomerular filtration rate (GFR) is about 125 ml/min. Thus, the rate of drug filtration will depend upon the plasma concentration of drug and also upon its molecular weight (MW). The glomerular capillary membrane contains a pore size approaching the molecular dimensions of albumin (MW approx. 68 000 daltons). Therefore all but a very few drugs can be filtered easily at the glomerulus provided that the drug is free, i.e. not bound to plasma protein. When it is partially bound to plasma protein then it is only the unbound fraction that is available for filtration. It should be noted that the rate of filtration is not dependent on either the lipid solubility or on the degree of ionization of the drug.

Drug excretion in the presence of renal impairment

When glomerular filtration is impaired this will have potentially serious implications for the excretion of any drug that is eliminated predominantly by the renal route. The clearance of creatinine (Cl_{cr}) is commonly used to measure GFR. Creatinine is a breakdown product derived from the amino acids of muscle and is eliminated by glomerular filtration at a rate equivalent to GFR. Thus, in a healthy adult, the Cl_{cr} is approximately 125 ml/min. In a patient suffering from renal impairment this figure will be reduced, and the prescriber will need to make appropriate allowance for this fact when calculating the dosage of a drug that depends mainly upon renal excretion. The simplest way to calculate the appropriate amended dosage is by means of nomograms, which are available in appropriate texts on clinical pharmacology.

Tubular reabsorption

The function of the renal tubules is to reabsorb appropriate amounts of selected ions, particularly sodium and chloride, along with water. Any molecules of drug that are present in the filtrate will be reabsorbed in accordance with their physico-chemical profile in just the same way as this profile determined their absorption. Thus, highly ionized drugs entering the glomerular filtrate will be excreted in the urine without significant reabsorption by the renal tubules. On the other hand, a drug that arrives in the filtrate in an un-ionized and therefore lipid-soluble form will be partially reabsorbed by the renal tubules and so re-enter the circulation. Non-polar lipid-soluble drugs (for example, thiopentone, inhalational anaesthetics, and phenytoin) will be almost completely reabsorbed from the tubular urine. Acidic drugs that have a pK_a ranging from 2 to 8 (for example, salicylic acid) will be excreted in a pH-dependent fashion. Thus, the ionized (lipid-insoluble) moiety will not be reabsorbed by the tubules whereas the un-ionized (lipid-soluble) moiety will readily pass through the tubular cell membrane and thus be reabsorbed. When it is desired to expedite excretion of acidic drugs this can be achieved by alkalinizing the urine to a pH of approximately 8, which is why the urine is alkalinized as part of the treatment of aspirin poisoning (see Chapter 5). Basic drugs with a pK_a ranging from 6–12 also exhibit pH-dependent excretion but, of course, in the opposite direction. Thus, the excretion of amphetamine can be expedited by acidyifying the urine through administration of ascorbic acid to the lowest attainable pH, which is usually about 5.

Tubular secretion

As we have outlined above, the renal tubules contain three secretory systems, two in the proximal tubule of low specificity and the third in the distal tubule, which appears to be concerned with the secretion of digoxin. Of the two systems in the proximal tubule, one is for anions—for example, benzylpenicillin ($pK_a = 2.8$), acetylsalicylic acid (aspirin $pK_a = 3.5$), hydrochlorothiazide ($pK_a = 7.9$)—and also conjugates of drugs with glucuronic acid, glycine, and sulphuric acid. Probenecid is a competitive antagonist to this transport system and can thereby slow the excretion of a drug such as benzylpenicillin. The other low-specificity system is for cations and is concerned with the secretion of bases such as morphine ($pK_a = 8$), atropine ($pK_a = 9.7$), and neostigmine ($pK_a = 12$).

Drugs that undergo tubular secretion have a renal clearance which usually is in excess of the GFR because this process occurs in addition to elimination via glomerular filtration. The sum of the two clearances may be as large as the renal plasma flow.

Pharmacokinetics of drug elimination

For a given unit of time, drug elimination occurs at either a constant rate or at a constant fraction. We must now consider these in a little more detail.

Constant rate elimination (zero-order kinetics)

Under these conditions a drug is eliminated at a constant rate irrespective of any changes in the rate of absorption and is therefore independent of the amount of drug in the body at any one time (Fig. 1.7(a)).

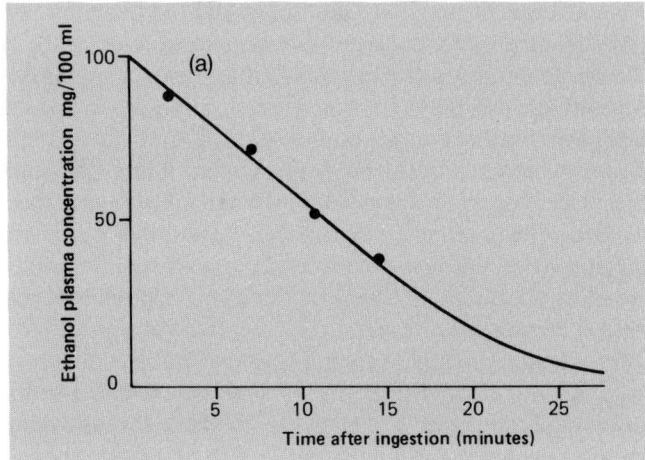

Fig. 1.7(a). Graph of zero-order kinetics as illustrated by the elimination of ethyl alcohol (ethanol). Note the linear relationship between time (abscissa) and concentration in plasma (ordinate) indicating a constant rate of elimination independent of plasma concentration (cf. first-order kinetics).

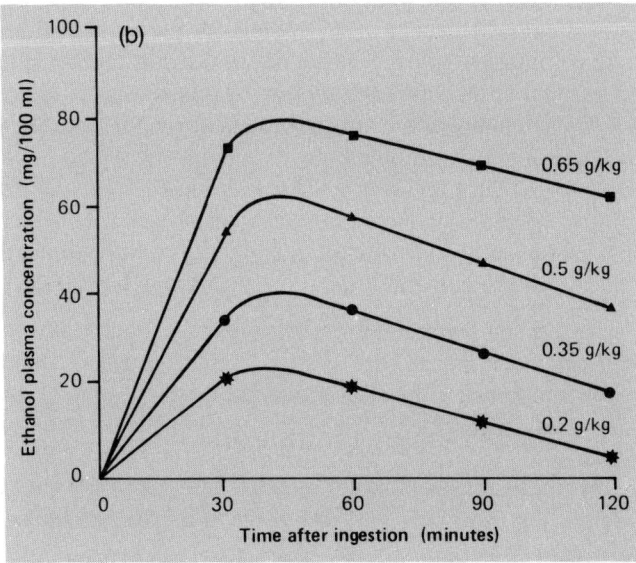

Fig. 1.7(b). Graph of the blood concentration of ethanol after taking four different doses of ethanol; each point is the mean of 40 subjects. Note that the curves are virtually parallel indicating that the rate of fall of blood concentration is the same and independent of the dose. The lowest dose is equivalent to about $\frac{3}{4}$ pint of beer or 1.5 whiskies and the largest dose to 3 pints of beer or 6 whiskies. (Reproduced from Drew *et al.* 1958 with permission.)

Mathematically, constant rate elimination (zero-order kinetics), for example mg/h, may be represented by the mathematical expression:

$$\text{Rate of movement} = K.$$

Thus the amount of drug in the body will decline at a constant rate, i.e. linear rate. If the rate of absorption exceeds the rate of elimination then the plasma concentration will increase, i.e. it will never reach a plateau. Drugs metabolized by readily saturable enzyme systems are likely to be treated in this way by the body. Thus, ethanol (ethyl alcohol) is metabolized by the enzyme, alcohol dehydrogenase, to acetaldehyde and subsequently to acetic acid. Figure 1.7(b) shows a family of blood concentrations of alcohol after taking four different doses of alcohol (Drew *et al.* 1958). The lowest dose (0.2 g/kg) is equivalent to about three-quarters of a pint of beer or 1.5 whiskies whilst the largest does (0.65 g/kg) is equivalent to 3 pints of beer or 6 whiskies. It should be noted that a graph plotted with linear coordinates (Fig. 1.7(b)) shows a series of virtually parallel curves thus indicating that the rate of elimination is constant and independent of the magnitude of the blood alcohol concentration. Although the rate of oxidation of ethyl alcohol varies in different individuals, the average value in a man of 70 kg body weight is 10 g or 12.5 ml per hour. The zero-order kinetics of ethanol explains why this drug readily accumulates if the rate of intake exceeds the rate of elimination.

The metabolism of certain other drugs may be initially first-order kinetics (see next section) but at therapeutic concentrations their metabolism is principally zero-order kinetics; examples of these are acetylsalicylic acid (aspirin) and the anticonvulsant drug, phenytoin. As a consequence of the saturation of first-order kinetics of such a drug, there is a switch to zero-order kinetics with the *clinically important result* that for a relatively small increase in the dose of the drug there may be a large increase in plasma concentration.

Constant fraction elimination (first-order kinetics)

Under these conditions the rate of elimination of the drug is proportional to the quantity of drug to be transferred. This process of elimination applies to the majority of drugs and it means that for any regular dosage a plateau is reached when the rate of clearance of the drug equals the rate of its entry; this is known as the steady state. Mathematically, the process can be expressed as:

$$\text{Rate} = K \times D.$$

where K = elimination rate constant with units of reciprocal time i.e. hours^{-1} or days^{-1} (for example, 0.1 h^{-1} = a tenth or 10 per cent of the drug eliminated per h); D = amount of drug to be transferred.

Figure 1.8(a) shows a graph of first-order kinetics plotted on linear coordinates, from which it can be seen that the slope of the curve is initially steep but becomes less so as elimination proceeds. If these data are now plotted semi-logarithmically, i.e. time against the *logarithm* of the dose, the result is a straight line (Fig. 1.8(b)).

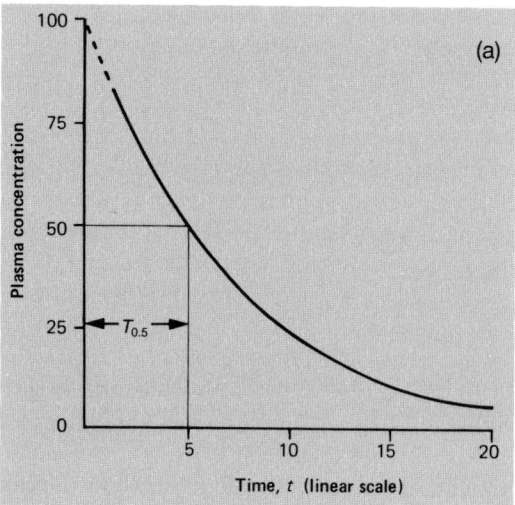

Fig. 1.8(a). Graph of first-order kinetics illustrating the elimination pattern typical for most drugs. Note (i) the exponential curve indicating that a constant fraction of drug is eliminated in unit time and (ii) the half-life which represents the time taken for the amount in the plasma to fall by half ($T_{0.5}$).

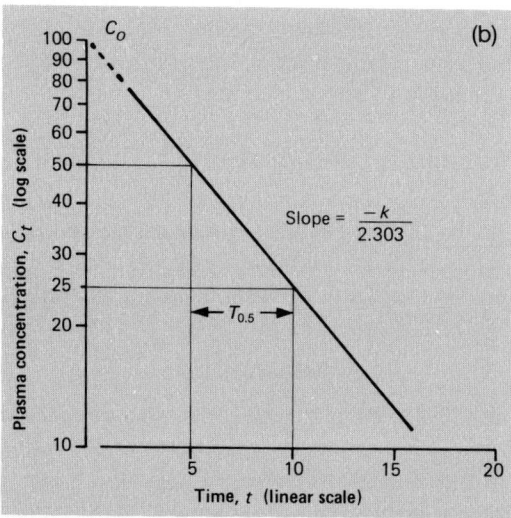

Fig. 1.8(b). Re-plot of (a) on semi-logarithmic scale resulting in linear graph thus confirming log-linear (exponential) relationship between coordinates. The half-life ($T_{0.5}$) can be measured between any two points that correspond to a change of plasma concentration of one-half.

If this is extrapolated backwards to time zero then the theoretical concentration of drug at zero time can be read from the graph.

Half-life

The half-life is the time required for the concentration of drug to decline to half of its original value. In Figs. 1.8(a) and (b) we are concerned with plasma concentration of a drug so, in this context, the half-life ($T_{0.5}$) is the time taken for the concentration in the plasma to decline to half of its original value. The measurement of $T_{0.5}$ from the graph can be made over any part of it (most conveniently from the semi-log plot).

The half-life may also be calculated from K (elimination rate constant) by the equation:

$$T_{0.5} = \log_e 2 = \frac{0.693}{K}$$

where K = elimination rate constant.

The half-lives of drugs vary greatly from less than an hour to many hours or even days. The following is a list of half-lives of drugs in common use:

Name	$T_{0.5}$ (h)	
	[Very short to short half-life]	
Tubocurarine	0.1	
Acetylsalicylic acid (aspirin)	0.3	(i) hydrolysis with deacetylation to salicylate
	2.0–4.5	(ii) salicylate
Benzylpenicillin	0.5	
Ampicillin	1.0–1.5	
Erythromycin	1.5–2.0	
Cortisol (hydrocortisone)	1.7	
Paracetamol	2.0	
	[Intermediate half-life]	
Pethidine	2.5	
Morphine	3.0	
Tetracycline	6–10	
Phenytoin	10–42	

Name	$T_{0.5}$ (h)
	[Long to very long half-life]
Warfarin	35–45
Nortriptyline	15–90
Digoxin	30–40
Desmethyldiazepam	36–200
(active metabolite of diazepam which has a $T_{0.5}$ of 20–100 h i.e. longer than the parent drug)	
Phenylbutazone	30–175

(Main source of data: Avery 1980)

Drug clearance

This is a more accurate measure of the efficiency with which a drug is eliminated by the body. It is based upon the apparent volume of distribution (AVD), and may be defined as the theoretical portion of the AVD that is cleared of the drug in unit time. Therefore, the clearance is the product of the volume of distribution (AVD) and the elimination rate constant. Thus it may be expressed as:

$$\text{Clearance} = \text{AVD} \times K = \frac{\text{AVD} \times 0.693}{T_{0.5}},$$

where K = elimination rate constant.

It is expressed in units of time, for example, ml/min, and where necessary this may be corrected for body weight, for example ml/kg. Clearance may be considered in relation to one organ (e.g. liver) or to the whole body (total body clearance). The total body clearance is equal to the sum of the clearances by the different routes of elimination involved for a particular drug. For practical purposes this may be divided into renal and non-renal clearance.

The advantage of measuring drug elimination in terms of clearance rather than half-life ($T_{0.5}$) is that unlike half-life it is unaffected by a change in the volume of distribution of the drug.

Routes of administration

Drugs may be administered locally in order to apply a high concentration to a particular site of action or may be administered systemically and thereby rely on the circulation to carry them to the required site of action.

Local

Local methods of administration include:

topical	intranasal	intra-articular
intradermal	intraconjunctival	intra-arterial
intrathecal	intra-oral	other special routes
	vaginal	

It is of particular importance for dental practitioners to note that locally administered drugs may be absorbed at a rate and to an extent sufficient to result in the production of systemic effects. This is even more likely to occur when the drug has been applied to diseased tissues where the natural barriers have been damaged and the blood supply increased by inflammatory changes.

Systemic

These routes are enteral or parenteral. The major enteral routes are sublingual, gastro-intestinal, and rectal.

Sublingual   administration is useful for the absorption of drugs that are given in small amounts and are relatively lipid-soluble. The high vascularity of the oral mucosa ensures rapid absorption directly into the general circulation and bypasses the liver. This route is thus particularly useful for drugs that undergo high 'first pass' metabolism by destruction in the gastro-intestinal tract and liver before reaching the general circulation.

The rate of absorption of ingested drugs (*gastro-intestinal* route) depends on a number of factors, particularly the rate of gastric emptying, which is itself dependent on both physiological and psychological factors.

Rectal   administration by means of a suppository is utilized when the oral route is unsuitable or unavailable, for example in a patient unable to take food by mouth or who is vomiting. The absorption of drugs from the rectum is slow and may be incomplete but can nevertheless be most useful in certain circumstances, such as when opioid suppositories are used in the treatment of terminal cancer patients.

The parenteral routes are subcutaneous, intramuscular, and intravenous.

The rate of absorption after *subcutaneous* or *intramuscular* administration depends on the local blood flow and also on whether vasoconstrictor substance has been added to the injection or not. It also depends upon the physico-chemical profile of the drug.

A drug administered by the *intravenous* route is obviously absorbed immediately and for this reason the rate of an intravenous injection should be slow enough for the injected bolus not to result in an excessively high plasma concentration, as this might produce undesirable local and systemic effects, particularly on the cardiovascular and central nervous systems.

It should be noted that the results of an intramuscular injection are inconstant and may give a pattern of absorption varying between that of a subcutaneous and an intravenous injection.

Plasma concentrations and clinical effects

The plasma concentrations (levels) achieved in different patients receiving the same oral dose of a given drug vary greatly. This is due mainly to intrinsic differences between individuals. The relationship between plasma concentration and clinical effect is less variable and has been studied in considerable detail for a large number of drugs. For drugs with a low therapeutic index (see page 40) the therapeutic range of plasma concentration and the toxicological range are in close proximity. Table 1.2 is a list of drugs and their plasma concentrations commonly associated with a therapeutic effect or likely to be associated with unwanted effects. It shows that with some drugs the gap between the two concentrations is very narrow whilst for others it is considerably wider.

Table 1.2. Therapeutic and toxic plasma concentrations of some drugs

Drugs	Normal half-life (hours)	Therapeutic range		Toxic level		Usual route of elimination[4]
Amitriptyline[2]	15–60	<200	µg/l	>200 µg/l		M
Carbamazepine	30–40	5–10	mg/l	>10	mg/l	M
Digoxin	30–40	1–2	µg/l	>2	µg/l	R
Disopyramide	4–8	3–6	mg/l	>8	mg/l	R
Lignocaine	2–4	2–5	mg/l	>8	mg/l	M
Lithium	7–20	0.8–1.3	mmol/l	>1.5	mmol/l	R
Mexiletine	4–8	1–2	mg/l	>3	mg/l	M&R
Nortriptyline	15–90	50–150	µg/l	>180 µg/l		M
Phenobarbitone						
plasma	20–100	15–40	mg/l	>40	mg/l	M
saliva	20–100	8–20	mg/l	>20	mg/l	
Phenytoin[1,3]						
plasma	10–42	10–20	mg/l	>20	mg/l	M
saliva	10–42	1–2	mg/l	>2	mg/l	
Procainamide	2–6	4–8	mg/l	>8	mg/l	M
Propranolol	2–4	>100	µg/l	—		M
Quinidine	3–6	3–6	mg/l	>6	mg/l	M
Salicylate[3]	2–4.5	150–300	mg/l	>400 mg/l		M&R
Theophylline[3]	8–20	5–20	mg/l	>20	mg/l	M
Valproate	6–12	>50	mg/l(?)	?		M

  1. Phenytoin binding (normally 90%) is reduced substantially in uraemia and the 'therapeutic' and 'toxic' ranges of plasma concentrations are reduced. Alternatively, monitor salivary levels (which correspond to unbound levels) and aim for a therapeutic range of 1–2 mg/l.
  2. Amitriptyline is metabolized to nortriptyline. The sum of the two concentrations should be added to yield the therapeutic range for amitriptyline.
  3. These drugs have 'non-linear' kinetics and increasing the dose is likely to produce a more than proportional increase in plasma levels.
  4. M = eliminated by metabolism; R = eliminated by renal excretion.
N.B. In the International System of Units (Système International d'Unités; SI) concentrations may be expressed either as mass concentration, e.g. mg/l, µg/l, as in this table, or as 'amount of substance' concentration, e.g. mmol/l, µmol/l. The two ways of expressing each concentration are readily interconverted by using the value of the appropriate molecular weight (MW) as follows: $mmol/l = \dfrac{mg/l}{MW}$ and conversely, mg/l = mmol/1 × MW. Example: phenytoin (MW = 252), 10 mg/l $= \dfrac{10}{252} = 0.04$ mmol/l = 40 µmol/l; m = milli; µ = micro; 1 m = 1000µ.

Plasma concentration–time curve

Plasma concentration–time curves obviously vary with the route of administration of a drug. Figure 1.9 illustrates the different shaped curves following the administration of penicillin by oral, intramuscular, and intravenous routes. With the oral route the peak plasma concentration is the lowest, with the intravenous route it is the highest, and with the intramuscular it is intermediate.

The effects of regular dosing as in normal therapeutic use are shown in Fig. 1.10(a) for the intravenous route and Fig. 1.10(b) for the oral route. In each case a dose is followed by a peak plasma concentration, which then falls to a trough to be followed by another peak plasma concentration, which then falls to a trough to be followed by another peak and trough and so on until a plateau is reached, i.e. the steady state. The major difference between these two routes is that with the intravenous route the rise of the plasma concentration is steeper and reaches a higher peak. It should be noted that the graphs (Fig. 1.10) have been drawn for the situation where each dose is given at intervals (6-hourly) equal to one-half of the half-life of the drug (12 h), and that it takes approximately five doses to reach steady state. Where there is a close correlation between the plasma concentration of a drug and its effect—for example, with the use of phenytoin for the control of epilepsy—it is essential to arrange that the doses are given at regular intervals so that not only the peak but also the trough concentrations are within the therapeutic range. If they are not, then as the plasma concentration falls between doses, the risk of a fit is increased. This is an important example of the application of the relationship between the plasma concentration and therapeutic effect of drugs (see Table 1.2). The same principle applies to the use of aspirin for the relief of dental pain.

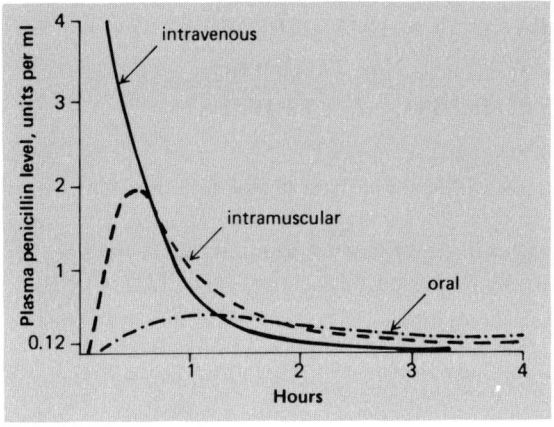

Fig. 1.9. Plasma concentration curves in a human subject after administration of 100 000 units = 60 mg benzylpenicillin by intravenous, intramuscular, and oral routes. (Reproduced from Creasey 1979 with permission of the publisher.)

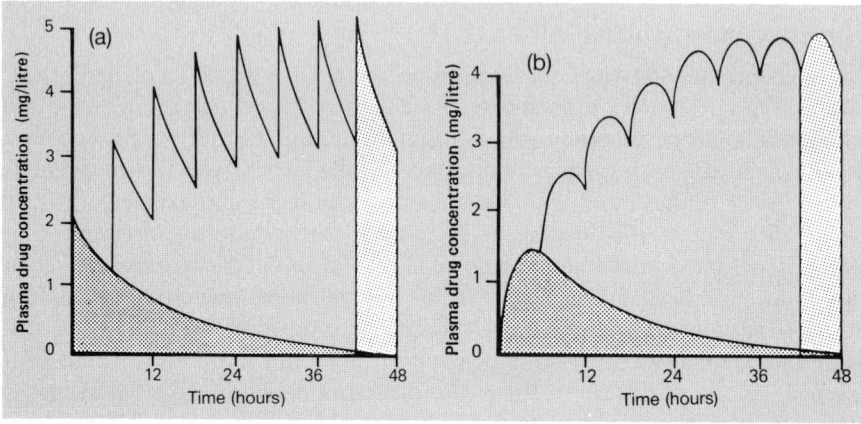

Fig. 1.10. Plasma concentrations of a drug given (a) intravenously and (b) orally on a fixed dose of 50 mg and fixed dosing interval of 6 hours. The half-life is 12 hours. Note that the area under the plasma concentration-time curve during a dosing interval *at steady state* is equal to the total area under the curve for a single dose. The fluctuation of the concentration is diminished when given orally (half-life of absorption is 1.4 hours) but the average steady-state concentration is the same as that after intravenous administration because the absorption of this drug is assumed to be complete.

Cumulation

This results when the intake of a drug exceeds its clearance from the body. It is obviously more likely to occur when drugs with long half-lives are used. It also occurs when the mechanisms for elimination are affected by disease, for example, renal failure. Thus the dose of the cardiac stimulant, digoxin, must be reduced when given to a patient who suffers from renal failure. If this step is not taken then the drug may accumulate and reach dangerously high concentrations in the body.

THE PHARMACODYNAMIC PROCESS: IS THE DRUG PRODUCING THE REQUIRED PHARMACOLOGICAL EFFECT?

Drugs modify the function of living cells. When a drug produces an effect on a certain tissue this is the end-result of an interaction between its molecules and some part of the cells of which that tissue is composed. It is now clear that drugs can be divided into two main types according as to whether or not they act on pharmacological receptors, special receptive sites situated on or within cells.

Drugs which act via pharmacological receptors:

(1) act at *low* concentrations;

(2) react with *specific* receptors;

(3) show *structure–activity relationships*;

(4) can be antagonized by *specific antagonists*.

Examples are acetylcholine, noradrenaline, adrenaline, and histamine.

Drugs which do NOT act via pharmacological receptors:

(1) act at *higher* concentrations;

(2) do *not* react with specific receptors;

(3) *tend not* to show structure–activity relationships;

(4) do *not* have specific antagonists.

Examples of drugs which belong to this group are general anaesthetics, e.g. diethyl ether, halothane; diuretics, e.g. thiazides; and non-specific destructants of cell membranes, e.g. detergents.

Drugs which act on specific pharmacological receptors

Historical

The concept of receptors grew out of the work of Paul Ehrlich (1854–1915), who was Director of the Institute for Experimental Therapy in Frankfurt from 1899 to 1915. He believed living matter was composed of large protoplasmic molecules that possessed side chains. He developed a side-chain theory of immunity, enzyme action, and drug action. The proposal that drugs may act upon special sites or 'receptive substances' was first made in 1905 by J. N. Langley (1852–1925), who was Professor of Physiology at Cambridge (Langley 1905). Over the ensuing 75 years, evidence for the existence of 'receptive substances', now renamed 'pharmacological receptors', grew steadily. Mathematical theories to explain the relationship between the dose of a drug and the response or effect produced were developed by other workers, especially A. J. Clark (1885–1941), who was Professor of Pharmacology at Edinburgh University, and also by J. N. Gaddum, E. J. Ariens, and H. Schild. More recently, with the development of new techniques, attempts have been made to visualize and to isolate receptors. The development of various binding techniques has made it possible to map out and to measure the density of receptors for drugs, hormones, and neurotransmitters on various tissues, including changes that take place during various disease processes.

Drug–receptor interaction

A pharmacological receptor is a macromolecule with special sites to which specific substances, i.e. drugs (sometimes called ligands) bind. Drug–receptor (ligand–receptor) binding leads to a change in the macromolecule, which in turn triggers a train of events resulting in the response of the tissue or organ—for example, contraction of smooth muscle, secretion of a gland, and stimulation (or inhibition) of nerve cells leading to release (or inhibition of release) of the chemical transmitter from their endings. In this context, we must now define other important terms relating to drugs and receptors.

An *agonist* is a drug (or hormone, or neurotransmitter) which combines with its specific receptor, activates it, and initiates a sequence of effects.

An *antagonist* is a drug which interferes with the action of an agonist. A *pure* antagonist has no action of its own but only by virtue of the fact that it interferes with the action of an agonist. An example of such a drug is the opioid antagonist, naloxone.

A *partial agonist* is a drug that acts on a receptor with an intrinsic activity or efficacy of < 1. In practical terms an activity of 1 means the ability of a drug to elicit a maximal response. By definition it follows that the largest response obtainable from a partial agonist is less than the maximum that can be achieved by a complete agonist acting on the same receptor. It will be appreciated that the term partial agonist is a comparative one; the degree of agonism is measured by comparing the maximum responses obtainable from a whole series of compounds acting on the same receptor. The one that produces the largest response is said to have an intrinsic activity or efficacy of 1 (the symbol α (alpha) is commonly used for this purpose so that in this case $\alpha = 1$) and the other compounds are ranked accordingly.

Mixed agonist–antagonist is a relatively new term that we must also mention. It is frequently confused (and thereby abused) with the term partial agonist. A mixed agonist–antagonist is a drug that acts simultaneously on a mixed group of receptors with an agonist action on one set and with an antagonist action on another set. There are two corollaries of this definition:

(1) The agonist action of such a drug may be complete or partial.

(2) With multiple receptor systems upon which this type of drug may act, numerous combinations of agonist or antagonist actions are theoretically possible.

At the present time, drugs with mixed agonist–antagonist activity are most likely to be found among the opioids (see Chapter 6).

Distribution of pharmacological receptors

Pharmacological receptors are found in two main sites and are named according to either (a) the principal endogenous agonist that activates them (adrenoceptors, cholinoceptors, glucocorticoid receptors, etc.) or (b) the first exogenous agonist found to activate them (for example, opioid receptors, benzodiazepine receptors, and so on) whether or not an endogenous agonist is subsequently discovered (Bowman *et al.* 1986).

The sites in which drug receptors are found are as follows:

(1) *On or within cell membranes*: these may be one of two types, those that:
   (i) act on membrane permeability to alter it with a very fast response time

measured in milliseconds such as produced by the nicotinic acetylcholine receptor, or;

(ii) act on intracellular second messenger with a fast response time of seconds or minutes such as is produced by adrenaline or noradrenaline.

(2) *Inside cells*: alter DNA transcription with a slow response time of hours such as that produced by steroids.

Evidence for the existence of pharmacological receptors

A substantial body of evidence now exists to support the concept of pharmacological receptors. This may be listed as follows:

1. Many drugs act in low concentrations (= high dilutions), for example, 10^{-3} to 10^{-5} mols per litre. For a drug with a molecular weight $= 200$ daltons this represents 200 μg per ml to 2 μg per ml. Some drugs, for example atropine, are active in very low concentrations (10^{-8} and 10^{-9} mols per litre).

2. The rate of the frog heart can be slowed 50 per cent by 0.02 μg of acetylcholine per gram of tissue. This dose of acetylcholine contains about 10^{14} molecules and Clark (1937) calculated that this amount would cover approximately 1/6000th of the total cell surface i.e. less than 0.02 per cent. This implies that only *part* of each cell needs to be covered with drug molecules in order to produce an effect.

3. In some tissues certain cells appear to possess areas specially sensitive to particular drugs: for example, the end plate of skeletal muscle normally only responds to acetylcholine.

4. Chemical alteration of many drugs alters their pharmacological activity (structure–activity relationship).

5. Where a drug exists in optically isomeric forms, the pharmacological activity of the isomeric forms usually differs greatly. Thus, L(R)-noradrenaline is more active than D(S)-noradrenaline, the ratio of activities depending upon the tissue under consideration.

6. Pharmacologically active substances produced in the body—for example acetylcholine, catecholamines (i.e. dopamine, noradrenaline, and adrenaline), histamine, 5-hydroxytryptamine (serotonin)—are found to act as endogenous ligands at their own specific receptors located on certain cells.

7. Not all cells in the body have a complete set of specific receptors for all endogenously produced pharmacological ligands. However, in cells where more than one type of receptor co-exists, the effects of activating them may produce the same or opposite effects depending upon the particular tissue.

8. Some endogenous ligands and drugs act on more than one type of receptor for a particular ligand. For example, adrenaline acts on both α- and β-adrenoceptors; histamine acts on H_1 and H_2 (histamine)-receptors.

9. The use of radio-ligand techniques has helped greatly to plot the distribution of receptors in tissues.

10. New techniques have made it possible to isolate certain receptors and to determine their chemical structures. Furthermore, some receptors have been isolated from cell membranes and then inserted into artificial membranes.

Some features of the receptor system

As indicated earlier, drugs that act on receptors, the neurotransmitters, and some hormones all exert their effects without entering the cell upon which they act. They interact with specific receptors that are coupled to various effector or amplifier systems, which then generate internal signals or so-called second messengers. The detailed mechanisms are still being worked out but the main components of the system, together with two examples, may be represented as follows (Berridge 1981):

(1) Agonist (drug, hormone, or neurotrans- mitter)	(2) Receptor	(3) Transducer	(4) Effector	(5) Second messenger	(6) Effect
		EXAMPLES			
Acetylcholine (Ach)	Ach receptor	Phospholipase C	Calcium gate	Ca^{2+}	Contraction of smooth muscle
Noradrenaline (NAd)	NAd receptor	Guanosine triphosphate (GTP)	Adenylate cyclase	Cyclic adenosine monophos- phate (cyclicAMP)	Metabolic changes

From the above it can be seen that there is a cascade of events that links the interaction of an agonist with its receptor and with the ultimate biological effect. This multi-stage system is analogous to an amplifier in that the initial molecular interaction leads to progressively larger numbers of interactions at each of the stages involved. Thus, just as a small signal from a microphone can be amplified in stages so that the output is capable of driving powerful loudspeakers, so small molecules of acetylcholine acting upon muscle endplate can ultimately result in powerful contraction of a large skeletal muscle. Although theoretically the complexity of receptor–response coupling mechanisms is very great, in reality the number of mechanisms is limited to three as follows:

1. *Receptor–ion channel coupling*   The interaction between agonist and receptor causes the cell membrane to undergo a conformational change with the result that an ion channel opens to allow the passage of a particular ion. An example (already referred to earlier) is the action of acetylcholine on nicotinic cholinoceptors, which results in an influx of sodium ions. This leads to depolarization of the muscle endplate, which in turn triggers off an action

potential. This brings about the release of calcium ions, which in its turn leads to a contraction of the muscle fibres.

2. *Receptor–enzyme coupling* Here the interaction between agonist and receptor leads to a conformational change in an enzyme. An example is the activation of β-adrenoceptors that are coupled to the enzyme adenylate cyclase in the cell membrane. Activation of this enzyme leads to the formation of cyclic AMP, which then phosphorylates a protein kinase and which in turn phosphorylates intracellular proteins so modifying the activity of the cell.

3. *Intracellular steroid receptor–protein synthesis coupling* Steroid hormones, which are highly lipid-soluble and therefore penetrate cell membranes with ease, combine with specific receptor-binding proteins in the cytosol. The hormone–receptor complex then enters the cell nucleus and triggers changes that are transcribed into messenger RNAs. These in turn signal the synthesis of specific proteins and by this means cellular activity is modified.

Receptor regulation

There is abundant evidence to show that neither the density nor the affinity of receptors are fixed quantities. Tissues normally innervated by the autonomic nervous system, for example, vascular smooth muscle, after sympathetic denervation show supersensitivity to the catecholamines, noradrenaline and adrenaline. This phenomenon is known as Cannon's Law of Denervation (Cannon and Rosenblueth 1949). The use of modern techniques has shown that the density and affinity of receptors are in a dynamic state subject to various physiological and pathological factors. Thus, alterations in the receptors will modify the effects produced by agonists (drugs, neurotransmitters, or hormones) acting on these receptors, and may play a role in the pathology of various diseases and in their therapy (Lefkowitz 1979; Lefkowitz and Hoffman 1981). Table 1.3

Table 1.3. Factors regulating α- and β-adrenoceptors

Regulatory agent or condition	Effect on number of receptors
α-adrenoceptors	
α-adrenergic catecholamines	Decrease
Denervation	Increase
Hyperthyroidism	Decrease (also decrease affinity)
β-adrenoceptors	
β-adrenergic catecholamines	Decrease
Propranolol	Increase
Denervation (chemical, pharmacological, or surgical)	Increase
Hyperthyroidism	Increase
Hypothyroidism	Decrease

(Lefkowitz 1979; Lefkowitz and Hoffman 1981.)

Table 1.4. Clinical implications of receptors (for drugs, hormones, and neurotransmitters

Disease	Receptor involved
Diabetes mellitus	Insulin
Male pseudohermaphrodism:	
Testicular feminization syndrome	Androgen
Reifenstein syndrome	Androgen
Vitamin D-resistant rickets	1,25-dihydroxy Vitamin D_3 (1,25-dihydroxy cholecalciferol; calcitriol)
Asthma, including desensitization to β-agonists	β-adrenoceptor
Hypothyroidism	β-adrenoceptor
Myasthenia gravis	Acetylcholine (nicotinic)

(Lefkowitz 1979; Lefkowitz and Hoffmann 1981.)

lists some factors regulating α- and β-adrenoceptors. Table 1.4 indicates the clinical implications of receptors by listing those diseases in which receptor abnormalities are known to be involved. Thus, the subject of pharmacological receptors is not only of academic interest to pharmacologists but has become of great practical importance in the pathology, diagnosis, and treatment of disease.

Relationships between the dose of a drug and the effect (response) it produces

Two types of relationship need to be considered.

1. *Quantitative (= graded) responses or effects*

Consider the situation where increasing doses of a drug are applied to a piece of isolated tissue—for example, small intestine. With the smallest doses no effect is seen until a certain threshold dose is reached when a detectable effect is recorded. Thereafter the effect increases as the dose is increased until a maximum is reached. Beyond this point any further increase in dose is not accompanied by an increase in the size of the response. When the relationship between the dose and effect is plotted as a graph it produces a hyperbolic shaped curve; see Fig. 1.11(a). Pharmacologists find it more useful to plot the logarithm of the dose of agonist (instead of the dose) against the effect because this transforms the hyperbolic curve (Fig. 1.11(a)) into a sigmoid curve; see Fig. 1.11(b). It can be seen that over the range 25–75 per cent maximum response the graph is a straight line and this is much more convenient to handle than the hyperbolic curve. This is particularly so when comparing a series of dose–effect curves that have been constructed from the results of testing varying concentrations of a drug in the presence of a series of fixed concentrations of a specific antagonist to that drug.

It is not necessary for the dental student or practitioner to be conversant with the detailed mathematical analysis of dose–effect curves. However, the present availability of personal microcomputers has encouraged many individuals to

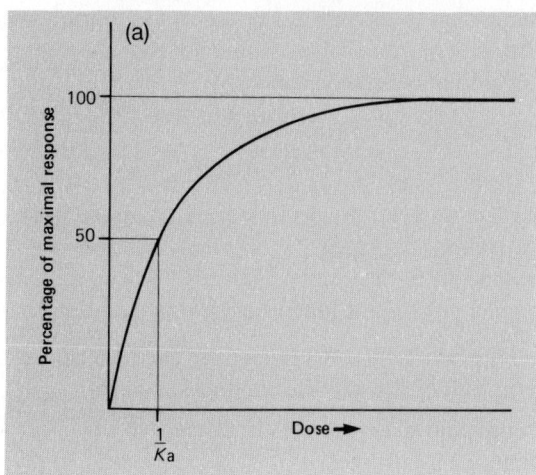

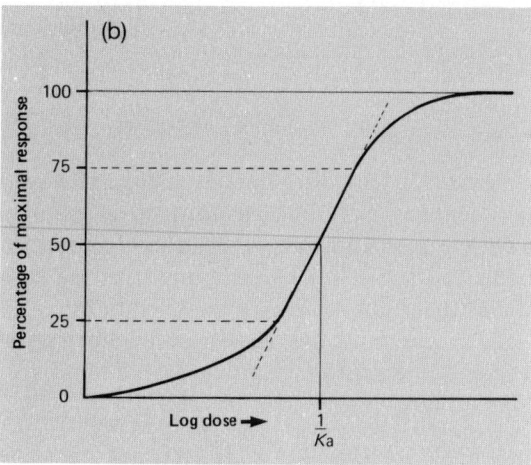

Fig. 1.11. Quantitative (graded responses: dose–response (dose–effect) curves. (a) Graph showing relationship between concentration of a drug and response (effect) plotted linearly. (b) Same data as in (a) but plotted semi-logarithmically. Note: (i) Hyperbolic curve in (a) transformed by semi-logarithmic plot into sigmoid curve (b), which is conveniently linear over the range 25–75% maximal response. (ii) Both curves have same maxima. (iii) If it is assumed that a half-maximal contraction occurs when 50% of receptors are occupied, then from equation 2 (see text)

$$(A) = \frac{1}{Ka}.$$

The Figure shows how the value of (A) is measured from the dose–response curve and from which the affinity constant (Ka) is obtained by calculating the reciprocal. Thus, the lower the concentration required to elicit a half-maximal response, the greater the affinity of the drug and the larger the numerical value of Ka.

become mathematically inquisitive. It thus seems appropriate to indicate that the relationship between the dose of a drug and the effect it produces can be represented by a mathematical equation:

$$Y = \frac{(A)Ka}{1+(A)Ka}.$$ Equation (1)

where Y = proportion of receptors occupied; (A) = molar concentration of drug; Ka = affinity (association) constant.

Thus, if it is assumed that the effect produced by a drug is related to the number of receptors occupied (Y) then it follows from this equation that:

(1) With no drug (i.e. when (A) = 0) there is no effect (because the expression on the right-hand side of the equation reduces to zero).

(2) As the concentration of drug (A) is increased, so the effect increases until it reaches a *limiting maximum*.
   Note: this statement may be verified by substituting the term $(A)Ka$ (which appears in both the numerator and denominator of the equation) with increasing numerical values, e.g. 1, 10, 100, 1000, etc.

(3) When 50 per cent of receptors are occupied:

$$(A) = \frac{1}{Ka}.$$ Equation (2)

The affinity constant (Ka) for a drug can be readily determined by carrying out a laboratory experiment in which sufficient doses are given to span the full range of the dose–response curve. The curve is then plotted and from this the dose required to produce 50 per cent of maximum response is read off and the reciprocal calculated; this value represents the Ka of the drug (see Fig. 1.11). This method can be used to determine the relative affinities of a series of drugs acting on the same receptor—for example, a group of β-adrenoceptor blocking drugs.

2. Quantal (all or nothing) responses or effects

In many situations the response to a drug is all or none. For example, in a toxicity test a dose of a drug will either kill or not, so that an animal is either alive or dead. When such a test is carried out, the animals are first divided into several groups. The dosage *within* groups is the same (on a dose for body weight basis) whereas the dose *between* groups is different. For example, there might be five groups of animals each containing six animals. The doses given to each group might be 2.5, 5, 10, 20, and 40 mg/kg (i.e. distributed logarithmically) and each animal in a particular group would receive the dose for that group adjusted for body weight. The percentage responding in each group is recorded and a graph is plotted of these values against the dose used for each group.

Similarly, the dose of an hypnotic needed to produce drowsiness can be expressed graphically. Figure 1.12 shows the results of a study in which amylobarbitone (a barbiturate) was used to produce drowsiness (given by slow intravenous injection) in 55 obstetric patients, and shows that these kind of data can be plotted in two ways. Figure 1.12(a) shows the data as a frequency histogram, and Fig. 1.12(b) shows them in the form of a cumulative distribution curve. Note that the data in Fig. 1.12(b) have been plotted linearly, i.e. it has not been necessary to carry out a semi-logarithmic transformation (although this may be necessary when data turns out to be skewed). From the foregoing it can be seen that quantal data can be treated in the same way as data representing quantitative (= graded) effects. When, as mentioned earlier in this section, the experiment concerns the measurement of drug toxicity in animals, the amount required to kill 50 per cent of animals can be determined, and this is known as the LD_{50} (lethal dose to kill 50 per cent). An analogous term used to describe the dose required to produce a given effect in 50 per cent of the population of animals is known as the ED_{50} (effective dose in 50 per cent of animals).

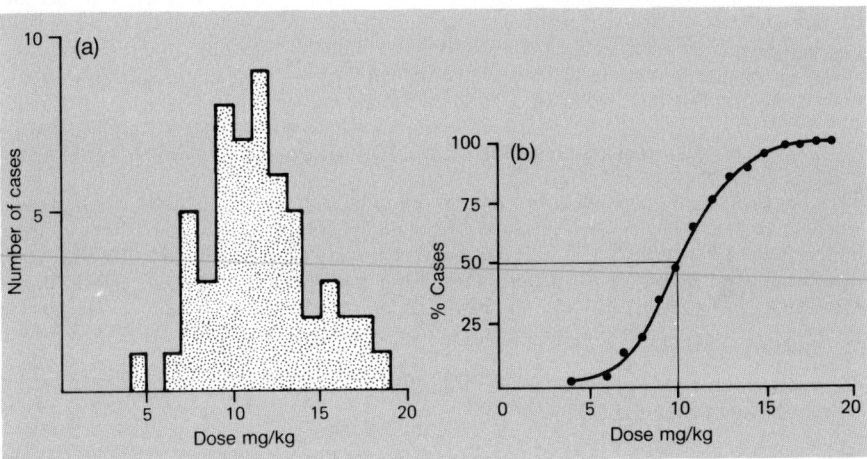

Fig. 1.12. Quantal (all or nothing) responses. Graphs showing the dosage of amylobarbitone sodium needed to produce drowsiness when given by slow intravenous injection to 55 obstetric patients. (a) The data have been expressed as a frequency histogram. (b) The same results plotted as a cumulative frequency distribution. Note: effective dose for 50% of patients (ED_{50}) is 10 mg/kg with a four-fold range extending from 4–19 mg/kg for all patients.

Therapeutic index

An 'ideal' drug would cure all patients in a dose that kills none. The therapeutic index gives a measure of the safety margin available, although it does not take into account the possible occurrence of an abnormal response, such as an allergic response or idiosyncracy (see Chapter 21). Figure 1.13 shows quantal responses

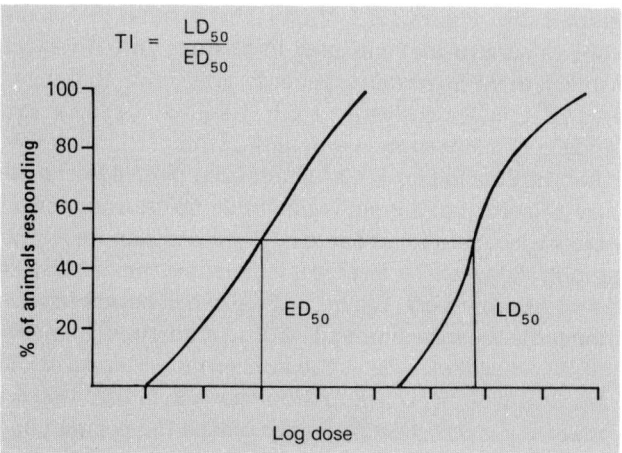

Fig. 1.13. Illustration of the concept of therapeutic index (TI). Abscissa shows the dose of drug (mg/kg) and ordinate shows percentage of animals responding. The left-hand curve indicates the percentage of animals that respond to various doses of drug from which the dose needed to produce the desired pharmacological effect in 50% of animals is found. The right-hand curve shows the relationship between the dose of drug and the number of animals that die from it, from which the dose required to kill 50% is then found.

$$\text{The Therapeutic Index (TI)} = LD_{50}/ED_{50}. \quad \text{For example:} \quad \frac{6.6}{3} = 2.2.$$

The drug that has the same pharmacological action but a higher TI than the one illustrated would (other things being equal) be a safer drug and vice versa. Graphically the TI is represented by the distance between the two curves, provided they are tolerably parallel. (Reproduced by permission from Clark, W. G., Brater, D. C., and Johnson, A. R. (1988). *Goth's Medical Pharmacology*, (12th edn). The C.V. Mosby Co., St Louis, MO, USA.)

for a therapeutic effect (for example, hypnosis) and a toxic effect (death) from which it can be seen that:

$$\text{Therapeutic index} = \frac{LD_{50}}{ED_{50}}$$

which in this case is 6.6 divided by $3 = 2.2$. The higher the numerical value of the therapeutic index, the safer the drug is likely to be.

Clinical implications

Whilst there is no such thing as a 'safe' drug, some are safer than others, i.e. have a higher therapeutic index than others. For example, if lignocaine is taken as a reference compound with a therapeutic index $= 1$, then cocaine has a therapeutic index of 0.6 whereas prilocaine has a therapeutic index of 1.18. This means that, all other things being equal, cocaine is substantially more toxic than lignocaine whereas prilocaine is about as toxic as the reference compound. When it is proposed to prescribe any drug its toxicity should always be taken into consideration and the risk of treatment weighed against the risk of the disease (risk: benefit ratio). An example of the application of this principle in practice is the use of a known highly toxic drug for the treatment of cancer.

Drug antagonism

Antagonism between two drugs can be said to occur when their biological effect is less than the expected sum of their individual effects. Therapeutically, drug action is commonly employed in order to reduce (or sometimes abolish) the action of (i) some endogenous compound—for example, a neurotransmitter or hormone; or (ii) another drug—for example, to counteract an unwanted effect or to treat an overdose effect. There are some five types of drug antagonism classified as follows:

Pharmacological antagonism

By convention the term 'pharmacological antagonism' implies antagonism by receptor blockade and is of two main types:

1. *Reversible competitive (equilibrium competitive) antagonism* This occurs when the action of an agonist is interfered with by an antagonist because both substances are competing dynamically for the same pharmacological receptor (see Fig. 1.14). A key feature, and one of both academic and clinical importance, is that of surmountability of the block by the addition of agonist. An example is atropine antagonizing the muscarinic actions of acetylcholine. As indicated earlier, with this type of antagonism the concentration of the agonist (in this example, acetylcholine) is not altered by the presence of atropine; but the effect of the atropine is to reduce the probability that a given molecule of acetylcholine will be successful in arriving at and activating a receptor. This will be because it has been prevented from so doing by a molecule of atropine that, having united with the receptor, is unable to inactivate it. This concept can be verified both experimentally and in certain clinical situations, where an existing degree of pharmacological block can be increased or decreased at will by administering additional doses of the appropriate antagonist or agonist (within reasonable limits). Other examples are H_1 and H_2 blockers antagonizing the actions of histamine; α- and β-adrenoceptors blocking the actions of noradrenaline and adrenaline.

2. *Irreversible competitive (non-equilibrium competitive) antagonism* Some drugs act as antagonists by forming very strong bonds—for example, covalent bonds with receptors—thereby occluding them for long periods of time (see Fig. 1.14). Thus the molecules of antagonist dissociate very slowly or not at all. Examples are: phenoxybenzamine which antagonizes the actions of noradrenaline and adrenaline.

Clinical implications

A reversible competitive antagonist has much greater clinical acceptability than an irreversible competitive antagonist because its action can, if necessary, be reversed (theoretically, if not in practice) by administering a dose of an

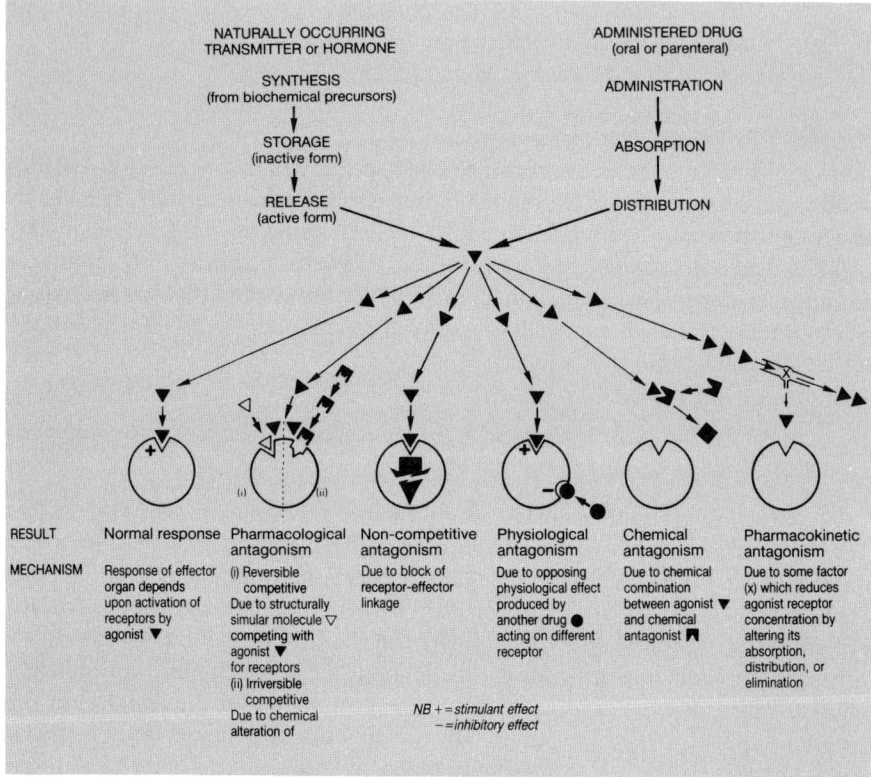

Fig. 1.14. Diagram to illustrate the different types of drug antagonism. The molecules of agonist are shown arising from alternative sources. Top left, endogenous: the stages in the synthesis of a naturally occurring transmitter or hormone are indicated. Top right, exogenous: the stages that follow the oral or parenteral administration of a drug are indicated. The action of agonist molecules on a single receptor of an effector organ under normal conditions is depicted as well as in the presence of pharmacological (reversible competitive or irreversible competitive), non-competitive, physiological, chemical, or pharmacokinetic antagonists. Note: in order to simplify the diagram, it has been assumed that the naturally occurring substance and the administered drug act on the same receptor and that all four types of antagonist exist for the same agonist. Reversible pharmacological antagonism occurs commonly; the second and third are uncommon, and the fourth is rare. Physiological antagonism and pharmacokinetic antagonism are less common, whilst the others are uncommon.

appropriate agonist. This cannot be done with an irreversible competitive antagonist because it binds on to the receptors tenaciously and remains static. Therefore if the patient is given too large a dose of an irreversible competitive antagonist no amount of agonist (which normally acts on the same receptor) can reverse the effect, although it may be possible to reverse it by using a physiological antagonist (see below).

Non-competitive antagonism

Some antagonists block the action of an agonist NOT at the receptor level *but* by interfering, in a non-specific way, with some point in the critical link between receptor and effector that normally leads to the action of the agonist. A good example is that of a calcium channel blocker, which will interfere with the action of any agonist that normally activates a response in which calcium ions (Ca^{2+}) play a critical role.

Physiological antagonism

This occurs when two drugs that act on *different* receptors produce opposite effects. A good example is when adrenaline antagonizes the constrictor effects of histamine on bronchial smooth muscle. Physiological antagonism is of clinical importance and can be life-saving in the treatment of bronchial asthma (due to endogenous bronchoconstrictor substances) with drugs such as adrenaline, isoprenaline, or salbutamol (the latter two given as inhalations). Physiological antagonism can also be used to deal with a clinical situation where an excessive dose of an irreversible competitive antagonist (see above) has been given.

Chemical antagonism

This occurs when one drug combines chemically with another to produce an inactive product; for example, as when dimercaprol (British Anti-Lewisite) forms relatively non-toxic complexes with compounds of mercury, arsenic, antimony, and gold and so can be used to treat poisoning with these substances. Thus, with sodium arsenite (a trivalent arsenical compound), dimercaprol, forms a cyclic thioarsenite by means of coupling with sulphydryl (SH) groups:

$$NaOAs=O \; + \; \begin{array}{c} HS-CH_2 \\ | \\ HS-CH \\ | \\ HO-CH_2 \end{array} \rightarrow \; NaOAs \begin{array}{c} S-CH_2 \\ | \\ S-CH \\ | \\ HO-CH_2 \end{array} \; + \; H_2O$$

Chemical antagonists that combine chemically with another substance (endogenous or exogenous) are also known as chelating agents (Gk. *khele* = claw). Other important examples are D-penicillamine (chelates Cu, cystine) and ethylenediamine tetra-acetic acid (EDTA) (chelates Ca).

Pharmacokinetic antagonism

This occurs when one drug effectively reduces the concentration of another at its site of action by altering its absorption, distribution, or elimination. For example, the effect of warfarin (an anticoagulant) may be reduced by certain drugs (e.g. phenobarbitone) that increase its rate of metabolism in the body.

Drugs which do NOT act on specific receptors

As indicated earlier, members of this group (i) act at higher concentrations; (ii) tend NOT to show structure–activity relationships; and (iii) do not have specific antagonists. Examples include general anaesthetics, e.g. halothane; diuretics, e.g. thiazides; and non-specific destructants of cell membranes, e.g. detergents.

Drugs in this group act by causing some change in cell membranes by virtue of their physico-chemical properties. It seems likely that general anaesthetics perturb cell membranes in such a way that they interfere with the normal passage of ions and other essential substances across these vital structures. Although general anaesthetic agents produce the same type of effect on all cells membranes, brain cells are more susceptible and can thus be reversibly depressed by these agents at concentrations that do not produce serious effects on cells of other tissues. Also of importance is the fact that cells within the vital centres of the brain (respiration, blood pressure) are more resistant than those in certain other parts of the nervous system. This produces a useful differential effect resulting in general anaesthesia without the loss of function of vital centres, except in overdose. (For further discussion on the mode of action of general anaesthetics see Chapter 8.)

THE THERAPEUTIC PROCESS: IS THE PHARMACOLOGICAL EFFECT BEING TRANSLATED INTO A DESIRED THERAPEUTIC EFFECT?

When drugs are used to treat disease it is important to try to understand the way in which the drug and its effects interact with the pathological processes

Table 1.5. Factors that determine the relationship between prescribed drug dosage and drug effect

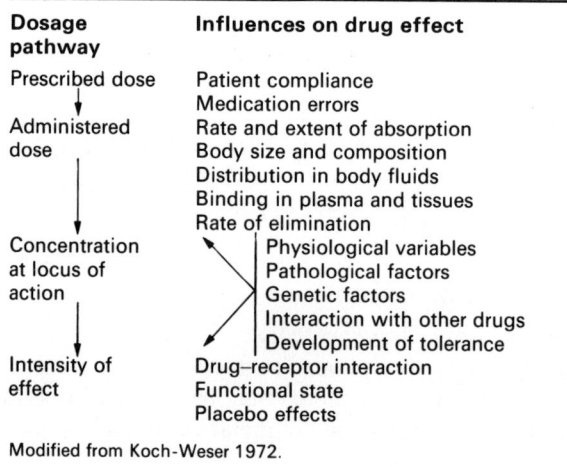

Dosage pathway	Influences on drug effect
Prescribed dose	Patient compliance
	Medication errors
Administered dose	Rate and extent of absorption
	Body size and composition
	Distribution in body fluids
	Binding in plasma and tissues
	Rate of elimination
Concentration at locus of action	Physiological variables
	Pathological factors
	Genetic factors
	Interaction with other drugs
	Development of tolerance
Intensity of effect	Drug–receptor interaction
	Functional state
	Placebo effects

Modified from Koch-Weser 1972.

underlying the disease. In some instances this is fairly obvious whilst in others it is far from clear. There are many factors concerned with the drug and with the patient that influence the final result and these vary from drug to drug and from patient to patient. The use of particular drugs for the treatment of particular diseases encountered by the dental practitioner are dealt with elsewhere within the appropriate chapters of this book. Nevertheless, each time a drug is prescribed the dental practitioner should bear in mind the main steps that lead from the prescription of the drug(s) to the end result. It is useful and important to have in mind a check list of the various stages involved and the factors that determine the relationship between prescribed drug dosage and drug effect. These have been usefully summarized by Koch-Weser (1972) in the form of a flow chart (Table 1.5).

REFERENCES

Alvares, A. P. [1978]. Interactions between environmental chemicals and drug biotransformation in man. *Clinical Pharmacokinetics*, **3**, 462.

Avery, G. S. (1980). *Drug treatment* (2nd edn). Adis Press, Sydney and New York.

Berridge, M. J. (1981). Receptors and calcium signalling. In *Towards understanding receptors* (ed. J. W. Lamble). Elsevier/North Holland, Amsterdam.

Bowman, W. C., Bowman, A., and Bowman, A. (1986). *Dictionary of pharmacology*. Blackwell Scientific Publications, Oxford.

Brodie, B. B. (1956). Review Article. Pathways of drug metabolism. *Journal of Pharmacy and Pharmacology*, **8**, 1–17.

Brodie, B. B. (1964). Physico-chemical factors in drug absorption. In *Absorption and distribution of drugs*. (ed. T. B. Binns). Livingstone, Edinburgh.

Cannon, W. S. and Rosenblueth, A. (1949). *The supersensitivity of denervated structures: law of denervation*. The Macmillan Company, New York.

Clark, A. J. (1937). General pharmacology. In *Handbuch der experimentelle Pharmakologie Vol. 4* (ed. A. Heffter and H. Henbner). Springer, Berlin.

Clark, W. G., Brater, D. C., and Johnson, A. R. (1988). *Goths Medical Pharmacology*, (12th edn). The C. V. Mosly Co., St Louis, MO, USA.

Creasy, W. A. (1979). *Drug disposition in humans*. Oxford Univesity Press.

Dost, F. H. (1953). *Der blutspiegel kinetik der konzentraztion-sablaufe in der kreislauffussigkeit*. Thieme, Leipzig.

Drew, G. C., Colquhoun, W. P., and Long, H. A. (1958). Effects of small doses of alcohol on a skill resembling driving. *British Medical Journal*, **2**, 993–9.

Gillette, J. R. (1967). In *Drug responses in man*. (ed. G. Wolstenholme and R. Porter). Churchill, London.

Goldberg, A. and Griffin, J. P. (1984). Functions of the Committee on Safety of Medicines. *Update* July 1984, 29–33.

Grahame-Smith, P. G. and Aronson, J. K. (1984). *Oxford textbook of clinical pharmacology and drug therapy*. Oxford University Press, Oxford.

Houslay, M. D. and Stanley, K. K. (1982). *Dynamics of biological membranes*. John Wiley and Sons, Chichester and New York.

Jusko, W. J. (1978). Role of tobacco smoking in pharmacokinetics. *Journal of Pharmacokinetics and Biopharmaceutics*, **6**, 7.

Kalow, W. (1962). *Pharmacogenetics: heredity and the response to drugs*. Saunders, Philadelphia.

Katzung, B. G. (1984). *Basic and clinical pharmacology* (2nd edn), Lange Medical Publications, Los Altos, CA.

Koch-Weser, J. (1972). Serum drug concentrations as therapeutic guides. *New England Journal of Medicine*, **287**, 227–31.

Langley, J. N. (1905). On the reaction of cells and of nerve-endings to certain poisons chiefly as regards the reaction of striated muscle to nicotine and to curari. *Journal of Physiology*, **33**, 374–413.

Lee, E. J. D. and Lee, L. K. H. (1982). A simple pharmacokinetic method for separating the three acetylation phenotypes: a preliminary report. *British Journal of Clinical Pharmacology*, **3**, 375–8.

Lefkowitz, R. J. (1979). Direct binding studies of adrenergic receptors: biochemical, physiologic and clinical implications. *Annals of Internal Medicine*, **91**, 450–8.

Lefkowitz, R. J. and Hoffman, R. J. (1981). New directions in adrenergic receptor research. Parts I & II. In *Towards understanding receptors*. (ed. J. W. Lamble). Elsevier/North Holland, Amsterdam.

Leonards, J. R. (1963). The influence of solubility on the rate of gastrointestinal absorption of aspirin. *Clinical Pharmacology and Therapeutics*, **4**, 476–9.

Lindemann, B. and Solomon, A. K. (1962). Permeability of luminal surface of intestinal mucosal cells. *Journal of General Physiology*, **45**, 801–10.

Ogilvie, R. I. (1978). Clinical pharmacokinetics of theophylline. *Clinical Pharmacokinetics*, **3**, 267.

Park, B. K. and Breckenridge, A. M. (1981). Clinical implications of enzyme induction and enzyme inhibition. *Clinical Pharmacokinetics*, **6**, 1–24.

Paton, W. M. D. (1963). *The early days of pharmacology*. In *Chemistry the service of medicine* (ed. F. N. L. Paynter). Pitman Medical, London.

Rawlins, M. D., James, O. F. W., Williams, F. M., Wynne, H., and Woodhouse, K. W. (1987). Age and the metabolism of drugs. *Quarterly Journal of Medicine, New Series*, **64**, 243, 545–7.

Rawlins, M. D. and Thompson, J. W. (1985). Mechanisms of adverse drug reactions. In *Textbook of adverse drug reactions*. (3rd edn) (ed. D. M. Davies). Oxford University Press, Oxford.

Routledge, P. A. (1986). Interactions that matter: 6. Warfarin. *Prescriber's Journal*, **26**(3), 71–5.

Schild, H. O. (1980). *Applied pharmacology*. Churchill Livingstone, Edinburgh.

Sjöqvist, B., Borga, A., and Orme, M. L'E. (1980). Fundamentals of Clinical Pharmacology. In *Drug treatment* (ed. G. S. Avery). Adis Press, Sydney and New York.

Smith, J. M. and Dodd, T. R. P. (1982). Adverse reactions to pharmaceutical excipients. *Adverse Drug Reactions and Acute Poisoning Review*, **i**, 93–142.

Smyth, D. H. (1964). In *Absorption and distribution of drugs*. (ed. T. B. Binns). Livingstone, Edinburgh.

Thompson, J. W. (1967). Pharmacology in perspective. An inaugural lecture, University of Newcastle upon Tyne.

Tyrer, J. H., Eadie, M. J., Sutherland, J. M., and Hooper, W. D. (1970). Outbreak of anticonvulsant intoxication in an Australian city. *British Medical Journal*, **iv**, 271–3.

2

The administration of drugs: the routes of administration

IN broad terms, the administration of drugs has already been considered in Chapter 1 under two headings: (a) local or topical administration; and (b) systemic administration. The purpose here is consider detail of these routes, their advantages and disadvantages.

LOCAL ADMINISTRATION

This route includes applications to the oral mucous membranes, the skin, and other epithelial surfaces. Topical application is instituted to obtain a local drug effect, such as the use of a local anaesthetic spray prior to insertion of a needle, or of a caustic stick to remove a wart from the skin. The intention behind such local applications is to restrict the activity of that drug to the point of application.

There is some danger in thinking of drugs in this static way for, although most drugs do not penetrate the unbroken skin, this is not universally true. However, many potentially toxic drugs may be applied topically to the skin without the worry of them causing general unwanted effects throughout the body. A good example of this are the potent synthetic corticosteroids, which have revolutionized the treatment of many skin diseases. Corticosteroid creams and ointments when applied locally to skin disorders will provide relief in properly selected cases. Some of the steroid drug may be absorbed into the body but fortunately the plasma levels so obtained are usually insufficient to produce systemic effects. Of course, if the skin is broken then drugs can be quickly absorbed from such damaged surfaces. In a child with extensive eczema there could be significant absorption of the applied steroid. An infant's skin is more permeable and in them steroids penetrate more completely.

The mucous membranes of the oral cavity differ from the skin in that they provide excellent surfaces for the *absorption* of a wide variety of substances. Indeed absorption may be very rapid and this fact has not always been utilized to advantage in pharmacy. Nevertheless, mucous absorption (see below) is made use of (e.g. sublingual glyceryl trinitrate for angina) as one of the enteral, systemic routes. What must be made clear is that when a drug is applied to the mucous membranes with the intention of producing a local effect, it may not only produce a local action but may also be rapidly absorbed (e.g. xylodase paste).

SYSTEMIC ADMINISTRATION

When a drug is given with the intention of being absorbed it is said to have been administered systemically. The systemic routes can conveniently be classified (see Chapter 1) as (a) enteral; and (b) parenteral.

Enteral routes

By these oral and rectal routes a drug is placed directly into the gastro-intestinal tract from where absorption occurs.

Oral route

This is probably the safest, most convenient, and economical method of administering drugs systemically. Drugs given by mouth are, for the most part, absorbed from the small intestine but alcohol is appreciably absorbed through the stomach—almost an unique substance. The ways of drug absorption have been discussed in Chapter 1. The oral route is probably the safest way because, if the patient is allergic to the drug, the reaction is likely to be less severe if administration is by this route than by some other routes. This does not imply that this route is absolutely safe; drugs given orally can produce some very severe reactions. However, it is a more convenient method for obvious reasons and much more economical, for patients can always take the dose themselves, and tablets and capsules are much less costly than an injection, which often has to be given by a nurse or doctor.

There are several disadvantages to the oral ingestion of drugs:

1. Irritant drugs cannot always be given by mouth for they may cause sickness, e.g. large doses (over 1.5 mg) of erythromycin will hardly be tolerated. Often the irritant effect can be mitigated by giving such a drug just before or with food, when absorption may be delayed, e.g. iron preparations on an empty stomach.

2. It is not feasible to give drugs by this route to patients who are vomiting or who are moribund.

3. Many drugs are destroyed by the action of the digestive ferments before they can be absorbed, e.g. benzylpenicillin.

4. Intestinal absorption may, at times, be somewhat irregular due to the influences of other substances in the gastro-intestinal tract. The timing of drug administration in relation to food, for instance, can influence the effectiveness of that drug. There may be enhanced absorption or reduced absorption. Generally speaking oral antibiotics should be given on an empty stomach to avoid impairment of absorption when food is present. On the other hand, oral hypoglycaemic agents should be taken with or just before meals in order that they can exert optimal control of blood sugar.

Rectal route

Drugs are sometimes given via the rectum, in a solid form as suppositories or in a liquid form as enemata. It is a route which can be used if the patient is unable to swallow, and it also avoids the acidity and enzymes of the gastric juice.

Parenteral routes

Parenteral administration is generally chosen when speed or reliability are especially desired.

Injection

In some instances injection of the drug is essential if the drug is to be absorbed in active form, e.g. streptomycin. Absorption is usually more predictable and more rapid than when the oral route is used. Injections have some obvious disadvantages:

(1) It can be difficult for patients to perform the injection themselves.

(2) Strict asepsis must be maintained if infection is to be avoided.

(3) Parenteral administration is usually more costly than oral administration and is generally less safe.

(4) Injections can cause pain whereas swallowing a tablet is usually an innocuous business.

Injections can be made into subcutaneous, intramuscular, and intravenous sites.

Subcutaneous (SC)   The subcutaneous route can only be used for drugs which are not irritant to tissues, otherwise a slough could be caused. It is a common way of giving such drugs as morphine sulphate, adrenaline, and insulin. The volume of most subcutaneous injections is usually 1 ml or less, and should seldom exceed 2 ml. Cutaneous blood flow is much slower than in muscle and so absorption is that much slower. Sustained effects can be obtained from drugs by the implantation of a pellet subcutaneously.

Intramuscular (IM)   The blood supply to muscle is good. Lipid-soluble drugs are able to diffuse rapidly through capillary walls and so absorption from this route is good. Even completely lipid-insoluble drugs can be rapidly absorbed provided their molecular weight is low enough for them to pass through the pores in the capillary membrane.

Strangely enough the intramuscular route can be more dangerous than the intravenous route. If an adverse effect occurs during intravenous injection, then the injection can be immediately discontinued but, if such an effect develops after an intramuscular injection, there is no way in which further absorption can be prevented. Larger volumes can be injected intramuscularly than subcutaneously, and the route is also better for irritant substances.

Occasionally, long acting depot preparations are used by deep intra-muscular injection, e.g. norethisterone ocnanthate. This is an oily preparation providing contraception for 8 weeks.

Intravenous (IV)   The advantages of this route are:

(1) Rapid action: the desired blood concentration is reached with an immediacy not obtained by any other route.

(2) It can be used for drugs which are irritant by intramuscular injection.

Disadvantages are:

(1) Once introduced, the drug cannot be recalled.

(2) Intravenous injections tend to produce more immediate unfavourable reactions.

(3) If injected rapidly a too high concentration of the drug is readily obtained.

(4) The chance of getting into an artery instead of a vein is a possibility.

Other routes of administration include (a) buccal and sublingual; (b) inhalation.

Buccal and sublingual

This enteral route is used infrequently but, as explained in Chapter 1, is useful in the case of a drug which has pronounced 'first-pass' hepatic metabolism. For example, glyceryl trinitrate is of proven use in an angina attack but if swallowed it is likely to be totally ineffective as its first-pass metabolism approaches 100 per cent. So it is used by sublingual administration, when there is no such effect.

Inhalation

Inhalant anaesthetics are the best example of this route of administration and are discussed in Chapter 8.

Aerosol inhalation has been used extensively in the treatment of obstructive airway disease, such as asthma. Inhalation is via the mouth; absorption will occur in the small bronchioles. An example is the use of disodium cromoglycate for inhalation via a 'Spinhaler'.

Other, less common sites of parenteral administration include intrathecal injection. Antimicrobials are sometimes given by this route in meningeal infections in order to by-pass the blood–brain barrier.

3

Prescribing and the law

THE dental surgeon does not prescribe a wide variety of drugs, but he must have knowledge of the regulations that govern prescribing. At one time pharmacists made up elaborate prescriptions to the order of the doctor; today most drugs are conveniently prepared in various forms (tablets, capsules, etc.). Drugs have chemical names, official/approved names, and proprietary names—the brand names provided by a manufacturer. Wherever possible it is sensible to use the official name rather than the proprietary name. If the proprietary name is used, then the pharmacist must supply that particular brand. If the official name is used, then the pharmacist is able to dispense whichever brand is available. After all, there may be many proprietary names and it would be impossible for any pharmacist to stock all of them. The official name is spelt with a small initial letter, and the proprietary name with an initial capital e.g. erythromycin (Erythrocin, Erycen, Erythroped).

Prescribing is governed by a number of regulations made under the Medicines Act of 1968 and the Misuse of Drugs Act of 1971.

THE MEDICINES ACT 1968

This Act deals with the manufacture, distribution, and importation of medicines for human use and of medicines for administration to animals. It also deals with things like the advertising and promotion of drugs, the registration of pharmacies, homeopathic medicines, containers and packages for drugs, labelling regulations, pharmacopoeias, formularies, and much else.

The Medicines Act is an enabling Act that allows, or enables, the appropriate Ministers (Health Ministers) to make orders or regulations interpreting the spirit of the Act in practical terms. The Health Ministers are advised by The Medicines Commission, which is a body appointed to advise them on matters related to medicines. The orders that are promulgated from time to time to interpret the meaning of the Act are known as Statutory Instruments (SI).

The Medicines Act is intended to ensure the safety, quality, and efficacy of medicines to be prescribed. The products subject to the Act are those which fall within the definition of a medicinal product, together with certain other articles and substances incorporated in an animal feeding stuff for a medicinal purpose, or brought within the licensing provision by statutory orders under the Act.

A basic principle of the Act is that it only applies when substances are used as medicinal products or as ingredients of medicinal products. A medicinal product is defined as a substance or article sold or supplied for administration to human beings or animals for a medicinal purpose, or as an ingredient for use in a preparation in a pharmacy or in a hospital, or by a practitioner, or in the course of a retail herbal remedy business.

There are three classes of medicinal products:

1. *General Sales List (GSL) Medicines*   This is really a list of substances that can be sold or supplied other than under the direction of a pharmacist. This list includes such things as aspirin, paracetamol, liquid paraffin, honeysuckle flowers, rock water, rose water, and much else. Such substances do not have to be sold in a pharmacy, although there may be a limit on the quantity supplied if sold other than in a pharmacy.

2. *Prescription Only Medicines (POM)*   These are medicinal products that can only be sold or supplied from pharmacies in accordance with a prescription given by an appropriate practitioner. For the purposes of the Act, a dental surgeon is regarded as an 'appropriate practitioner', as is a doctor and veterinary surgeon. The order that specifies such medicines includes things like lignocaine, antimicrobials, psychotropic drugs, and many other substances.

3. *Pharmacy Medicines (P)*   There is a host of substances, ill-defined, which are called pharmacy medicines. These are medicinal products that are not listed as General Sales List Medicines or as Prescription Only Medicines. These are substances which can be sold over the counter to the general public without prescription but which have to be sold from a pharmacy and with the pharmacist present at the time of the sale.

The prescription for a Prescription Only Medicine

This has to follow certain rules, for example:

(1) It must be written in indelible ink, or be typewritten.

(2) It must contain the following particulars:

    (i) the address and usual signature of the practitioner giving it

    (ii) the appropriate date on which it was signed by the practitioner giving it

    (iii) such particulars as indicate whether the practitioner giving it is a dentist, a doctor, or a veterinary surgeon

    (iv) where the practitioner is a dentist or a doctor, the name, address, and the age (if under 12) of the person for whose treatment it is given.

(3) The prescription shall not be dispensed later than 6 months after the appropriate date.

The form of the prescription

Prescriptions should be written clearly in English. There are a number of abbreviations that have commonly been used and may still be used—for example,

IM(i.m.) = intramuscular injection; IV (i.v.) = intravenous injection; SC (s.c.) = subcutaneous injection. Many other abbreviations are best discarded— such as o.m. = every morning; o.n. = every night; t.d.s. = three times a day; q.d.s. = four times a day. Multiplicity of abbreviations leads to confusion and error.

Doses of drugs are to be found in official books of reference, such as the *Dental Practitioners' Formulary* (DPF). The recommendations contained in these guides are not binding on the prescriber but are obviously sensible indications based on experience and deliberation. A prescription is the authority for a pharmacist to supply specified drugs to any particular patient. A sample of a completed prescription is shown in Fig. 3.1.

The general form of the prescription should be clear from the sample provided. The main body of the prescription refers to the actual drugs to be prescribed, in this instance penicillin V. The name and strength of the drug is first indicated (e.g. penicillin V tablets 250 mg), and this is followed by the amount of the drug to be

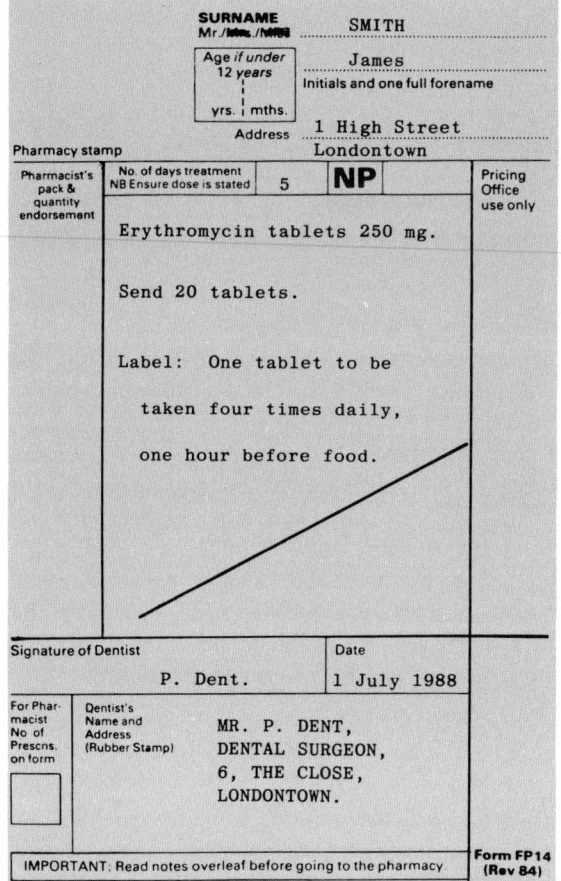

Fig. 3.1. Prescription writing. Layout for a prescription only medicine (POM).

supplied (e.g. 20 tablets). This information is immediately followed by instructions to the pharmacist as to what information is to be written on the labelled medicine and, on the prescription form, follows the word 'Label'. Such directions should be written in English without abbreviation and it is of the utmost importance that these instructions are clear. There must be no possibility of confusion on the part of the dispenser, for it is these instructions that are transcribed by the dispenser to the label on the package to be received by the patient. A phrase like 'as directed' should never appear as this is far too vague and open to misinterpretation.

It is not always necessary to give the strength of the drug to be supplied, prescribing can be by 'title'. Drugs that are of fixed composition and are included in the *British National Formulary* (BNF) or the *Dental Practitioners' Formulary* (DPF) may be prescribed by title. For example, instead of writing penicillin V tablets, 250 mg, it is in order to write penicillin V tablets DPF. Here the amount in each tablet is not specified because the inclusion of the abbreviation DPF indicates a standard preparation. Prescriptions for other and non-standard preparations must be written out in full.

Although the dental surgeon may issue a prescription for such drugs, he may wish to keep some in his surgery for supply to the patients as needed. The dental surgeon is a person who is able to purchase such medicines. In this case, the seller, i.e. the chemist, has to keep a record of supply of Prescription Only Medicines (POM) in his Prescription Only Register. The following details are required:

(1) the date on which the Prescription Only Medicine was sold or supplied

(2) the name, quantity, and pharmaceutical form and strength of the medicine

(3) the name and address, trade, business, or profession of the person to whom the medicine is sold or supplied.

No entry is required in the Prescription Only Register where the drug is a 'controlled drug' (see Misuse of Drugs Act below) as a separate entry has then to be made in another register.

The dental practitioner is able to prescribe drugs listed in the *Dental Practitioners' Formulary* as a charge to the Health Service. For this purpose Form F.P.14 is used in England and Wales, and Form E.C.14 in Scotland. Prescribing is not limited to those drugs listed in the *Formulary* but if a drug is prescribed which is not so listed it will have to be prescribed privately. A prescription must be signed by the prescribing practitioner and an assistant must also add the name of the practitioner by whom he or she is employed.

SOME FACTORS INFLUENCING PRESCRIBING

Age

The dose of a drug should bear some relationship to body weight. The reaction to drugs is markedly different in children, especially in the new born, to that of adults. In the very early days of life there is limited renal filtration and detoxification of drugs is inadequate. Although doses for children based on body weight or body surface area are to be preferred, an age-related dosage can be used when prescribing drugs with a high therapeutic index (see Chapter 1).

Age	Percentage of adult dose
Birth	12–13
1 year	25
3 years	33
7 years	50
10 years	60
14 years and over	Adult dose

Dosage for the in-between years can be adjusted accordingly. An important point to remember is that drugs should not be prescribed in liquid preparations containing sucrose, particularly if this is to be over a long period. Clearly the presence of sucrose will encourage dental caries.

The elderly also present a problem for the prescriber. In old age many factors may be changed, for instance the speed of absorption of drugs may be altered, and so may the metabolism and excretion. These were explained in Chapter 1 but bear repetition here. Of especial importance is the decrease in renal clearance which occurs from mid-life onwards. This will invariably increase the concentration of the drug in the body because of the reduction in the rate of elimination. At the same time the liver may not be so efficient in metabolizing drugs as it is in earlier life. The *British National Formulary* suggests that 'when prescribing drugs in the elderly, it is a sensible policy to limit the range of drugs used to a minimum' and that 'it is good practice to initiate treatment in aged patients with doses of little more than half that recommended for younger subjects'.

Prescribing in pregnancy and during breast-feeding

Care must be exercised in prescribing drugs to the pregnant patient because of the possibility of fetal damage. In fact, it is better not to prescribe drugs to the pregnant patient at all unless this is absolutely imperative, and new drugs should be viewed with extreme caution. This subject is extensively reviewed in the combined *National Formulary*, which should be possessed by all dental practitioners. Prescribing during breast-feeding is also reviewed in the combined *Formulary*.

The letters NP appear on National Health Service prescription forms. NP (*nomen proprium*) means that the drug(s) listed in the prescription will be named on the label automatically. This is invaluable in that it makes for ready identification of the drug(s). If, for any reason, the prescriber does not want the drugs so labelled, then the NP must be crossed out.

Prescribing in renal disease

Some drugs should be avoided when the patient has reduced renal function, whilst others should be prescribed at reduced dosage (Table 3.1). In the presence of renal impairment a drug, or its metabolites, may not be excreted and the accumulation of the drug may produce a toxic effect.

Table 3.1. Drugs in the DPF to be avoided or used with caution in renal impairment

Drugs	Dosage recommendations	Comments
Central nervous system		
Anti-inflammatory analgesics	Avoid if possible	Fluid retention and deterioration in renal function
Aspirin	Avoid	As above. Also increased risk of gastro-intestinal bleeding
Diflunisal	Avoid	Excreted by kidney
Hypnotics and anxiolytics	Start with small doses	Increased cerebral sensitivity
Narcotic analgesics		
Codeine, dihydrocodeine	Avoid	Increased and prolonged effect
Pethidine	Avoid	Increased CNS toxicity
Infections		
Acyclovir	Reduce dose	May produce transient increase in plasma urea
Amphotericin	Use only if no alternative	Nephrotoxic
Cephalosporins		
Cephalexin	Max. 500 mg daily when GFR<10	
Cephradine	Reduce dose	
Co-trimoxazole	Max. 960 mg daily when GFR<10	Rashes and blood disorders
Lincomycin	Use clindamycin instead	
Penicillins		
Amoxycillin	Reduce dose	Rashes more common
Ampicillin	Reduce dose	Rashes more common
Benzylpenicillin	Max. 6 g daily when GFR<10	Neurotoxicity
Tetracyclines (except doxycyline and minocycline)	Avoid	Anti-anabolic effect, increased plasma urea, further deterioration in renal function

Source: Dental Practitioners' Formulary 1986–8. (Published by kind permission of The Pharmaceutical Society of Great Britain.)

Prescribing in liver disease

Many factors may alter the patient's response to drugs in liver disease. Although metabolism by the liver is probably the principal route whereby drugs are metabolized (see Chapter 1), liver disease has to be very severe before significant effects are produced on drug metabolism. Prothrombin and fibrinogen are formed in the liver and, in the presence of liver disease, there may be reduced synthesis of such clotting factors, which may lead to overactivity of oral anticoagulants such as warfarin. Furthermore, some drugs are hepatotoxic, and this may be dose-related or idiosyncratic. Drugs that should be used with caution or avoided in liver disease, and which are drugs listed in the DPF, include anti-inflammatory analgesics (e.g. aspirin, paracetamol), opioid analgesics, psychotropic drugs, and antimicrobials such as clindamycin, metronidazole, and i.v. tetracyclines.

Cardiovascular disease

The problems associated with the use of vasoconstrictors in cardiovascular disease will be dealt with elsewhere (see Chapter 7).

STANDARD REFERENCE BOOKS AND DATA SHEETS

The Dental Practioners' Formulary (DPF)

This is perhaps the most useful book of reference for the dental surgeon. It is revised every 2 years and comes out as a supplement to the *British National Formulary*, which is itself issued every 6 months. The *Dental Practitioners' Formulary* is issued free to all practising dentists and lists all those preparations that the dental surgeon can prescribe as a charge to the Health Service. Information is provided on each drug listed, on adverse effects of drugs used in dentistry, and on medical problems.

Dental surgeons are not limited in their prescribing to those drugs listed in the *Formulary*—they can prescribe other drugs provided that they observe the appropriate regulations. The patient will have to bear the full cost of the prescription. The hospital dental surgeon is not limited to the DPF in NHS prescribing.

The British National Formulary (BNF)

This is an index of preparations in common use in medicine. It contains useful information on the actions and adverse effects of important drugs. It is a useful publication for the dental practitioner because identification of a drug that the patient is taking on medical prescription, and details about that drug, provide information about the nature of the disease from which the patient is suffering.

MIMS (Monthly Index of Medical Specialties)

A quote from the cover of MIMS (July 1988) reads: 'MIMS is designed as a reference and prescribing guide for doctors in general practice and lists proprietary preparations which may be prescribed or recommended. The inclusion of products in the index does not necessarily mean that they are available at NHS expense.'

MIMS is a useful reference booklet because of its monthly revision. It is sent free of charge to all general medical practitioners, heads of hospital pharmacy departments, and on rotation to selected doctors and consultants in the UK. It is not supplied free of charge to dental practitioners and all payments and enquiries about subscriptions should be addressed to: MIMS Subscriptions, 12–14 Ansdell Street, London, W8 5TR.

Data sheets

Before an advertisement is forwarded to a practitioner (dental or medical), or any representation made to him about a medicinal product, a data sheet relating to the product must have been provided. A data sheet is simply an information sheet about a drug, which has to conform to certain particulars as regards size, printing, etc. The data sheet must contain the following information about the product:

(1) name of the product

(2) presentation: e.g. a description of appearance and pharmaceutical form of the medicinal product;

(3) uses: the main action of the medicinal product and the purpose for which it is to be recommended in treatments;

(4) dosage and administration; methods and routes of administration must be specified,

(5) contraindications and warnings.

There is other information that must be contained on the sheet, but the above indicates the main categories. The data sheet is produced for each product of a manufacturer and the information contained must be factual and not promotional.

Data Sheet Compendium

Data sheets are prepared by the individual pharmaceutical manufacturers. A *Data Sheet Compendium* is compiled each year and is published by Datapharm Publications Limited in association with the Association of the British Pharmaceutical Industry (ABPI). This joint compendium is prepared other than by persons or organizations concerned with manufacturing medicinal products. The individual data sheets are prepared by the companies concerned and participation in this joint compendium is open to all producing medicinal products for use under medical or dental supervision.

THE MISUSE OF DRUGS ACT 1971

Prior to 1971 drugs that were regarded as subject to abuse were regulated by the Dangerous Drugs Act in particular. The present legislation has tidied up what had become a somewhat confused legislation.

The Misuse of Drugs Act of 1971 and its associated orders control those drugs that are liable to abuse, e.g. morphine, amphetamines, etc. These are described as 'controlled' drugs, whereas at one time they would have been referred to as 'dangerous' drugs.

Under this Act an Advisory Council has been set up to advise the appropriate Minister (in this instance, the Secretary of State for the Home Office) on those drugs that are, or appear likely to be, misused and that may thereby cause a social problem. The Council consists of 20 members representing various interested parties, including dentistry and medicine.

Controlled drugs are classified in the Act as 'Class A drugs', 'Class B drugs', and 'Class C drugs', and this division refers to the penalties for misuse awarded under the Act. Penalties for illegal use or possession of Class A drugs tend to be more severe than for the other two classes. Class A drugs (over 100 preparations) include substances such as cocaine, diamorphine, lysergide, methadone, opium, pethidine. Class B drugs include oral amphetamines, barbiturates, cannabis, codeine, and pentazocine, for example. Class C drugs include most benzodiazepines.

The Misuse of Drugs Regulations, which interpret the spirit of the Act, allow certain persons or classes of persons (e.g. dentists) to possess, supply, prescribe, or administer controlled drugs in the *practice of their profession*. They also apply selective controls in relation to record-keeping, custody of drugs, and prescription writing. The regulations to the Act were originally stated in 1973 and have been revised in 1985, Statutory Instrument No. 2066. These regulations include five schedules listing different categories of drugs to which varying requirements as to supply, prescribing, and record-keeping apply. A further schedule, Schedule 6, is simply a form of register indicating details to be kept when drugs listed under Schedules 1 and 2 are received or supplied (see p. 61 later).

Schedule 1   includes such drugs as cannabis, lysergide, and mescaline. A licence from the Home Secretary is required to possess, supply, administer, or cause to be administered, any drugs specified in this Schedule.

Schedule 2   lists those drugs that are used medicinally and are subject to the strictest controls. The list includes amphetamine, cocaine, codeine, dihydrocodeine, dextropropoxyphene, methadone, morphine, pethidine, and many others.

Unless exempted in Schedule 5, these drugs are subject to the full control exercised by the regulations regarding prescriptions, safe custody, and record-keeping.

Schedule 3 includes the barbiturates and pentazocine. These drugs must fulfil the special prescription requirements for controlled drugs, but not the special requirements for safe custody. The Schedule 6 type of register need not be kept for drugs so listed.

Schedule 4 includes over 30 benzodiazepines, which are not subject to the strict controls regarding prescriptions, safe custody, or record-keeping indicated for drugs in the previous schedules. The benzodiazepines are Prescription Only Medicines (POM) and the form of prescription is as indicated on p. 53.

Schedule 5 includes preparations that, because of their strength, are exempt from nearly all the Controlled Drug requirements. The substances so exempt are not preparations for injection. Included in this list are certain preparations of dihydrocodeine or codeine. For instance, dihydrocodeine tartrate 30 mg tablet, because of the strength used, is classed simply as a Prescription Only Medicine (POM), whereas dihydrocodeine for injection is a Schedule 2 drug and therefore strictly controlled. Similarly, codeine, as contained in Codis tablets, has even less control than does dihydrocodeine tartrate tablets, being classified as a Pharmacy Medicine (P). On the other hand, codeine phosphate injection would come under the strict regulations governing Schedule 2 drugs.

A doctor or dentist may administer to a patient any drug specified in Schedule 2, 3, or 4. Furthermore, the dentist may direct another person, other than a doctor or a dentist, to administer such a drug to a patient under his/her care. Any person may administer to another any drug specified in Schedule 5.

The form of the prescription for a Schedule 2 or 3 drug

A prescription containing a controlled drug listed in Schedule 2 or 3, and issued by a dentist or doctor, must be written in ink or otherwise indelible material. Its layout is shown in Fig. 3.2. The whole of the prescription must be in the handwriting of the prescriber and it must be signed by him/her with his/her usual signature and be dated by him/her. Except in the case of a NHS prescription, the address of the person issuing the prescription must be given, but this need not be in handwriting. To minimize the possibility of forgery or alteration of the prescription, the following details should be in the dentist's or doctor's own handwriting:

(1) the name and address of the person for whose treatment the prescription is issued;

(2) the dose to be taken and, in the case of a prescription that is a preparation, the form, e.g. tablet, capsule, etc.;

(3) the total quantity of the drug to be supplied must be stated in both words and figures;

Schedule 6

THE MISUSE OF DRUGS REGULATIONS 1985

'FORM OF REGISTER'

PART 1
Entries to be made in case of obtaining

Date on which supply received	NAME ADDRESS of person or firm from whom obtained	Amount obtained	Form in which obtained

PART 2
Entries to be made in case of supply

Date on which the transaction was effected	NAME ADDRESS of person or firm supplied	Particulars as to licence or authority of person or firm supplied to be in possession	Amount supplied	Form in which supplied

Fig. 3.2. Prescription writing.
Layout for a controlled drug
(CD).

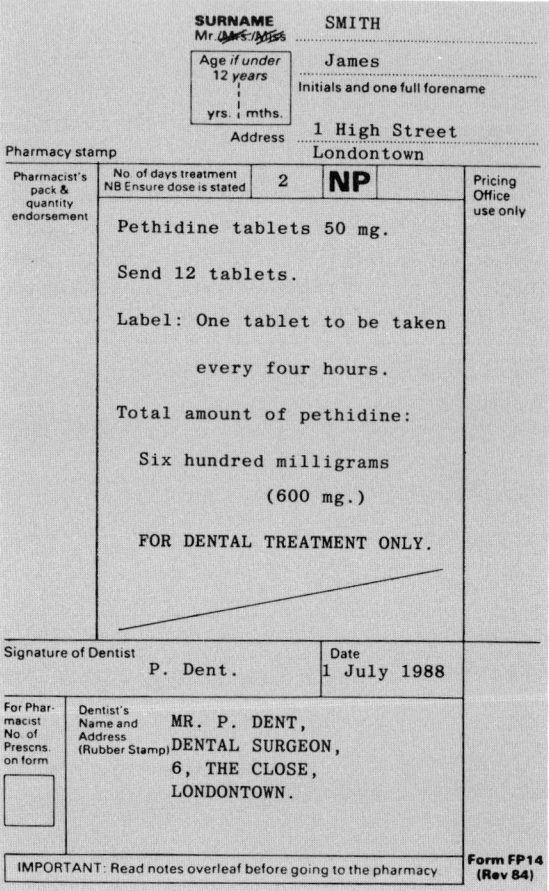

(4) a dental prescription for Schedule 2 or 3 drugs must be endorsed with the words 'for dental treatment only'.

It must be seen that the requirement of providing a prescription in the handwriting of the prescriber, and the necessity of writing the total quantity of the drug in both words and figures, is to prevent alterations of the prescription. This elaboration is only required for drugs listed in Schedules 1, 2, and 3, and even here there is some modification in that phenobarbitone is exempt from the handwriting requirement, other than for the prescriber's usual signature.

A dental surgeon working in a general hospital may wish to instruct staff to administer a fully controlled drug to a patient under his/her care. Any such drug prescribed to an in-patient in a NHS hospital must conform to standard prescribing procedures of the ward.

Requisition of controlled drugs

In order to obtain supplies of such drugs for use in practice, the practitioner must provide the supplier (pharmacist) with a signed requisition form giving the practitioner's name, address, profession or occupation, the purpose for which the drug is required, and the total quantity of the drug to be supplied.

The supplier must be satisfied that the signature on the requisition form is genuine and that the signatory is engaged in the profession or occupation stated.

Registers for controlled drugs (Schedule 6)

Registers must be kept for all drugs specified in Schedules 1 and 2 of the Regulations. A register must be kept for receipt of drugs and another for the issue of these drugs. The 'Form of Register' is shown on p. 61. The register must be a bound book, loose-leaf books will not do. All entries must be in chronological order giving particulars of every quantity of a drug received and every quantity of a drug supplied, whether by way of administration or otherwise.

Entries must be made on the day the drugs are obtained or supplied and, if this is not possible, then the entries must be made not later than the next day. Entries must be made with some indelible material and must not be erased or changed in any way. If a correction is necessary, then this must be made by means of marginal or footnote, and the date of correction indicated. A separate part of the Register must be used for each substance specified in the Act.

The Registers must be kept on the premises to which they relate, in other words separate Registers must be maintained for each set of premises. The record must be preserved for 2 years from the date of the final entry, and the Registers must be available for scrutiny by appropriate authority when required.

Storage of controlled drugs

A controlled drug must be kept in a locked receptacle, the key of which is in the possession of the dentist.

It will be seen that the acquiring, possession, and storage of Schedule 1 and 2 drugs does pose problems and it is unlikely that many dentists will feel the effort is worthwhile. The use of opioids and like drugs in hospital practice is, of course, another matter.

LIMITED LIST REGULATIONS

From 1 April 1985 the range of drugs available for prescription on the NHS was limited (The 'Selected List Scheme'). The Government had concluded that there were two areas in which action should be taken. Firstly, action concerning simple remedies for the relief of minor ailments and self-limiting complaints which were often bought over the counter by patients, without recourse to the medical practitioner, e.g. antacids, laxatives, analgesics. Secondly, action over the use of benzodiazepines, which had escalated in recent years, very often with expensive proprietary preparations being prescribed rather than generic compounds. The limitation was introduced to deal with these two areas and the categories of drugs involved were listed as:

> laxatives
> antacids
> mild analgesics
> cough and cold remedies
> vitamins
> benzodiazepines

So there came into being what has come to be known as a 'white list' and a 'black list' of drugs. The list of drugs available for the medical practitioner to prescribe under the NHS is the 'white list' and the 'black list' comprises those drugs no longer prescribable under the NHS, as shown above. Doctors and pharmacists were provided with a complete list of drugs not prescribable as from 1 July 1986. This list is amended from time to time.

FURTHER READING

Anon. (1978). The Medicines Act 1968 and other legislation. *British Dental Journal*, **145**, 174–7.

Duxbury, A. J., Leach, F. N., and Duxbury, J. T. (1984). Common prescribing problems. *Dental Update*, **11**, 101–10.

Dental Practioners' Formulary 1986–8. British Dental Association, the British Medical Association and the Pharmaceutical Society of Great Britain.

Medicines Act, 1968. HMSO, London.

Misuse of Drugs Act, 1971. HMSO, London.

The Misuse of Drugs Regulations, 1985. Statutory Instrument 1985 No. 2066. HMSO, London.

The Medicines (General Sale List) Order, 1977. Statutory Instrument 1977 No. 2129. HMSO, London.

The Medicines (Prescription Only) Order, 1977. Statutory Instrument 1977 No. 2127. HMSO, London.

The Medicines (Prescription Only) Amendment Order, 1978. Statutory Instrument 1978 No. 189. HMSO, London.

PART I

DRUGS USED IN DENTISTRY

4

Pharmacology of inflammation

INFLAMMATION is a complex process that can be defined as 'the reaction of the vascular and supporting elements of a tissue to injury, and results in the formation of a protein-rich exudate, provided the injury has not been so severe as to destroy the area' (Walter and Israel 1980).

The clinical features that accompany inflammation have been known since antiquity; they include swelling (tumor), redness (rubor), hotness (calor), and pain (dolor). Inflammation is under the control of a variety of endogenous biochemical mediators produced at or near the site of injury. The biochemical and pharmacological properties of these mediators will be considered in this chapter, together with drugs that can affect the inflammatory response.

CHEMICAL MEDIATORS OF INFLAMMATION

Histamine

This vasocative amine is found in most tissues of the body, but the major source is in the granules of mast cells. Histamine is formed by the decarboxylation of the amino acid, histidine. Trauma, either mechanical or chemical, causes the release of histamine from the mast cells into the extracellular fluid. Once released, histamine is rapidly metabolized by one of two enzyme systems (histamine-N-methyltransferase and diamine oxidase) to metabolites with little or no pharmacological activity (Fig. 4.1).

Pharmacological properties

Many of the properties of histamine are related to its action on smooth muscles, including relaxation of the vascular smooth muscle and contraction of the bronchi and gut wall. It is also a very potent stimulus to secretion of the exocrine glands, particularly those in the gastric mucosa. Histamine also has a direct effect on free nerve endings and is important in the production of pain and itch.

H_1 and H_2-receptors

There are two types of histamine receptors termed H_1 and H_2. H_1-receptors are

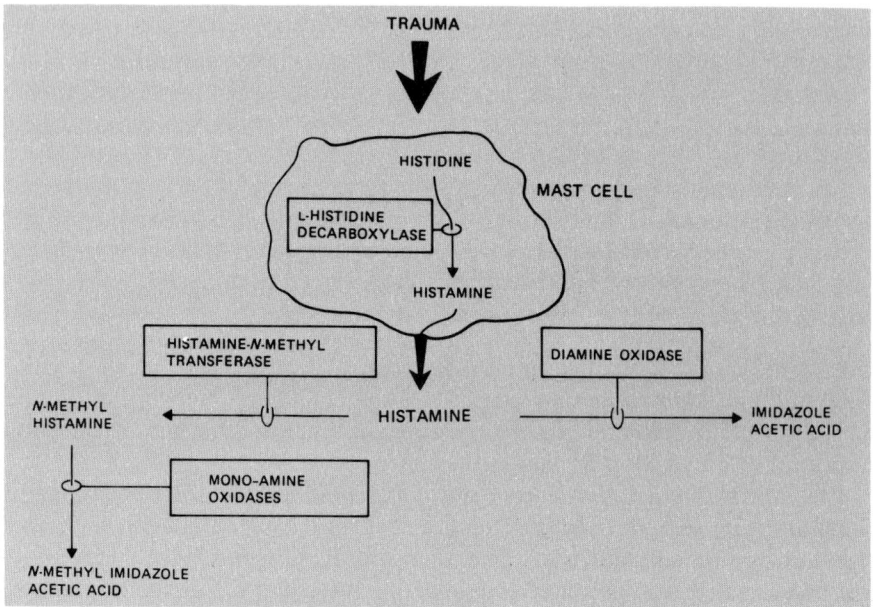

Fig. 4.1. The synthesis and metabolism of histamine.

primarily related to smooth muscle activity, i.e. vasodilatation and bronchial constriction (Ash and Schild 1966). H_2-receptors are mainly involved with the stimulation of gastric secretion (Black et al. 1972).

Cardiovascular effects

Histamine causes dilation of the small blood vessels, an effect mediated principally by the H_1-receptor, that leads to flushing, a lowered peripheral resistance, and a drop in blood pressure. The vasodilatation is accompanied by an increase in capillary permeability that results in oedema. The effect of histamine on the vasculature is best demonstrated by the 'triple response' described by Lewis and Grant in 1924.

The effect of histamine on the heart is variable: the response depends, in part, upon concentration, the simultaneous release of catecholamines, or the reduction in blood pressure causing stimulation of the baroreceptor reflex. Cardiac effects include an increase in heart rate and force of contraction, which result in an increase in cardiac output. Higher concentrations of histamine may cause arrhythmias due to slowing of the A-V conduction.

Smooth muscles

The bronchial muscles are the most important group of smooth muscles affected by histamine. Bronchoconstriction results from activation of the H_1-receptor. Patients who suffer from asthma are particularly sensitive to the action of histamine on the bronchial musculature. However, antihistamines are of no value in the treatment of asthma because histamine is not the principal causative agent in this condition.

Gastric secretion

The gastric secretory cells are very sensitive to the action of histamine, with even low concentrations causing a copious secretion of the gastric juices. This effect is mediated by the H_2-receptor.

Pain and itch

Histamine directly stimulates free nerve endings, which accounts for its ability to produce pain and itch when injected into the skin. A subcutaneous injection of histamine causes a sharp pain of short duration, similar to a wasp's sting. When injected into the more superficial layers of the skin, histamine causes itching.

Anaphylaxis and allergy

The release of histamine from mast cells plays a crucial role in both anaphylactic and allergic reactions. The active release is due to an antigen combining with a specific antibody attached to the surface of the mast cell. The combination of antigen with antibody causes the extrusion of histamine from the secretory granules in the mast cells (degranulation). Histamine release is accompanied by the liberation of many other endogenous substances (see below) that contribute to the varied responses seen in such reactions.

Many substances can act as antigens and cause anaphylactic or allergic reactions. Common examples include penicillin, animal fur, and pollen. Anaphylactic reactions can be fatal; their management is discussed in Chapter 21.

The eicosanoids

The term eicosanoids has been used to denote the metabolites of certain 20-carbon polyunsaturated fatty acids, mainly arachidonic acid. These precursors can be converted into a range of compounds that have a variety of effects as regulators and mediators of the functions of various cells.

A considerable number of different products of arachidonic-acid metabolism have been identified, but they can all be conveniently divided into two main groups on the basis that they are ultimately derived from the action of one of two enzymes (cyclo-oxygenase or lipoxygenase enzyme systems) on arachidonic acid. Thus they may all be considered as either cyclo-oxygenase products or lipoxygenase products.

Cyclo-oxygenase products can be further subdivided into three groups, the prostaglandins, the thromboxanes, and prostacyclin. Lipoxygenase products consist mainly of the leukotrienes and various compounds based on eicosatetraenoic acid. The synthesis of the eicosanoids is illustrated in Fig. 4.2.

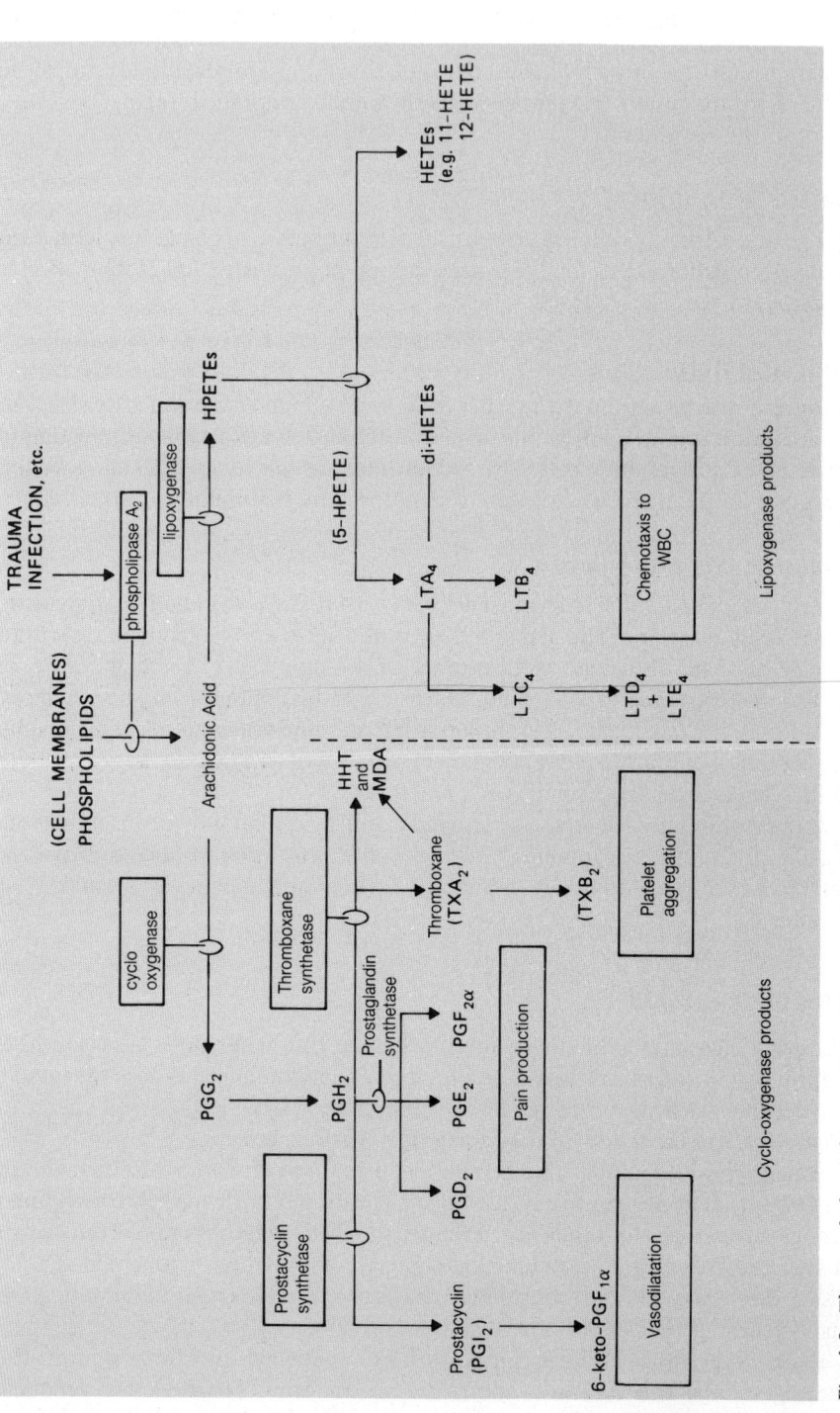

Fig. 4.2. The metabolic pathways of arachidonic acid and the synthesis of the eicosanoids. (WBC = white blood cells; other abbreviations, see text.)

Arachidonic acid

This is a 20-carbon polyunsaturated fatty acid. It has been suggested that there are two sources, the metabolic pool and the cell membrane pool (Crawford 1983). The endogenous synthesis of arachidonic acid appears to be from the metabolic pool by metabolism of dietary linoleic acid, whereas stimulated synthesis (e.g. from trauma) comes from the cell membrane pool. The membrane pool would seem to be the major source of the eicosanoid precursor in inflammation.

In most cells and tissues it is thought that the phosphatide fraction constitutes the major source of arachidonic acid (Blackwell and Flower 1983), and therefore the first step in eicosanoid synthesis is the liberation of arachidonic acid from that fraction. Arachidonic acid is liberated from cell membrane phospholipids (phosphate fraction) by the action of a group of enzymes collectively known as the phospholipases. In particular, the action of phospholipase A_2 is responsible for the bulk of arachidonic-acid synthesis.

Cyclo-oxygenase products

The next step in the formation of cyclo-oxygenase products is the action of the enzyme cyclo-oxygenase on free arachidonic acid. This action results in the insertion of two oxygen molecules into the fatty-acid carbon chain to form PGG_2, which is rapidly transformed by the peroxidase-like activity of cyclo-oxygenase into the hydroxyperoxide, PGH_2 (Bakhle 1983). Following this, and depending on the particular cell and circumstances involved, one or more of the three main groups mentioned earlier may be formed—the prostaglandins, thromboxane, or prostacyclin.

Prostaglandins

These were first identified in 1930, but it was not until the 1960s that their structure and function were elucidated. Prostaglandins occur in every tissue and body fluid; their pharmacological properties are listed later.

Thromboxane and prostacyclin

As we have seen, cyclo-oxygenase activity converts arachidonic acid to an intermediate compound, PGH_2. Further enzyme activity (thromboxane and prostacyclin synthetase) on PGH_2 results in the formation of thromboxane (TXA_2) and prostacyclin (PGI_2). The main synthesis of thromboxane occurs in platelets, whereas prostacyclin is synthesized in vessel walls. Thromboxane A_2 plays an important role in platelet aggregation. Prostacyclin is a potent vasodilator and acts as an antagonist of platelet aggregation. It would appear that thromboxane A_2 and prostacyclin represent biologically opposite poles of the mechanism for regulating the platelet–vessel wall interaction and the formation of a haemostatic plug (Moncada and Vane 1978). Both thromboxane A_2 and prostacyclin are unstable with very short half-lives. Thromboxane A_2 is broken down to thromboxane B_2 whereas prostacyclin is further metabolized to 6-keto-PGF_1 (Fig. 4.2). Further details of the mechanisms of haemostasis are given in Chapter 12.

Lipoxygenase products (leukotrienes)

The pathways resulting in the synthesis of lipoxygenase products have only recently been elucidated (Samuelsson 1981). The action of the lipoxygenase enzyme system on arachidonic acid forms a range of hydroperoxyeicosatetrae-noic acids (HPETEs), which may then be reduced to form the corresponding hydroxyeicosatetraenoic acids (HETEs). The leukotrienes are derived from 5-lipoxygenase acting on arachidonic acid to form 5-HPETE, which may then be reduced to 5-HETE or rearranged to form LTA_4 (Taylor and Morris 1983). The LTA_4 can be hydrolysed enzymatically to produce LTB_4, or non-enzymatically to produce various di-HETEs. Alternatively, LTA_4 may undergo nucleophillic attack by glutathione to produce LTC_4 from which LTD_4 and LTE_4 are generated.

The role of the leukotrienes in inflammation has not been fully elucidated. Lipoxygenase products have potent chemotactic properties and are probably involved in the process of cellular infiltration that accompanies inflammation.

Pharmacological properties of prostaglandins

Cardiovascular system

The prostaglandins are potent vasodilators and hence cause a fall in blood pressure (Robinson *et al.* 1973). Cardiac output is increased by prostaglandins E and F.

Smooth muscles

Prostaglandins of the F series contract bronchial muscles, whereas prostaglandins of the E series relax them (Cuthbert 1973). An intravenous infusion of PGE_2 or $PGF_{2\alpha}$ causes severe contractions of the uterus.

Inflammation and immune response

Prostaglandins play an important role in the inflammatory process and the immune response (Larsen and Henson 1983). Prostaglandins of the E series cause a long-lasting vasodilatation accompanied by an increase in vascular permeability. PGE_1 appears to regulate the function of the B-lymphocyte and the activity of the T-lymphocyte by inhibiting the production and release of lymphokines from sensitized T-cells (Goldyne 1977).

Pain

Prostaglandins contribute to the pain that often accompanies inflammation, either by directly stimulating sensory nerve endings or by sensitizing the nerve endings to other stimuli. They also produce pain when given either intravenously or intramuscularly (Vane 1976). The intradermal administration of histamine, bradykinin (see below), and PGE_2 produces pain of short duration, but hyperalgesia is only produced by PGE_2 (Ferreira 1972). Histamine, bradykinin, or PGE_2, when given singularly via the subcutaneous route, produce slight pain of short duration. However, the effect of the addition of PGE_2 to bradykinin or to histamine is overtly painful, whereas the further addition of bradykinin or histamine is not. In areas already 'sensitized' by prostaglandins, subsequent infusions of bradykinins or histamine cause pain. It would appear that prostaglandins, particularly of the E series, are able to sensitize pain receptors (free nerve endings) to mechanical and chemical stimulation.

Bradykinin

Bradykinin is a polypeptide formed from $alpha_2$-globulins in plasma by a complex series of proteolytic reactions. Trauma, in particular cell damage, causes the release of proteolytic enzymes that act on plasma kininogen to form bradykinin. The half-life of bradykinin is very short (30 s), with the compound being rapidly inactivated by carboxypeptidases (Fig. 4.3).

Pharmacological properties

Bradykinin is a very potent vasodilator and increases capillary permeability leading to oedema. In this respect, bradykinin, on a molar basis, is approximately ten times more active than histamine. The role of bradykinin in pain has been discussed under 'Pain' above.

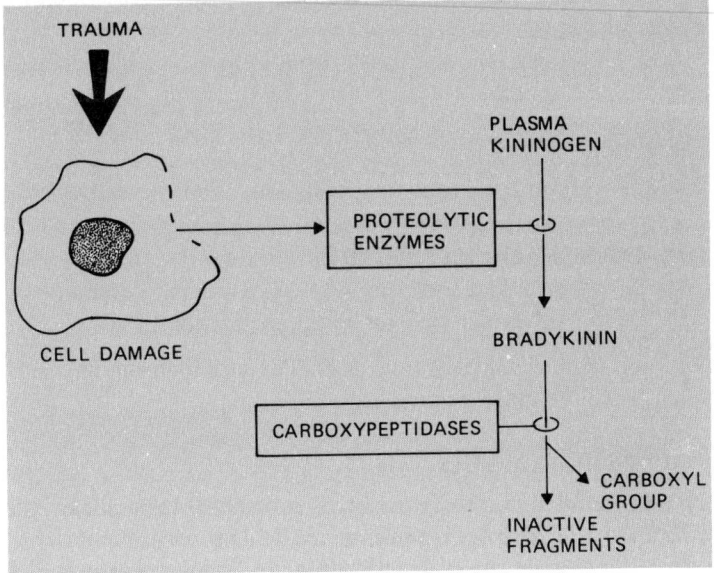

Fig. 4.3. The synthesis and metabolism of bradykinin.

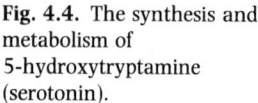

Fig. 4.4. The synthesis and metabolism of 5-hydroxytryptamine (serotonin).

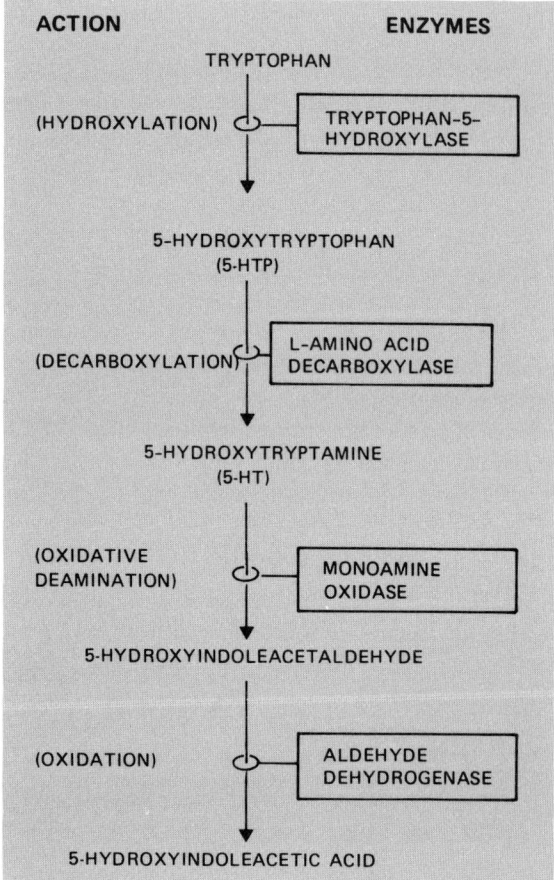

5-Hydroxytryptamine (serotonin)

5-Hydroxytryptamine (5-HT) is an amine formed by the hydroxylation of tryptophan, which is then decarboxylated to form 5-HT. After release, 5-HT is oxidized by monoamine oxidases (Fig. 4.4). The enterochromaffin cells of the gastric mucosa are the main storage site of 5-HT.

Pharmacological properties

The role of 5-HT in inflammation is uncertain and may be insignificant. However, it has a wide and variable range of pharmacological properties that not only vary between species but also in the same individual. An important property of 5-HT is its effect on blood vessels—dilatation of arteries and constriction of veins.

Complement

The complement system consists of a series of proteins that react in a cascade fashion (Fig. 4.5). One stimulus for the cascade reaction is the combination of antigen with antibody on a cell surface (this is known as the 'classical pathway'). An 'alternate' pathway can be triggered by bacterial toxins or large polysaccharides.

Fragments produced during the complement cascade are important in the inflammatory process. Fragments C3a and C5a induce the release of histamine from mast cells which, as described earlier, causes increased capillary permeability. Other components of the complement cascade are chemotactic to white blood cells (C5a, C5b, C567 complex) and enhance phagocytosis (C3b, C5b). Damage to cell membranes, followed by cell lysis, occurs when factors C8 and C9 are activated.

Lymphokines

These are a series of factors, presumably proteins, produced by the sensitized T-lymphocyte and to a lesser extent by the B-lymphocyte. The stimulus for

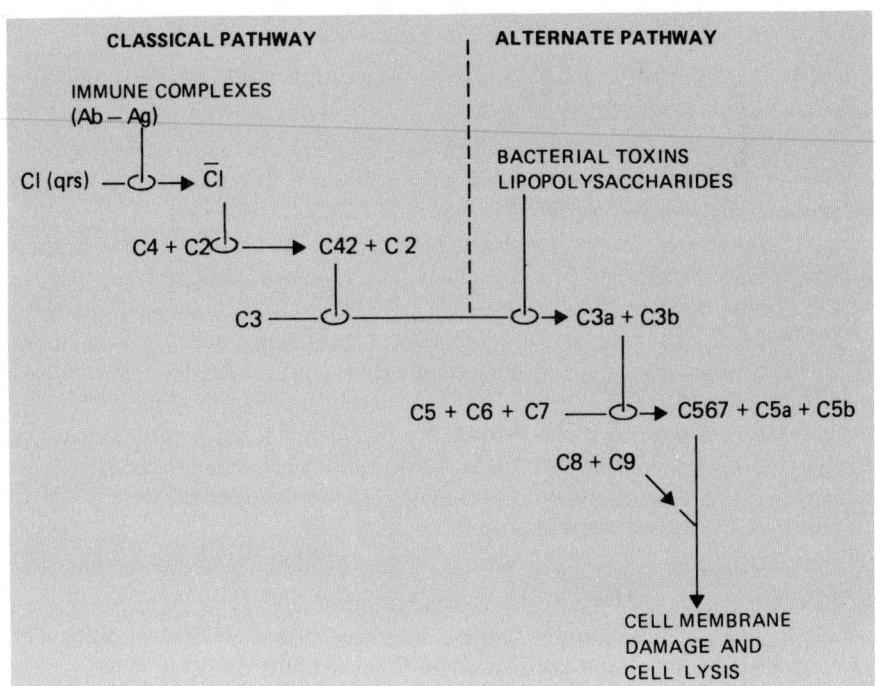

Fig. 4.5. The complement cascase.

production is antigenic challenge. The functions of lymphokines in inflammation are as follows:

(1) chemotactic for macrophages;

(2) macrophage activation;

(3) macrophage inhibition—promotes accumulation of macrophages at the site of inflammation;

(4) chemotactic for other mononuclear white blood cells;

(5) mitogenic for other lymphocytes;

(6) increases vascular permeability;

(7) activates osteoclasts.

ANTIHISTAMINES

These competitively antagonize histamine at the receptor sites: they do not alter the formation or release of histamine from tissues or mast cells. Antihistamines are conveniently classified as H_1- or H_2-receptor blockers.

H_1-blocking agents

These are sometimes referred to as the classical antihistamines and examples are chlorpheniramine and promethazine.

Pharmacological properties

H_1-blockers are competitive antagonists, that is they interact with H_1-receptors on cell membranes, which results in a decrease in the availability of these receptors for the actions of histamine. Hence, H_1-blockers will antagonize the action of histamine on smooth muscles, vasodilatation, capillary permeability, and the flare and itch components of the 'triple response'. Furthermore, H_1-blockers have central effects, including sedation and the reduction of nausea and vomiting, that are not related to the antagonism of histamine.

H_1-blockers are well-absorbed from the gastro-intestinal tract. Therapeutic effects can be observed within 15 to 30 minutes after dosage. The drugs are widely distributed throughout the body and broken down in the liver.

Therapeutic uses

H_1-blockers are widely used in the treatment (prevention) of a variety of allergic conditions, for example rhinitis, hay fever, and certain allergic dermatoses such as acute urticaria. Topical application of H_1-blockers is useful in relieving the itching associated with insect bites, but such application is not without problems (see below). H_1-blockers are widely used in common cold remedies—usually combined with a decongestant (e.g. Actifed). However, there is no evidence to suggest that H_1-blockers prevent or shorten the duration of the common cold.

The central effects of H_1-blockers make them useful in the prophylaxis of motion sickness and as a sedative, especially in children.

H_1-blockers have no effect on bronchospasm or the severe hypotension associated with anaphylactic shock. Similarly, this group of drugs is of no value in the treatment of asthma.

Unwanted effects

Sedation is the major unwanted effect associated with the H_1-blockers, but the degree of sedation does vary between different preparations, and indeed some may cause stimulation (e.g. Thephorin). Alcohol should be avoided whilst taking H_1-blockers as it will enhance the sedative effect. Other unwanted effects include xerostomia (dryness of the mouth) and a variety of gastro-intestinal disturbances. The incidence of these disturbances can be reduced by taking the H_1-blockers with meals.

Topical application of antihistamines

Antihistamine creams and lotions are widely used to relieve itching in skin conditions and after insect bites. However, these preparations are liable to produce a contact dermatitis (Type IV reaction) (see Chapter 21) and their use is contra-indicated. Under these conditions, topical antihistamines act as haptens and probably conjugate with some protein of epidermal origin. If these drugs were to be applied topically in certain oral conditions, a similar sensitization might occur. Such sensitization to antihistamines is not only highly undesirable but may be fatal because at some future time a patient so sensitized might be in urgent need of systemic treatment with antihistamines. If it were known that the patient was hypersensitive to antihistamines, they could not be treated with systemic antihistamine; if this vital fact were not known, treatment with antihistamines would be potentially dangerous.

H_2-blocking agents

These competitively antagonize the action of histamine at the H_2-receptor. The two most widely used H_2-blockers are cimetidine and ranitidine.

Pharmacological properties and therapeutic uses

The most important property of H_2-blockers is their ability to reduce gastric secretion in both volume and hydrogen ion concentration. Hence their main therapeutic use is in the treatment of duodenal ulcers and gastric hypersecretion such as occurs in the Zollinger–Ellison syndrome. Unwanted effects are slight and include headache, dizziness, constipation or diarrhoea, and skin rashes.

Dental applications of antihistamines

Only H_1-blocking agents have any dental applications, and it is rather for their central actions that they are used in dentistry. Promethazine has both sedative and weak atropine-like properties, and is used as a pre-operative sedative, particularly in children. H_1-blockers may be of some value in the treatment of allergic lesions on the face and lips.

Antihistamines have been evaluated in the control of pain, swelling, and other sequelae of oral surgery, but appear to be of little value in this application (Seymour and Walton 1984).

5-HT ANTAGONISTS

The ergot alkaloids are a group of related compounds that are antagonists for 5-HT. Ergotamine is the most widely used of the ergot alkaloids and is an important drug in the relief of migraine. The treatment of migraine is discussed in more detail in Chapter 14.

STEROIDS

Corticosteroids and synthetic steroids have potent anti-inflammatory properties. The general pharmacology and physiology of the steroids is discussed in Chapter 18.

Anti-inflammatory properties

Steroids inhibit many of the processes associated with inflammation. In its early stages they reduce the capillary permeability caused by histamine and bradykinin, which in turn reduces oedema. They also inhibit both bradykinin formation and the migration of white blood cells into the site of inflammation. In its later stages, steroids reduce granulation-tissue formation by inhibiting the proliferation of fibroblasts and blood vessels. There is also evidence that steroids can affect eicosanoid synthesis by inhibiting the conversion of fatty acids to arachidonic acid (see above). It is suggested that steroids induce the formation of an intermediate protein (macrocortin) that inhibits the phospholipase A_2 enzyme system. We have seen that this system acts on cell membrane phospholipids to form arachidonic acid, which in turn serves as a substrate for the precursor of prostaglandins and leukotrienes (Blackwell et al. 1980; Hirata et al. 1980).

When steroids are used to suppress inflammation, such therapy is palliative for the underlying cause of the inflammation still remains. Steroids should not be used where an infection is suspected.

Topical corticosteroid therapy

Such topical application is extensively used in the treatment of most dermatological conditions. However, this use of corticosteroids is not without unwanted effects, the most common of which, atrophy of the skin, can occur as early as three to four weeks after commencement of treatment. Atrophy is especially common on the face where the skin is normally thin. Both epidermis and dermis are affected: in the epidermis there is a reduction in cell size and number, and in the dermis there is decreased fibroblast activity and collagen synthesis. These latter two decreases give rise to a loss of dermal support, which in turn leads to dilatation of small blood vessels and to telangiectasia; the telangiectactic vessels rupture easily and produce ecchymosis.

Absorption of topical corticosteroids may lead to adrenal suppression (see Chapter 18). The extent of suppression is dependent upon the steroid potency, the duration of treatment, the amount used, and the skin area treated. Although isolated cases of severe adrenocortico-suppression have been reported (Miyachi 1982), the suppressive effect of topical steroids on cortisol levels is of little clinical significance with normal usage (Munro and Clift 1973). As a general rule, little adverse effect on cortisol production is likely to occur with the application of up to 50 g weekly for an adult or 15 g weekly for a child of a potent steroid ointment (Dahl 1985).

Allergic contact dermatitis due to topical steroids is very rare and is more commonly due to a constituent of the base (e.g. lanolin).

Use of steroids in dentistry

Oral ulceration and oral mucosal lesions

Steroids are widely used in the treatment of recurrent oral ulceration and other oral mucosal lesions such as erosive lichen planus, erythema multiforme, and pemphigus. Many of these conditions are treated by topical applications and optimal results are achieved when the period of contact between steroid and lesion is maximal. Severe oral ulceration may require systemic steroids. In some instances, injection of a steroid into the lesion may be of benefit. Topical steroid preparations include triamcinolone acetonide 0.1 per cent; hydrocortisone sodium succinate 2.5 mg; betamethasone 17-valerate (topical spray). Intralesional steroids are triamcinolone hexacetonide and hydrocortisone acetate. Prednisolone is the most widely used systemic steroid.

Pulpal inflammation

Steroids are often applied over a carious exposure of the dental pulp. One such preparation, Ledermix, contains triamcinolone and a tetracycline (demeclocycline hydrochloride); however, its efficacy is not established.

Temperomandibular-joint pain

Intra-articular injections of hydrocortisone or prednisolone have been shown to be of value in certain inflammatory joint conditions. However, such use can cause deterioration of the articular surface of the joint and it is unwise to repeat the procedure more than twice (Toller 1977).

Bell's palsy

This is a unilateral facial paralysis affecting one or more branches of the facial nerve. It is of unknown aetiology but may accompany a viral infection. Prednisolone is the treatment of choice and therapy must be started within five to six days of onset of the paralysis. It is usual to start off steroid administration with a high dose, tailing this off over 10 days.

Postoperative pain and swelling after dental surgery

There has been much interest in the use of steroids to reduce pain, swelling, and other sequelae after removal of impacted lower third molars and after orthognathic surgery (Lyuk *et al.* 1985). For this, a course of steroids is usually short so unwanted effects are minimized. Methylprednisolone and betamethasone are used for this purpose and, for optimal effect, the steroids are given intramuscularly just before surgery.

Anaphylactic and allergic reactions

The use of steroids in the treatment of anaphylacic and allergic reactions is dealt with in Chapter 21.

REFERENCES

Ash, A. S. F. and Schild, H. O. (1966). Receptors mediating some actions of histamine. *British Journal of Pharmacology*, **27**, 427–39.

Bakhle, Y. S. (1983). Synthesis and catabolism of cyclo-oxygenase products. *British Medical Bulletin*, **39**, 214–18.

Black, J. W., Duncan, W. A. M., Durant, C. J., Ganellin, C. R., and Parsons, E. M. (1972). Definition and antagonism of histamine H_2-receptors. *Nature*, **236**, 385–90.

Blackwell, G. J., Carnuccio, R., Dirosa, M., Flower, R. J., Parente, L., and Persico, P. (1980). Macrocortin: a polypeptide causing the anti-phospholipase effects of glucocorticoids. *Nature*, **287**, 1147–9.

Blackwell, G. J. and Flower, R. J. (1983). Inhibition of Phospholipase. *British Medical Bulletin*, **39**, 260–4.

Crawford, M. A. (1983). Background to essential fatty acids and their prostanoids derivatives. *British Medical Bulletin*, **39**, 210–13.

Cuthbert, M. F. (1973). Prostaglandins and respiratory smooth muscle. In *The prostaglandins: pharmacological and therapeutic advances* (ed. M. F. Cuthbert), pp. 253–86. Lippincott, Philadelphia.

Dahl, M. G. C. (1985). Hazards of topical steroid cream. *Advance Drug Reactions Bulletin,* **115**, 428–31.

Ferreira, S. H. (1972). Prostaglandins, aspirin-like drugs and analgesia. *Nature New Biology,* **240**, 200–3.

Goldyne, M. E. (1977). Prostaglandins and the modulation of the immune responses. *International Journal of Dermatology,* **16**, 701–12.

Hirata, F., Schiffmann, E., Venkatasubamanian, K., Salomon, D., and Axelrod, J. (1980). A phospholipase A_2 inhibitory protein in rabbit neutrophils induced by glucorticoids. *Proceedings of the National Academy of Sciences U.S.A.,* **77**, 2533–6.

Larsen, G. L. and Henson, P. M. (1983). Mediators of inflammation. *Annual Review of Immunology,* **1**, 335–59

Lewis, T. and Grant, R. T. (1924). Vascular reactions of the skin to injury; the liberation of histamine-like substance to injured skin; the underlying cause of factitious articaria and of weals produced by burning; and observations upon the nervous control of certain skin reactions. *Heart,* **11**, 209–18.

Luyk, N. H., Anderson, J., and Ward-Booth, P. W. (1985). Corticosteroid therapy and the dental patient. *British Dental Journal,* **159**, 12–17.

Miyachi, Y. (1982). Adrenal axis suppression caused by a small dose of a potent topical corticosteroid. *Archives of Dermatologoly,* **118**, 451–2.

Moncada, S. and Vane, J. R. (1978). Unstable metabolites of arachidonic acid and their role in haemostasis and thrombosis. *British Medical Bulletin,* **34**, 129–36.

Munro, D. D. and Clift, D. C. (1973). Pituitary–adrenal function after prolonged use of topical corticosteroids. *British Journal of Dermatology,* **88**, 381–7.

Robinson, B. F., Collier, J. G., Karim, S. M. M., and Somers, K. (1973). Effect of prostaglandins A_1, A_2, B_1, E_2 and F_2 on forearm arterial bed and superficial hand veins in man. *Clinical Science,* **44**, 367–76.

Samuelsson, B. (1981). Prostaglandins, thromboxane and leukotrienes: formation and biological roles. *Harvey Lectures,* **75**, 1–40.

Seymour, R. A. and Walton, J. G. (1984). Pain control after third molar surgery. *International Journal of Oral Surgery,* **13**, 457–85.

Taylor, G. W. and Morris, H. R. (1983). Lipoxygenase pathways. *British Medical Bulletin,* **39**, 219–22.

Toller, P. A. (1977). Use and misuse of intra-articular corticosteroids in treatment of temporomandibular joint pain. *Proceedings of the Royal Society of Medicine,* **70**, 461–3.

Vane, J. R. (1976). Prostaglandins as mediators of inflammation. *Advances in Prostaglandin and Thromboxane Research,* **2**, 797–801.

Walter, J. B. and Israel, M. S. (1980). *General pathology* (5th edn). Churchill Livingstone, Edinburgh.

5

Aspirin and other non-steroidal anti-inflammatory drugs

THIS group of analgesics, the non-steroidal anti-inflammatory drugs (NSAIDs) or aspirin-like drugs, acts at the site of inflammation by interfering with the biochemical mediators of inflammation (Chapter 4), especially those associated with pain. Most of these drugs, as described later, inhibit the synthesis of the prostaglandins by blocking the cyclo-oxygenase enzyme system (Vane 1971) and they have, in addition to their analgesic properties, anti-inflammatory and central antipyretic activity. All these properties are important in the treatment of dental pain.

The prostaglandins, particularly PGE_2 and $PGF_{2\alpha}$, sensitize free nerve endings to the nociceptive properties of histamine and bradykinin, which produce pain (see Chapter 4). Therefore any analgesic that inhibits the production of prostaglandin will primarily reduce pain occurring at the site of inflammation.

ASPIRIN

Aspirin (acetylsalicylic acid) is the most wisely used medicinal agent in the Western world. It is a weak organic acid structurally related to salacin, a natural product found in willow bark (*Salix alba*). The drug is nearly always taken orally and soluble preparations are more efficacious than tablet formulations (Seymour *et al.* 1986).

Pharmacokinetics

Aspirin is rapidly absorbed from the gastro-intestinal tract, partly from the stomach, but mainly from the upper small intestine. On absorption, it is quickly hydrolyzed to salicylate by esterase enzymes (aspirin esterases) in the gut wall, blood, and liver. The half-life of aspirin in man is 20 to 30 minutes, whereas that of salicylate is two to three hours.

Salicylate is excreted in the urine mainly as salicyluric acid and glucuronides. In the liver, salicylate is conjugated with glycine and glucuronic acid to form

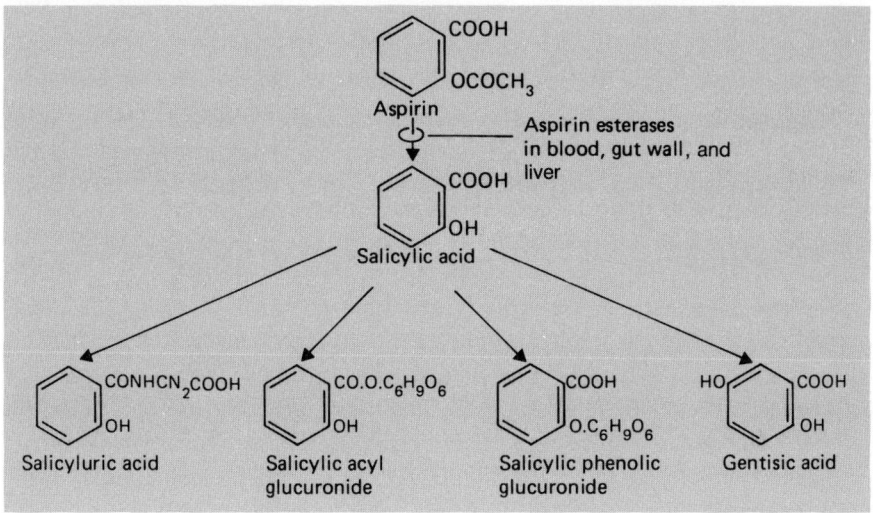

Fig. 5.1. The metabolism of aspirin.

salicyluric acid, and acyl and phenolic glucuronides, respectively. A very small fraction of salicylic acid is converted to gentisic acid. The metabolism of aspirin is illustrated in Fig. 5.1.

Pharmacodynamics

There is now convincing evidence that many of aspirin's pharmacological properties come from its ability to inhibit the synthesis of the important chemical mediators—the eicosanoids (prostaglandins, prostacyclin, thromboxane, and the leukotrienes). The eicosanoids, formed from fatty acids, have been discussed in Chapter 4. Aspirin is an irreversible inhibitor of the cyclo-oxygenase system by acetylating the active site of the enzyme (Roth *et al.* 1975), thus reducing its activity.

Pharmacological properties

Analgesia

Aspirin is usually classified as a mild analgesic and is effective against pain associated with inflammation, such as dental and rheumatic pain. The drug is also widely used to relieve headaches, migraines, and dysmenorrhoea. Aspirin's analgesic properties are mainly due to the inhibition of the synthesis of prostaglandins PGE_2 and $PGE_{2\alpha}$. Suitable dose regimes for aspirin are in the range 600–1200 mg every four to six hours.

Anti-inflammatory

These properties are again related to its ability to inhibit eicosanoid synthesis. In addition, salicylate, the major metabolite of aspirin, blocks the lipoxygenase enzyme system, the products of which are important mediators of the inflammatory response (Siegel *et al.* 1979). Thus, aspirin may have a dual action whereby acetylsalicylic acid blocks the synthesis of cyclo-oxygenase products and salicylate blocks the synthesis of lipoxygenase products.

Antipyretic

Aspirin effectively and rapidly lowers an elevated body temperature but has no effect on normal body temperature. Pyrexia, of course, usually accompanies an acute infection or acute inflammation. Many bacterial endotoxins can cause the synthesis and release of pyrogens from neutrophils. These pyrogens are proteins with a large molecular weight that stimulate the release of prostaglandins within the brain (particularly in the hypothalamic area). Prostaglandins PGE_2 and $PGE_{2\alpha}$ are pyrogenic and hence cause fever. The antipyretic properties of aspirin are therefore due to its inhibition of the synthesis of prostaglandins as stimulated by pyrogens.

Unwanted effects

Aspirin has many of these and they show marked individual variation; some of them are related to dosage and chronic usage.

Gastro-intestinal

Aspirin causes a high incidence of gastro-intestinal disturbances including epigastric pain, nausea, and gastric erosions leading to blood loss. Faecal blood loss is often related to dose and can be in the range of 3–10 ml per day. Because of these effects, aspirin should not be given to patients who suffer from peptic ulceration or inflammatory disease of the gut.

Haemostatic effects

Aspirin causes a prolongation of bleeding time (O'Brien 1969; Weiss *et al.* 1968) and this effect can occur after ingestion of a single aspirin tablet (300 mg). The prolonged bleeding time is due to impaired platelet aggregation caused by aspirin inhibiting the synthesis of platelet thromboxane (Roth and Majerus 1975). The increase in bleeding time will continue until the platelet population has been replaced (7–10 days), because platelets are incapable of regenerating the cyclo-oxygenase enzyme (see Chapter 12).

High doses of aspirin (i.e. 4–6 g/day), over a long time, will reduce plasma prothrombin levels and cause an increase in clotting time. This effect can be reversed by Vitamin K. Aspirin should be avoided in any patient with a haemorrhagic disorder (e.g. haemophiliacs) and in patients taking anticoagulants, as it may potentiate the anticoagulant effect.

Tinnitus

High doses of aspirin cause tinnitus and hearing loss due to a rise in labyrinthine pressure. Reducing the dose of aspirin reverses this problem in 2 to 3 days.

Uricosuric effect

Aspirin at the dosage of 1–2 g per day decreases uric acid secretion, which results in an increase in plasma uric-acid concentrations. Aspirin should not be given to patients suffering from gout, a disorder of uric-acid metabolism.

Metabolic effects

Oxidative phosphorylation

Aspirin causes the uncoupling of oxidative phosphorylation, which results in the inhibition of a number of ATP-dependent reactions. At normal therapeutic doses, this uncoupling has little untoward effect, but becomes serious in overdose (see below).

Carbohydrate metabolism

Aspirin in high doses (> 5 g/day) may cause hypoglycaemia and was indeed once used as a treatment of diabetes. In even higher doses (> 10 g/day) aspirin depletes the liver of its glycogen stores and causes hyperglycaemia.

Aspirin hypersensitivity

True hypersensitivity is rare as many patients confuse unwanted effects such as nausea and tinnitus with an allergic response. In a true hypersensitivity reaction, clinical manifestations occur within minutes of ingestion of aspirin and may range from a rhinitis to life-threatening laryngeal oedema. The management of aspirin hypersensitivity and other drug hypersensitivity reactions is discussed in Chapter 21. The underlying mechanism for hypersensitivity to aspirin is unknown. Although the response resembles anaphylaxis, it does not appear to be immunological in nature. However, the incidence of aspirin hypersensitivity is much higher in patients who suffer from general allergic conditions such as asthma and hay fever, hence aspirin should be avoided in such subjects (Settipane et al. 1974). Other drugs that inhibit the cyclo-oxygenase enzyme (e.g. ibuprofen and mefenamic acid) may cause a hypersensitivity reaction in patients allergic to aspirin.

Drug interactions

Aspirin binds firmly to plasma proteins and so may displace other drugs from the binding sites, especially warfarin (Pullar and Cappell 1983), methotrexate, and sulphonylureas. If such drugs are displaced, then their pharmacological properties will be enhanced. The problem with warfarin can be further compounded by the antihaemostatic properties of aspirin, which can lead to a fatal haemorrhage.

Aspirin overdose

As aspirin is widely used and readily available to the public, it is not surprising that it is one of the most common drugs for attempted suicide and is so often a cause of accidental poisoning in children. Doses of 10 to 30 g can be fatal.

Overdose of aspirin will cause an increase in CO_2 production in skeletal muscles due to deranged metabolism. Initially, this increase will stimulate respiration and cause some degree of hyperventilation. However, CO_2 production then outstrips its alveolar excretion causing a rise in plasma P_{CO_2} and hence blood pH falls; this is referred to as metabolic acidosis. The acidosis is further compounded by the high plasma concentrations of aspirin metabolites being themselves acidic, and also causing impairment of renal function, which will lead to the accumulation of acidic waste products. Hyperthermia and dehydration accompany the aspirin intoxication. If left untreated, death will occur as a result of coma and respiratory depression. Treatment is aimed at preventing further absorption of aspirin by gastric lavage and at restoring blood pH by intravenous infusion of bicarbonate.

Aspirin and Reye's Syndrome

Reye's syndrome is a rare disorder, occurring in childhood, that comprises an acute encephalopathic illness and fatty degeneration of the viscera, especially the liver. Its main feature is that it arises after an infectious illness, often chickenpox or influenza. The precise aetiology is unknown, but there is now accumulating evidence of a link between aspirin consumption during the course of the viral infection and the syndrome (Tarlow 1986). As a result of this association, paediatric aspirin preparations are no longer available to the public.

Aspirin in dentistry

Aspirin is widely used as an analgesic in postoperative dental pain, and many studies support the efficacy of this drug (Seymour 1983). Furthermore, the efficacy of aspirin is dose-related, with 1000 to 1200 mg providing greater analgesia than 500 to 600 mg (Seymour and Rawlins 1982) and related to the rate at which an individual hydrolyses aspirin to salicylate (Seymour et al. 1984). Postoperative dental pain is of short duration and usually patients only take analgesics for the first 24 to 48 hours after surgery (Seymour et al. 1983; 1985). As analgesics are only required for a short duration, it is unlikely that certain unwanted effects, for example, tinnitus, will occur.

If a patient has taken even a single dose of aspirin or an aspirin-containing analgesic *before* tooth extraction or other dental surgical procedure, then there is the real risk of postoperative haemorrhage (Lemkin et al. 1974; McGaul 1978). It would be a wise precaution to pack and suture extraction sockets in such patients. However, when aspirin is given postoperatively, there is little risk of haemorrhage as the haemostatic mechanism will be well-established.

Some toothache sufferers may try and relieve their pain by placing an aspirin tablet in the buccal sulcus against the offending tooth. This practice is of no value for pain relief, but will cause severe sloughing and ulceration of the buccal mucosa.

PARA-AMINOPHENOLS

These so-called coal-tar analgesics are all analine derivatives. Phenacetin and acetanalid were first introduced in 1887 but, in 1949, it was realized that the active metabolite of both these drugs is N-acetyl-p-aminophenol or paracetamol, which is now the most widely used of this group of analgesics.

Pharmacokinetics

Paracetamol is well-absorbed from the small intestine after oral ingestion. Peak plasma concentrations usually occur between 30 and 60 minutes after dosage, and the half-life is approximately 2 hours. Paracetamol is conjugated in the liver and the conjugates excreted in the urine.

Pharmacodynamics and pharmacological properties

Paracetamol has both analgesic and antipyretic properties similar to those of aspirin; however, the drug has little or no anti-inflammatory action, for which there is no satisfactory explanation. Neither the site nor the mechanisms of the analgesic action of paracetamol have been clearly established. Different workers have concluded that the site of action is purely peripheral, purely central, or both (Koch-Weser 1976). It is very much less effective than aspirin as a peripheral cyclo-oxygenase inhibitor, but has the same potency as aspirin in inhibiting brain prostaglandin synthetase (Ferreira and Vane 1974). The antipyretic property of paracetamol probably has a similar mechanism to that of aspirin.

Unwanted effects and overdose

Paracetamol has remarkably few unwanted effects and at normal therapeutic doses is probably the safest analgesic. Skin rashes and white blood-cell disorders have occasionally been reported. However, the most serious problem with paracetamol is hepatotoxicity after overdose (Prescott *et al.* 1971). At normal doses, paracetamol is broken down in the liver to metabolites that are normally innocuous. In overdose, one of the metabolites (probably N-acetyl-p-benzoquinone), which is usually reduced by glutathione and eliminated, accumulates and renders liver cells incapable of synthesizing protein. Acute liver damage can occur after a single dose of 10 to 15 g; a dose of 25 g is invariably fatal. The problem of paracetamol overdose is further compounded by the absence of untoward effects in the first 24 hours after overdose, during which time serious and perhaps fatal liver damage will have occurred. Hence the overdose victim may take further tablets but, more seriously, their relations or friends will have seen little obvious signs of illness and so may not seek help. Signs and symptoms of liver damage manifest themselves between 2 to 6 days after overdose. Jaundice and coagulation disorders accompany the hepatotoxicity, which leads to coma and death.

Early treatment is essential for success in paracetamol overdose. Gastric lavage will prevent further absorption, provided it is in the first hour after dosage. If less than 12 hours has elapsed, then N-acetylcysteine is the treatment of choice. This drug can be given orally and treatment should persist until there is a significant reduction of plasma paracetamol concentrations. N-acetylcysteine will conjugate with the metabolite and thus protect the liver cells from further damage (Prescott et al. 1979).

If the patient is seen after 24 hours, then the success of treatment will depend upon the magnitude of the initital overdose. If large quantities of paracetamol have been consumed, then they will invariably suffer a slow and often distressing death.

Use in dentistry

Paracetamol is a useful analgesic in patients where aspirin is contraindicated (e.g. those with a haemorrhagic diathesis). The efficacy of paracetamol in postoperative dental pain has not been shown to be dose-related, therefore increasing the dosage may not cause an equivalent increase in analgesia.

Paracetamol elixir is extensively used in the treatment of 'teething', although its efficacy in this poorly defined condition has not been established. Teething is often accompanied by systemic disturbances, particularly pyrexia, which may be due to some other infection. The combined antipyretic and analgesic properties of paracetamol, together with its few unwanted effects, thus make this drug popular for the relief of teething problems although it may be the symptoms of the underlying infection that are palliated and this may require medical attention. Paracetamol elixir also contains a high proportion of sugar, and its regular use may increase the incidence of dental caries. The problem of caries is compounded because the medicine is often given last thing at night.

OTHER NSAIDS

This group of analgesics is sometimes referred to as aspirin-like drugs, for they share many of aspirin's pharmacological properties. Like aspirin, they are anti-inflammatory and analgesic because they can inhibit the synthesis of the eicosanoids (see Chapter 4). However, many NSAIDs will produce unwanted effects similar to those of aspirin, such as gastro-intestinal disturbances and impaired platelet aggregation. The incidence of unwanted effects varies markedly between the different groups of these analgesics. Furthermore, a patient who is hypersensitive to aspirin is likely to have a similar reaction when given another NSAID. These analgesics are mainly used in rheumatic and other musculo-skeletal disorders. However, because of their combined analgesic and anti-inflammatory properties, they are becoming widely used for the treatment of dental pain.

Propionic-acid derivatives

Examples of these include ibuprofen, naproxen, and fenoprofen. Ibuprofen is the most widely used analgesic in this group and is becoming increasingly popular in dentistry.

Pharmacological properties and unwanted effects

Ibuprofen is rapidly absorbed following oral administration; peak plasma concentrations occur within 1.5 hours after dosage, and the plasma half-life is 2 hours. The drug is broken down in the liver and the metabolites excreted in the urine.

Ibuprofen has similar unwanted effects to those of aspirin. About 15 per cent of patients taking it find these effects so severe that they have to discontinue the drug (Davies and Avery 1971). Ibuprofen and other propionic-acid derivatives should be avoided in patients with a gastro-intestinal disorder, haemostatic problems, or a history of hypersensitivity to aspirin.

The fenamates

Mefenamic acid (Ponstan) is the only member of this group of drugs that is used in dentistry.

Pharmacological properties and unwanted effects

Mefenamic acid is rapidly absorbed after oral dose and peak plasma concentrations occur after two hours; the half-life is three to four hours. The drug is metabolized in the liver; half of the metabolites are excreted in the urine, and the other half in the faeces. Mefenamic acid is about as active as aspirin as an analgesic and anti-inflammatory agent. However, the incidence of unwanted effects, especially gastro-intestinal disturbances, is high. Troublesome diarrhoea occurs in 25 per cent of patients on this drug (Chadwick et al. 1976; Marks and Gleeson 1975). As with other NSAIDs, mefenamic acid should not be given to a patient for whom aspirin is contra-indicated.

Indomethacin (Indocid)

This is an indole derivative developed in 1963. The use of this drug in dentistry is limited because of the high incidence of unwanted effects.

Pharmacological properties and unwanted effects

Indomethacin is one of the most potent inhibitors of the cyclo-oxygenase enzyme, and a powerful anti-inflammatory agent. A high proportion of patients (30–50 per cent) receiving this drug experience unwanted effects; these include gastro-intestinal complaints, and central nervous system disturbances such as dizziness, headache, confusion, and vertigo. The precise mechanism of these central actions is unknown, but they may be due to prostaglandin inhibition within brain tissue, or to salt and water retention (Carney 1977). Severe depression of the activity of the bone marrow and hypersensitivity reactions have been associated with this drug.

Diflunisal

This is a difluorophenyl derivative of salicylic acid with similar pharmacological properties to aspirin. The main advantage of this drug is its long plasma half-life (approx. 8 h) so the dose regime is only twice a day. Diflunisal is a comparatively new analgesic with a low incidence of unwanted effects, but it has not been established if this low incidence persists with chronic usage.

Efficacy of NSAIDs in dental pain

This group of analgesics has been extensively evaluated in postoperative dental pain and many trials support their efficacy (for review, see Seymour and Walton 1984). However, the incidence and severity of unwanted effects sometimes outweighs the advantages of analgesia obtained from these drugs. Ibuprofen and diflunisal appear to have the lowest incidence of unwanted effects. It has not been established whether these two analgesics offer any advantage over 1 g aspirin in the treatment of postoperative dental pain.

REFERENCES

Carney, M. W. P. (1977). Paranoid psychoses with indomethacin. *British Medical Journal*, 2, 994.

Chadwick, R. G., Hossenbocus, A., and Colin-Jones, D. G. (1976). Steatorrhoea complicating therapy with mefenamic acid. *British Medical Journal*, 1, 397.

Davies, E. F. and Avery, G. S. (1971). Ibuprofen, a review of its pharmacological properties and therapeutic efficacy in rheumatic disorders. *Drugs*, 2, 416–34.

Ferreira, S. H. and Vane, J. R. (1974). New aspects of the mode of nonsteroidal anti-inflammatory drugs. *Annual Review of Pharmacology*, 14, 57–73.

Koch-Weser, J. (1976). Drug therapy—acetaminophen. *New England Journal of Medicine*, **295**, 1297–300.

Lemkin, S. R., Billesdon, J. E., Davee, S. S., Leake, D. L., and Kattlove, H. E. (1974). Aspirin-induced oral bleeding: correction with platelet transfusion: a reminder. *Oral Surgery*, **37**, 498–501.

McGaul, T. (1978). Postoperative bleeding caused by aspirin. *Journal of Dentistry*, **6**, 207–9.

Marks, J. S. and Gleeson, M. H. (1975). Steatorrhoea complicating therapy with mefenamic acid. *British Medical Journal*, **4**, 442.

O'Brien, J. R. (1968). Effects of salicylates on human platelets. *Lancet*, **1**, 779–83.

Prescott, L. F., Wright, N., Roscoe, P., and Brown, S. S. (1971). Plasma-paracetamol half-life and hepatic necrosis in patients with paracetamol overdosage. *Lancet*, **1**, 519–22.

Prescott, L. F., Illingworth, R. N., Critchley, J. A. H. J., Stewart, M. J., Adam, R. D., and Proudfoot, A. T. (1979). Intravenous N-acetylcysteine; the treatment of choice for paracetamol poisoning. *British Medical Journal*, **2**, 1097–100.

Pullar, T. and Capell, H. A. (1983). Interaction between oral anticoagulant drugs and non-steroidal anti-inflammatory agents: a review. *Scottish Medical Journal*, **28**, 42–7.

Roth, G. J. and Majerus, P. W. (1975). The mechanism of the effect of aspirin on human platelets. I Acetylation of a particular fraction protein. *Journal of Clinical Investigation*, **56**, 624–32.

Roth, G. J., Stanford, N., and Majerus, P. W. (1975). Acetylation of prostaglandin synthetase by aspirin. *Proceedings of the National Academy of Sciences U.S.A.*, **72**, 3073–6.

Settipane, G. A., Chafee, F. H., and Klein, D. E. (1974). Aspirin intolerance—a prospective study in an atopic and normal population. *Journal of Allergy and Clinical Immunology*, **53**, 200–4.

Seymour, R. A. (1983). Aspirin in dentistry. *Australian Journal of Pharmacology*, **16**, 19–21.

Seymour, R. A. and Rawlins, M. D. (1982). The efficacy and pharmacokinetics of aspirin in postoperative dental pain. *British Journal of Clinical Pharmacology*, **13**, 807–10.

Seymour, R. A. and Walton, J. G. (1984). Pain control after third molar surgery. *International Journal of Oral Surgery*, **13**, 457–85.

Seymour, R. A., BLair, G. S., and Wyatt, F. A. R. (1983). Postoperative dental pain and analgesic efficacy. II Analgesic usage and efficacy after dental surgery. *British Journal of Oral Surgery*, **21**, 298–303.

Seymour, R. A., Williams, F. M., Ward, A., and Rawlins, M. D. (1984). Aspirin metabolism and analgesic efficacy in postoperative dental pain. *British Journal of Clinical Pharmacology*, **17**, 697–701.

Seymour, R. A., Meechan, J. G., and Blair, G. S. (1985). An investigation into postoperative pain after third molar surgery under local anaesthesia. *British Journal of Oral and Maxillofacial Surgery*, **23**, 410–18.

Seymour, R. A., Williams, F. M., Luyk, N., Boyle, M. A., Whitfield, P. M., Nicholson, E., Ward-Booth, P., and Rawlins, M. D. (1986). Comparative efficacy of soluble aspirin and aspirin tablets in postoperative dental pain. *European Journal of Clinical Pharmacology*, **30**, 495–8.

Siegel, M. I., McConnell, R. T., and Cuatrecasas, P. (1979). Aspirin-like drugs interfere with arachidonic acid metabolism by inhibition of the 12-hydroperoxy-5,8,10,14-eicosatetraenoic acid peroxidase activity of the lipoxygenase pathway. *Proceedings of the National Academy of Sciencies*, **76**, 3774–8.

Tarlow, M. (1986). Reye's syndrome and aspirin. *British Medical Journal*, **292**, 1543.

Vane, J. R. (1971). Inhibition of prostaglandin synthesis as a mechanism of action for aspirin-like drugs. *Nature New Biology*, **231**, 232–5.

Weiss, H. J., Aledort, L. M., and Kochwa, S. (1968). The effect of salicylates on the haemostatic properties of platelets in man. *Journal of Clinical Investigation*, **47**, 2169–80.

6

Opioids and opiates

OPIOIDS and opiates exert their analgesic effect within the central nervous system by modifying neural activity associated with pain, hence they are sometimes referred to as centrally acting analgesics.

The therapeutic properties of the milky exudate obtained from the seed pod of the white poppy *Papaver somniferum* have been known since the third century BC. The exudate is dried and is known as opium, which contains the alkaloids morphine and codeine. These drugs, together with many synthetic compounds, are known as opioids, that is they have an opium- or morphine-like activity. The opioids are mainly used as analgesics through their interaction with specific opioid receptors within the central nervous system (CNS). Their other important therapeutic properties are the suppression of cough, and the reduction of gastrointestinal mobility.

TERMINOLOGY

The term 'opiate' is used to designate drugs derived from opium, i.e. essentially morphine and codeine, although it has been loosely applied to morphine derivatives. The term 'opioid' refers to any directly acting compound, the effects of which are antagonized by naloxone. Narcotics and major analgesics are now obsolete terms that have been used to describe this group of drugs.

OPIOID RECEPTORS

These were first isolated in 1973 (Pert and Snyder 1973), and four types have been described, μ (mu), κ (kappa), δ (delta) and σ (sigma), but there are also subtypes of these receptors. The effects of stimulating the various opioid receptors together with the endogenous ligard are summarized in Table 6.1.

Morphine and related compounds appear to have different affinities for the three types of receptors, which may account for many of the differing pharmacological properties of this group of drugs. Opioid receptors are found throughout the central nervous system; there are high concentrations in the limbic system, the substantia gelatinosa, the spinal nucleus of the fifth cranial nerve (V), and the thalamus. The receptors appear to be the site of action of the endogenous opioids (opioid peptides)—the enkephalins, dynorphins, and endorphins (Chang and Cuatrecasas 1981; Martin 1983).

Table 6.1. Opioid receptors, endogenous ligands and the effect of receptor stimulation

Receptor	Endogenous ligand	Effect of receptor stimulation
μ (mu)	Endorphin	Analgesia (μ_1) Dependence (μ_2) Miosis (μ_2) Respiratory depression (μ_2) Constipation (μ_2)
κ (kappa)	Dynorphin	Spinal analgesia Sedation
δ (delta)	Enkephalins	Respiratory depression
σ (sigma)	Unknown	Dysphoria

PAIN-RELATED NEUROTRANSMITTERS AND NEUROHORMONES

Enkephalins

These are a series of peptides originally identified from pig brain extracts by Hughes *et al.* (1975). Two structurally similar peptides were found—methionine enkephalin (met-enkephalin) and leucine enkephalin (leu-enkaphalin)—each of which is derived by enzyme cleavage from a larger and independent precursor, proenkephalin A. The identification of the enkephalins was followed by the realization that the met-enkephalin amino-acid sequence was present in the pituitary peptide, β-lipotropin, as residues 61 to 65. Soon afterwards, it was shown that the C-fragment of β-lipotropin (residues 61 to 91) interacts specifically with opioid receptors; this is now known as β-endorphin.

All of these peptides have properties in common with morphine, such as production of analgesia, physical dependence and tolerance, and the contraction of smooth muscle. Their actions can be reversed or blocked by the specific opioid antagonist, naloxone (see Terminology above). There is now evidence that the enkephalins are neurotransmitters of specific nerve fibres in the brain that modulate sensory information pertaining to pain and emotional behaviour. Regional variations in enkephalin levels parallel the distribution of opioid receptors. The highest levels of enkephalins are found in brain fractions containing nerve terminals, the distribution of which is likewise similar to that of the opioid receptor (Akil *et al.* 1984).

The dynorphins

These may act as neurotransmitters or neurohormones; they are produced by enzyme cleavage from the precursor, prodynorphin. The dynorphins are larger peptides than the enkephalins but their physiological role is uncertain.

The endorphins

These comprise at least four different peptides designated α-, β-, γ-, and δ-endorphins, of which β-endorphin is the most significant. All are derived by enzyme cleavage from the precursor pro-opiomelancortin, which also serves as the precursor for β-lipotropin (see Enkephalins above) and corticotropin.

The endorphins appear to be neurohormones that are released into the blood stream and have a variable duration of action. They are found mainly in the anterior pituitary gland, in the same cells as corticotropin and β-lipotropin. All of these hormones are secreted in parallel during stress, possibly as an adaptive mechanism: the endorphins may help to relieve any pain the individual might then incur.

β-endorphin has potent and long-lasting analgesic activity (Oyama et al. 1980). The analgesia produced by β-endorphin was also shown to be reversed by the opioid antagonist, naloxone. It was thus anticipated that the long-sought, non-addictive analgesic had finally been found, as it appeared a reasonable assumption that man is not likely to become addicted to endogenously produced substances. However, in experimental animals, repeated injections of β-endorphin have produced symptoms of tolerance and dependence.

If there is such a pain-suppressing system, why is it that the human being experiences pain? The answer may be connected with the fact that a painful stimulus activates both A-delta and C-fibres. Pain transmitted by A-delta fibres (first pain) acts as a warning system; this type of pain is hardly affected by morphine or other opioids. C-fibre-induced pain is perhaps the more clinically relevant, and it is affected by morphine. It may be inferred that pain of a protracted nature (suffering) is more likely to be modulated by endorphin release than warning pain. It is not difficult to conceive that suppression of protracted post-traumatic pain may serve a sensible purpose.

Further properties of the endorphins

The human placenta produces β-endorphin (Houck et al. 1980), which may be distributed to the fetus, so exposing it to high perinatal endorphin levels, but the significance of this is unclear. From behavioural investigations, it has been shown that pain sensitivity in the new-born child is relatively low, although pain reactions can be evoked, and that the sensitivity becomes much greater after a few days of life. This pattern of reaction to pain in neonates may be related to residual maternal levels of β-endorphin in the central nervous system.

Pain sensitivity varies between many ethnic groups. Research has demonstrated certain correlations between experimental measures of pain and β-endorphin levels in the cerebrospinal fluid (CSF). Patients with high endorphin levels have high pain thresholds and pain tolerance levels. At the risk of oversimplification, it would seem as if constitutional differences in response to pain, and differences in attitude to potentially painful or other noxious stimuli, may be related to endorphin activity (von Knorring et al. 1978).

Certain pathological conditions are characterized by abnormal insensitivity to pain. One such is congenital analgesia, in which there may be a central defect, and two cases have been reported of patients who responded to naloxone, with a lowering of pain threshold and return of pain responsiveness (Dehen *et al.* 1978; Yanagida 1978). This response suggests that these patients may have excessive endorphin production and activity. Patients with schizophrenia seldom complain during venepuncture. lumbar puncture, or other painful diagnostic procedures. Furthermore, their pain sensitivity increases after they have received naloxone. Various studies have shown that schizophrenics, as well as patients with endogenous depression, frequently show elevated CSF levels of endorphins (Bellenger *et al.* 1979; Geschwind 1975).

Placebo analgesia, acupuncture, hypnosis, and the endorphin system

It is a well-known clinical observation that psychological and emotional factors are important in the control of pain. Placebos are pharmacologically inert substances and it is estimated that some 30 to 40 per cent of the population will show a therapeutic response when, unknown to them, they are given placebo. Such subjects are known as 'placebo responders'. The placebo effect is prominent in the testing of any analgesics and its magnitude seems to be related to the potency of the analgesic drug under evaluation. Levine *et al.* (1978) have studied the effect of naloxone on the placebo response in patients undergoing removal of their impacted lower third molars. Postoperatively, these received intravenously either an analgesic or placebo in random, double-blind order. One-third of those who received placebo reported a significant reduction in pain. When these 'placebo-responders' were subsequently given naloxone, their pain returned to its original pre-injection level. The remaining patients, who did not respond to the placebo injection, failed to show any response after naloxone. These findings would suggest a link between endorphin production and activity, and the placebo response.

The derivation of the analgesia that may be induced by hypnosis is controversial. There have been conflicting reports of the effect of naloxone on hypnosis-induced analgesia (Barber and Mayer 1977; Goldstein and Hilgard 1975; Nasrallah *et al.* 1979; Stephenson 1978). However, the overwhelming impression from the literature is that naloxone does not appear to reverse hypnotic analgesia. But this may not be true for every type of hypnotherapy and it has not yet been ruled out that purely mental activation of a neuronal process could lead to endorphin release. If mental control over endorphin production and activation could be proven, this might lead to methods for the self-regulation of pain.

Acupuncture analgesia has been used for centuries in China, and recent studies have confirmed that it does induce an increase in the pain threshold in man. How acupuncture works remains uncertain, but the finding that naloxone can reverse the analgesia induced by acupuncture suggests that release of endorphins may be a factor (Mayer *et al.* 1977; Sjölund *et al.* 1977). Both the time delay before the onset of acupuncture analgesia, and the prolonged effect afterwards, indicate the release of some hormonal factor.

Closely related to acupuncture are electrical stimulation methods for controlling pain. Essentially, two procedures are in use. The first is high-frequency (100–200 Hz) stimulation, which is apparently not endorphin-mediated, but may work by activating the gate-control (see below) mechanisms. The second is low-frequency (1–2 Hz) stimulation, which is associated with a rise in CSF endorphin levels and is reversed by naloxone (Sjölund *et al.* 1977; 1979).

The detection of an endogenous opioid system (the opioid receptors, endorphins, dynorphins, and enkephalins) has created a great deal of interest in pain mechanisms. Furthermore these findings have given a rational background for the understanding and use of various stimulation techniques for pain relief.

Substance P

Substance P (so-called because it was a 'P'owder) is a polypeptide, originally discovered by von Euler and Gaddum (1931). The evidence suggests that substance P is a neurotransmitter in small-diameter fibres, particularly C-fibres. Staining techniques have shown that substance P is found in the following areas related to pain:

(1) cell bodies of posterior root ganglia projecting to the substantia gelatinosa of the spinal cord;

(2) caudal division of the trigeminal (V) spinal nucleus;

(3) nucleus raphe pallidus and magnus;

(4) periaqueductal grey area.

That substance P is specifically related to pain is indicated by the disappearance of nerve endings containing it (sited in the caudal division of the trigeminal nerve) after removal of tooth pulps in cats. The tooth pulp is innervated almost exclusively by pain fibres.

In general, endogenous opioid peptides suppress pain, whereas substance P promotes it (Sweet 1980). However, application of substance P to the exposed tooth pulp does not excite sensory neurones and its role in the pulp is still obscure (Gazelius *et al.* 1977). Substance P and enkephalins (see above) do interact: the release of substance P is inhibited not only by met-enkephalin, but also by β-endorphin and morphine.

The role of substance P and enkephalins in pain transmission

The discovery of the interaction between substance P, enkephalins, and opioid receptors (Jessel and Iversen 1977) can, in part, help to explain neuropharmacological aspects of Melzack and Wall's gate-control theory of pain (Melzack and Wall 1965).

Within the substantia gelatinosa, a nociceptive impulse transmitted via small C-fibres causes release of substance P at the synapse (Fig. 6.1). Substance P binds with specific receptors postsynaptically and the impulse is further transmitted. Synapsing with the small C-fibre terminal is an enkephalinergic fibre that, on excitation, releases met-enkephalin. The met-enkaphalin binds to opioid receptors on the terminal of the C-fibre, depolarizes the membrane, and inhibits the release of substance P. Consequently, the nerve impulse carrying nociceptive sensations does not progress beyond the synapse.

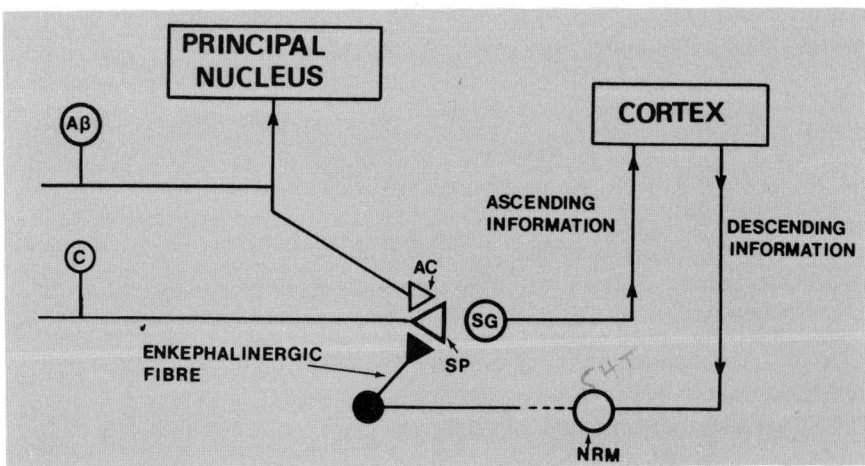

Fig. 6.1. Schematic representation of the organization of inhibition in the substantia gelatinosa (AC = acetyl-choline; SG = substantia gelatinosa; SP = substance P; NRM = nucleus raphe magnus; C = cell body of C-fibre; Aβ = cell body of a beta fibre).

The enkephalinergic fibres are, in turn, connected to the cortex via the nucleus raphe magnus. The transmitter substance in raphe neurones is not enkephalin, but 5-hydroxytryptamine. Their terminals synapse with and activate enkephalinergic interneurones in the substantia gelatinosa (Fig. 6.2). Activity in the nucleus raphe magnus is under the descending control of the cortex.

In addition to the pain-suppressing system brought about by activity in the enkephalinergic fibres, activity in the large sensory A-beta fibres can cause presynaptic inhibition (depolarization) of activity in small-fibre (C-fibre) terminals. This mechanism constitutes the gate-control. Clinically, it can be applied in the form of transcutaneous nerve stimulation, which consists of high-frequency, low-intensity electrical pulses passing through pad electrodes. Analgesia brought about by such stimulation is not naloxone-reversible.

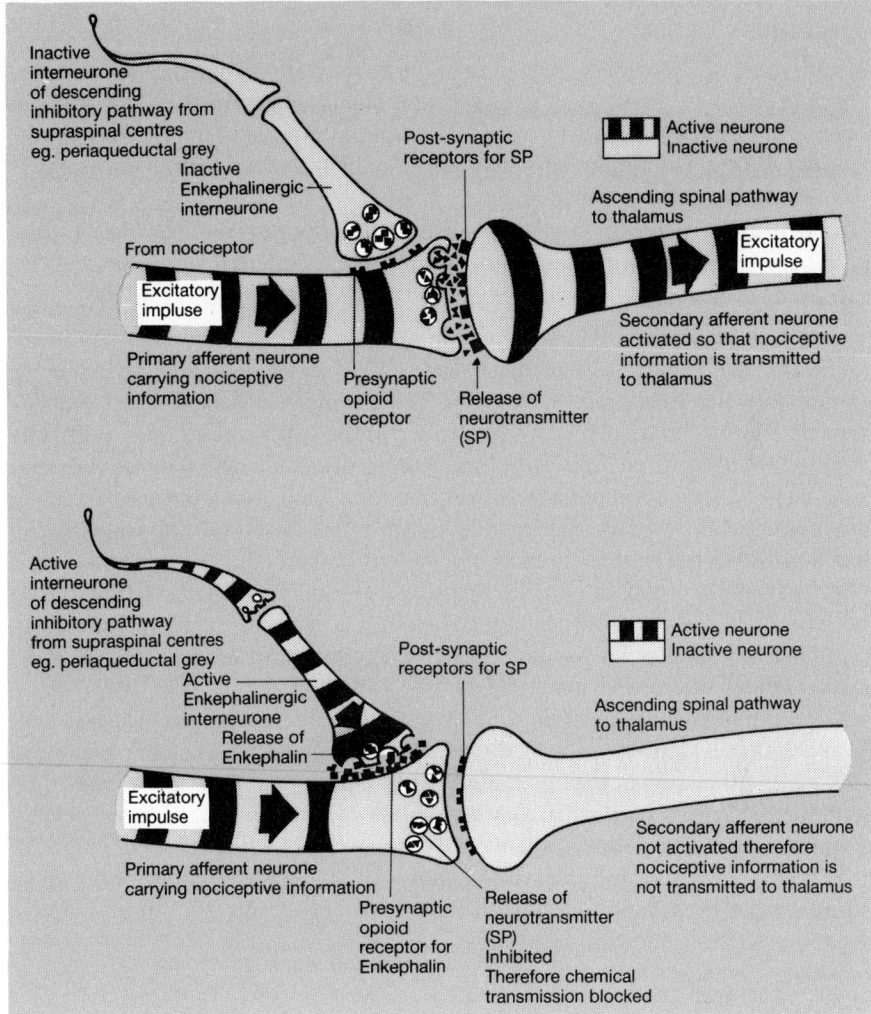

Fig. 6.2. Diagrammatic representation of the interaction between an enkephalinergic fibre and a C-fibre.

SPECIFIC OPIOIDS AND OPIOID ANTAGONISTS

Morphine

Morphine, named after Morpheus, the Greek god of dreams, was first isolated in 1803. This drug is the most widely used of the opioids and is considered to be the most potent analgesic in use for the relief of pain.

Pharmacokinetics

As with most of the opioids, morphine undergoes extensive first pass metabolism in the liver when given via the oral route. Hence for optimal use, it is given parenterally. Morphine is conjugated with glucuronic acid in the liver and is excreted via the kidney; its half-life in man is approximately three hours.

Pharmacodynamic and pharmacological properties

Analgesia

Understanding of how morphine works as an analgesic must be accompanied by more detailed information about the pain experience. This experience comprises the initial sensation together with emotional, psychological, and suffering components that the sensation evokes. For example, coronary chest pain or cancer pain will have a different significance to the sufferer than, say, toothache or pain from a fractured limb. Morphine is particularly effective against pain that has a large suffering component. In addition to its analgesic properties, the drug also produces other central effects, such as drowsiness, sedation, and euphoria, all of which add to the general comfort of a patient in pain. Morphine does not alter other sensations such as touch, pressure, vision, or hearing. Those given morphine will feel a pinprick as normal though it may be less unpleasant. Also, morphine is considered to be more effective against continuous, dull pain than against sharp, intermittent pain.

Although the precise mechanism of morphine-induced analgesia is uncertain, there is much evidence to suggest that the drug combines with opioid receptors (μ and κ) in the substantia gelatinosa, the spinal nucleus of V, and the periaqueductal and periventricular grey matter. By activating these receptors, morphine alters the central release of neurotransmitters (probably substance P) from nerve fibres transmitting painful stimuli. A 10 mg dose of morphine given intramuscularly will provide adequate pain relief within 30 minutes and a duration of effect of four to five hours.

Gastro-intestinal tract

Opium has been used for centuries to treat diarrhoea and dysentery. All the opioids produce a degree of constipation and some are used solely for this purpose (e.g. loperamide hydrochloride and diphenoxylate hydrochloride). These drugs act on the smooth muscles of the gastro-intestinal tract by increasing muscle and sphincter tone. This results in delayed emptying of the gut, diminished peristalsis, and a decrease in propulsive motility. The constipating properties of the opioids show marked variation between patients, with some experiencing painful muscle spasms, particularly of the smooth muscles of the biliary tract.

Cough suppression

Morphine and many of the opioids, especially codeine (see below), are effective antitussives. The opioids have a direct effect on the cough centre in the medulla. Cough suppression occurs with low doses of morphine.

Cardiovascular effects

Morphine at therapeutic doses has an insignificant effect on blood pressure, cardiac output, and heart rate. However, it does cause the release of histamine, which produces vasodilatation of the peripheral vessels and causes the sensation of warmth that many experience after receiving morphine.

Unwanted effects

Respiratory depression

Morphine and many of the other opioids depress respiration by a direct effect on the respiratory centres in the brain stem. Some degree of respiratory depression occurs with normal therapeutic doses but, in overdose, the respiratory depression can be life-threatening. Morphine decreases the response of the respiratory centre to the concentration of CO_2 (P_{CO_2}) levels in the blood; it also depresses the pontine and medullary centres that control respiratory rhythm. Thus, after morphine, there is a reduction in respiratory rate, minute volume, and tidal exchange.

Dependence

One of the main draw-backs of the opioids is the development of tolerance and physical dependence with repeated use. The problem of drug abuse is dealt with in more detail in Chapter 23. Tolerance develops to the depressant actions of the opioids—analgesia, euphoria, drowsiness, and respiratory depression. Both physical dependence and tolerance will depend upon the dose and frequency of administration. Similarly, the degree of physical dependence will determine the intensity of the withdrawal syndrome.

Nauseant and emetic effects

Nausea and vomiting are common unwanted effects associated with morphine and many of the other opioids. This is due to a direct stimulation of the chemoreceptor trigger zone in the medulla. The incidence of nausea and vomiting is much higher in ambulatory patients, which suggests that a vestibular component is active. The administration of an anti-emetic, such as cyclizine tartrate or prochlorperazine, may reduce this problem.

Effects on the pupil

Morphine, together with many of the more potent opioids, causes a constriction of the pupil (miosis), due to an excitatory action on the autonomic segment of the nucleus of the oculomotor nerve (Edinger–Westphal nucleus). Because of the miosis, it is unwise to give morphine to patients with a suspected head injury as the drug will mask the pupillary constriction reflex, which is an important indicator of brain damage.

Overdose

Death from overdose of the opioids is due to respiratory depression. The subject who has taken an overdose, either accidentally or intentionally, will invariably be asleep and difficult to arouse, The respiratory rate will be very low; there will be a drop in blood pressure; the pupils will be constricted and show no response to light. The skin will be cold and clammy, and all skeletal muscles will be flaccid, including the tongue, which may fall back and block the airway.

Treatment is to establish and maintain an airway and then administer an opioid antagonist such as naloxone. The usual dose of naloxone is 0.4 mg intravenously, which can be repeated after two to three minutes if required. The half-life of naloxone is short (about 1 h) and further repeated doses may be necessary to avoid a relapse into a coma state.

Uses of morphine

Although morphine is widely used in the treatment of postoperative pain after general surgery, its main use is in the relief of cancer pain and other pains of terminal illness. The combined analgesic, euphoriant, and sedative properties of morphine are a considerable advantage in reducing the pain and suffering that often accompany a terminal illness. A variety of other opioids are used for this purpose, particularly those that are effective by mouth, thus avoiding repeated injections in frail patients.

As morphine suppresses the cough reflex and respiratory activity, the drug should not be used indiscriminately in postoperative pain after general surgery, where such suppression can lead to pneumonia.

Codeine

Codeine, or methyl morphine, is a naturally occurring alkaloid present in opium; like all the opioids, it binds to opioid receptors within the central nervous system. The drug is metabolized in the liver to form nor-codeine and morphine, so morphine may acount for codeine's analgesic properties. About half the drug is excreted in the urine unchanged or conjugated with glucuronide; about 10 per cent is excreted as morphine glucuronide and the remainder as nor-codeine glucuronide.

Pharmacological properties

Codeine is one of the few opioids that is effective when taken by mouth, but it is only useful in treating mild to moderate pain. Peak plasma concentrations occur one hour after oral dosage, and the duration of analgesia is two to four hours. On a dose per dose basis, codeine has about one-twelth the potency of morphine, but it is appreciably more effective than morphine when given by mouth. There are many proprietary analgesics that contain mixtures of codeine and either paracetamol or aspirin. Combining both a peripherally and a centrally acting analgesic appears to enhance the efficacy of the combination—an effect that is often more than additive.

Codeine is a very effective antitussive, and so is contained in many proprietary cough medicines.

Unwanted effects

Codeine is capable of producing all the unwanted effects of the opioids as a group, such as nausea, vomiting, sedation, and dizziness. As with morphine, these effects are more often observed in ambulatory patients than those in bed. When the drug is administered orally in the usual therapeutic doses (30–60 mg), the incidence of unwanted effects is low, and those that do occur are annoying rather than serious. Codeine can depress respiration to a measurable extent, but the degree of respiratory depression is of little clinical significance except in overdose. Constipation is frequently noted when repeated doses are administered, and so the drug has been used as an antidiarrhoeal.

The risk of dependence or addiction to codeine is small. The usual dose regime of codeine (30–60 mg × 4 daily), even when given for several months, does not induce significant dependence. Most addicts who have resorted to codeine have done so because nothing better was available.

Pethidine

This is a synthetic opioid, first manufactured in 1939. It can be given orally, but optimal analgesia is obtained when given intramuscularly. Pethidine is hydrolysed in the liver to meperidinic acid, which is conjugated and excreted in the urine. The half-life of pethidine is about three hours.

Pharmacological properties

Pethidine provides rapid analgesia when given via the parenteral route, with the maximum analgesic effect occurring one hour after dosage. The duration of analgesia obtained from 50 mg is approximately two to four hours; this is slightly less than that obtained from morphine. It has been estimated that 80–100 mg pethidine have the same potency as 10 mg morphine.

Unwanted effects

These are similar to those of morphine and include respiratory depression, dependence, and pupillary constriction. The effect of pethidine on the muscles of the gastro-intestine tract is considerably less than that of morphine or codeine. At normal therapeutic doses, it has little effect on the cardiovascular system but intravenous administration causes an alarming increase in heart rate. In overdose, pethidine sometimes produces excitation of the central nervous system resulting in tremors, muscle twitching, seizures, and an atropine-like action causing an increase in heart rate.

Drug interactions

Pethidine should not be given to patients receiving monoamine oxidase inhibitors as this may cause convulsions, hypothermia, hyperpyrexia, and severe

respiratory depression. These reactions are totally unlike the normal pharmacological effects of pethidine and are therefore of the Type B reactions (see Chapter
22).

Concurrent administration of pethidine with either tricyclic antidepressants or
chlorpromazine will enhance its sedative properties.

Pentazocine

This is a benzomorphan derivative that has both agonistic and weak opioid
antagonistic activity. The drug acts as an antagonist on the μ-receptor, but as an
agonist on the κ- and σ-receptors. This agonism accounts for the high incidence of
hallucinations associated with pentazocine. Because of the antagonistic action on
the μ-receptor, pentazocine should not be used with an opioid agonist. It was
originally thought that it would have little or no abuse potential but, with
widespread use, physical dependence and abuse have become apparent.
Pentazocine can be administered both orally and parenterally; however, repeated
injections should be avoided as the drug causes a local irritation and extensive
fibrosis. Pentazocine is well absorbed from the site of administration and
undergoes extensive first pass metabolism (80 per cent). The drug is metabolized
in the liver and the metabolites are excreted in the kidney; the rate of metabolism
shows marked individual variation, which may account for inter-individual
differences in pharmacological properties (Beckett *et al.* 1970). The half-life of
pentazocine is two to three hours. An intramuscular dose of 30–50 mg
pentazocine is approximately equivalent to 10 mg morphine. When given orally,
50 mg pentazocine produces analgesia equivalent to 60 mg codeine.

Unwanted effects.

There is a high incidence of these (Forrest 1974)—including hallucinations,
nightmares, sedation, dizziness, sweating, and nausea—and their frequency
increases with dose. High doses of pentazocine cause an increase in blood
pressure and heart rate. The effect on blood pressure may be due to an increase in
plasma concentration of catecholamines (Tammisto *et al.* 1971). The effects of
pentazocine on the gastro-intestinal tract and respiration are similar to those of
the other opioids. Pentazocine raises pulmonary artery pressure (Alderman *et al.*
1972) and therefore should not be used to reduce chest pain following a
myocardial infarction.

Dihydrocodeine

This is considered to be a moderately potent analgesic and is in wide clinical use. It
is derived from codeine and was first manufactured in 1911. Structurally,
dihydrocodeine is related to both codeine and morphine and so may be expected
to share some of the properties of either or both of these drugs. It can be given

orally or parenterally and has a half-life of three to four hours. When given orally, the drug undergoes extensive first pass metabolism. Dihydrocodeine is metabolized in the liver to dihydromorphine, which is further conjugated with glucuronide and excreted via the kidneys. Dose regimes of dihydrocodeine are 30 mg every four to six hours.

Unwanted effects

Dihydrocodeine is associated with a high incidence of such effects, which include nausea, dizziness, and constipation. It is estimated that 25 per cent of patients who take dihydrocodeine experience side-effects of sufficient unpleasantness to prevent them from taking further doses (Langdon 1969).

Dextropropoxyphene

This is a tertiary amine ester, both chemically and pharmacologically related to methadone and other opioids. However, its efficacy as an analgesic agent is questionable, and as an individual compound the drug is not used in dentistry. However, co-proxamol, which is a combination of dextropropoxyphene (32.5 mg) and paracetamol (325 mg), is the most widely prescribed analgesic preparation in the UK (Skegg et al. 1977).

The toxicity of co-proxamol presents a serious problem in overdose, and death has been reported from as few as 15 tablets taken with alcohol (Whittington 1977). The effects of overdose of dextropropoxyphene are similar to those of other opioids, but a particularly worrying feature is the rapid onset of respiratory depression. Patients surviving the effects of dextropropoxyphene in co-proxamol may develop hepatic necrosis from the paracetamol. The continuing popularity of preparations containing dextropropoxyphene is difficult to understand; controlled studies have failed to show that dextropropoxyphene is any more effective than paracetamol or aspirin alone. (Hopkinson et al. 1976).

Combination analgesics

Combination analgesics (see co-proxamol above) contain both a peripherally acting (e.g. aspirin or paracetamol) and a centrally acting (e.g. codeine or dextropropoxyphene) analgesic. The rationale for combined analgesics is that they will block pain at the site of the injury as well as alter the transmission of pain within the central nervous system.

Evidence from clinical trials would suggest that combined analgesics are more effective than when the individual constituents are used singularly. The efficacy of the preparations is often more than additive. Although combined analgesics are widely used, there is also a high incidence of unwanted effects; this may be due to a synergistic effect of the two component drugs (Parkhouse 1975).

Naloxone

This is a competitive opioid antagonist, mainly used to treat opioid overdose, and in particular to reverse the effect of an opioid on respiration. In the treatment of opioid-induced respiratory depression, naloxone must be given intravenously (0.4–0.8 mg) for immediate effect. If the depression is not reversed, the dose is repeated after two minutes. The half-life of naloxone is only one hour and further repeated administration may be required. Naloxone can also be used if there is a problem in diagnosing physical dependence or addiction to the opioids for, in such subjects, naloxone will induce symptoms of withdrawal.

Buprenorphine

This is a semi-synthetic opioid derived from thebaine. An intramuscular dose of 0.4 mg buprenorphine has an analgesic potency equivalent to 10 mg of intramuscular morphine; the duration of analgesia with this dose of buprenorphine is about six hours. The drug is particularly well-absorbed when given sublingually. Buprenorphine is extensively bound to plasma protein (96 per cent) and has a plasma half-life of about three hours. Most of the drug is excreted unchanged in the faeces.

Receptor binding studies suggest that buprenorphine is a partial agonist for the μ-receptor but may well act as an antagonist at other opioid receptors.

Unwanted effects of buprenorphine are similar to those of morphine and include sedation, nausea, vomiting, dizziness, sweating, and dependence (Heel *et al.* 1980).

Methadone

This is a synthetic opioid, first manufactured during the early 1940s. It is well absorbed from all routes of administration, and is effective when given orally. Methadone is broken down in the liver and the metabolites are excreted in the urine; the plasma half-life is one to one-and-a-half days. Methadone is a μ-agonist and on a dose per dose basis is as effective an analgesic as morphine. However, the advantages of methadone over morphine are its longer duration of action and efficacy when given orally. The main uses of methadone are relief of pain, treatment of opioid abstinence syndrome, and treatement (by substitution) of heroin users.

USE OF OPIOIDS IN DENTISTRY

Although morphine and related analgesics are widely used in relieving pain, their dental application is limited. Most types of dental pain, such as in pulpitis, dry socket, or pericoronitis, can be effectively treated by local measures, and the dental surgeon is unlikely to prescribe opioids for these conditions.

Postoperative pain after a dental surgical procedure is the main indication for recommending or prescribing analgesics. Such pain has a major inflammatory component, and as the opioids possess no anti-inflammatory action, their efficacy is doubtful in this context. Clinical trials to evaluate codeine, dextropropoxyphene, and pentazocine, have all shown that the efficacy of these drugs in relieving pain after removal of impacted lower third molars is poor (Seymour and Walton 1984). One study (Seymour *et al.* 1982) showed that dihydrocodeine, when given intravenously, increased the severity of postoperative dental pain when compared to a placebo.

Critical reappraisal of evidence supporting the efficacy of opioids in dental pain indicates that these drugs are of virtually no value. However, the opioids are particularly effective in the treatment of postoperative pain after general surgery, and of cancer pain. Cancer pain, as described earlier, has emotional and suffering components that would be alleviated by the euphoriant properties of the opioids together with alteration of the pain reaction. Pain after general surgery, as after dental surgery, will have a similar, but greater, inflammatory element, but the patient's reaction to their pain may differ because of their own expectations: for example one undergoing major abdominal surgery as an in-patient is likely to have a different view of their circumstances from one who has had impacted lower third molars removed in an out-patient clinic. The difference between out-patient and in-patient surgery may be reflected in different levels of anxiety, particularly if the surgery has been undertaken for a life-threatening condition. The apparent lack of pain relief afforded by the opioids after dental surgery may be accounted for by the relative absence of any significant emotional component of the pain, a factor likely to be present after major in-patient surgery.

Thus analgesics with an established anti-inflammatory property (such as aspirin) appear to offer more advantages in the treatment of dental pain than the opioids.

REFERENCES

Akil, H., Watson, S. J., Young, E., Lewis, M. E., Khachaturian, H., and Walker, J. M. (1984). Endogenous opioids: biology and function. *Annual Review of Neuroscience*, **7**, 223–55.

Alderman, E. L., Barry, W. H., Graham, A. F., and Harrison, D. C. (1972). Haemodynamic effects of morphine and pentazocine differ in cardiac patients. *New England Journal of Medicine*, **287**, 623–7.

Barber, J. and Mayer, D. (1977). Evaluation of the efficacy and neural mechanisms of a hypnotic analgesia procedure in experimental and clinical dental pain. *Pain*, **4**, 41–8.

Beckett, A. H., Taylor, J. F., and Kourounakis, P. (1970). The absorption, distribution and excretion of pentazocine in man after oral and intravenous administration. *Journal of Pharmacy and Pharmacology*, **22**, 123–8.

Bellenger, J. C., Post, R. M., Sternberg, D. E., Kammen, D. P., Cowdry, R. W., and Goodwin F. K. (1979). Headaches after lumbar puncture and insensitivity to pain in psychiatric patients. *New England Journal of Medicine*, **30**, 110.

Chang, K. W. and Cuatrecasas, P. (1981). Heterogeneity and properties of opiate receptors. *Federation Proceedings*, **40**, 2729–34.

Dehen, H., Willer, J. G., Prier, S., Boureau, F., and Chambier, J. (1978). Congenital insensitivity to pain and the morphine-like analgesic system. *Pain*, **5**, 351–8.

Forrest, W. H. (1974). Oral pentazocine. *Annals of Internal Medicine*, **8**, 644–6.

Gazelius, B., Olgart, L., Edwall, L., and Trowbridge, H. O. (1977). Effects of substance P on sensory nerves and blood flow in the feline dental pulp. In *Pain in the trigeminal region* (ed. D. J. Anderson and B. Matthews) pp. 95–101. Elsevier, Amseterdam.

Geschwind, N. (1975). Insensitivity to pain in psychotic patients. *New England Journal of Medicine*, **296**, 1480.

Goldstein, A. and Hilgard, E. R. (1975). Failure of the opiate antagonist naloxone to modify hypnotic analgesia. *Proceedings of the National Academy of Sciences U.S.A.*, **72**, 2041–43.

Heel, R. C., Brogden, R. N., Speight, T. M., and Avery, G. S. (1980). Buprenorphine: a review of its pharmacological properties and therapeutic efficacy. *Drugs*, **17**, 81–110.

Hopkinson, J. H., Blatt, G., and Cooper, M. (1976) Effective pain relief: comparative results with acetaminophen in a new formulation, propoxyphene, a napsylate–acetaminophen combination and placebo. *Current Therapeutic Research*, **19**, 622–30.

Houck, J. C., Kimball, C., Chang, G., Pedigo, N. W. Y., and Yamamuraz, H. I. (1980). Placental β-endorphin-like peptides. *Science*, **207**, 78–9.

Hughes, J. H., Smith, T. W., Kosterlitz, H. W., Fothergill, I. A., Morgan, B., and Morris, H. R. (1975). Identification of two related pentapeptides from the brain with patient opiate agonist activity. *Nature*, **258**, 577–9.

Jessel, T. M. and Iversen, L. L. (1977). Opiate analgesics inhibit substance P release from rat trigeminal nucleus. *Nature*, **268**, 549–51.

Langdon, K. (1969). Adverse effects of dihydrocodeine. *British Dental Journal*, **126**, 494.

Levine, J. D., Gordon, N. C., and Fields, H. L. (1978). The mechanisms of placebo analgesia. *Lancet*, **ii**, 654–7.

Martin, W. R. (1983). Pharmacology of opioids. *Pharmacology Review*, **35**, 283–323.

Mayer, D. J., Price, D. D., and Rafii, A. (1977). Antagonism of acupuncture analgesia in man by the narcotic antagonist naloxone. *Brain Research*, **121**, 368–72.

Melzack, R. and Wall, P. (1965). Pain mechanisms: a new theory. *Science*, **150**, 971–9.

Nasrallah, H. A., Holley, T., and Janowsky, D. S. (1979). Opiate antagonism fails to reverse hypnotic-induced analgesia. *Lancet*, **i**, 1355.

Omaya, T., Jin, T., Yamaya, R., Ling, N., and Guillemin, R. (1980). Profound analgesic effects of β-endorphin in man. *Lancet*, **i**, 122–6.

Parkhouse, J. (1975). Simple analgesics. *Drugs*, **10**, 366–93.

Pert, C. B. and Snyder, S. H. (1973). Opiate receptor: demonstration in nervous tissue. *Science*, **179**, 101–14.

Seymour, R. A. and Walton, J. G. (1984). Pain control after third molar surgery—a review. *International Journal of Oral Surgery*, **13**, 457–85.

Seymour, R. A., Rawlins, M. D., and Rowell, F. J. (1982). Dihydrocodeine-induced hyperalgesia in postoperative dental pain. *Lancet*, **i**, 1425–6.

Sjölund, B. H. and Eriksson, M. B. E. (1979). The influence of naloxone on analgesia produced by peripheral conditioning stimulation. *Brain Research*, **173**, 295–301.

Sjölund, B. H., Terenius, L., and Eriksson, M. B. E. (1977). Increased cerebrospinal fluid levels of endorphins after electro-acupuncture. *Acta Physiologica Scandinavica*, **100**, 382–4.

Skegg, D. G., Doll, R., and Perry, J. (1977). Use of medicines in general practice. *British Medical Journal*, **ii**, 1561–3.

Stephenson, J. B. P. (1978). Reversal of hypnosis-induced analgesia by naloxone. *Lancet*, **ii**, 991–2.

Sweet, W. H. (1980). Neuropeptides and monoaminergic neurotransmitters: their relation to pain. *Journal of the Royal Society of Medicine*, **73**, 482–91.

Tammisto, T., Jaatela, A., Nikki, P., and Takki, S. (1971). Effects of pentazocine and pethidine on plasma catecholamine levels. *Annals of Clinical Research*, **3**, 22–9.

von Euller, U. S. and Gaddum, J. H. (1931). Unidentified depressor substance in certain tissue extracts. *Journal of Physiology*, **72**, 74–87.

von Knorring L., Almay, B. G. L., Johansson, F., and Terenius, L. (1978). Pain perception and endorphin levels in cerebrospinal fluid. *Pain*, **5**, 359–67.

Whittington, R. M. (1977). Dextropropoxyphene (Distalgesic) overdose in the West Midlands. *British Medical Journal*, **ii**, 172–3.

Yanagida, H. (1978). Congenital insensitivity and naloxone. *Lancet*, **ii**, 520–1.

7

Local anaesthetics
(local analgesics)

LOCAL anaesthesia may be produced by four methods:

(1) by the application of cold;

(2) by the application of pressure to nerve trunks;

(3) by rendering the tissues anaemic;

(4) by paralysing sensory nerve endings or nerve fibres with drugs.

The last of these methods is the most important therapeutically; method (1) has a limited application whilst (2) and (3) are unsafe for therapeutic use. Many different substances can interfere with the transmission of nerve impulses (method (4)), but for a drug to be clinically acceptable as a local anaesthetic, it must be able to produce a fully reversible block of nerve conduction at concentrations that do not damage the tissues. For example, procaine or lignocaine satisfy these criteria, whereas phenol abolishes the transmission of nerve impulses by causing irreversible damage to nerve fibres. Since 1884 when Karl Koller first introduced cocaine into clinical use (for historical review, see Koller 1928), much effort has been expended in trying to produce better and safer local anaesthetics. The perfect local anaesthetic does not exist and all of those in clinical use are capable of producing a variety of unwanted effects, which are discussed later.

CHEMISTRY

As a group, local anaesthetics are organic bases and as such are insoluble in water; but they can be converted into soluble salts, for example hydrochlorides, and these are the form in which they are used clinically. Their detailed chemical structures vary, but as Löfgren (1948) points out, the formulae of most local anaesthetics are built on a common plan, which is composed of three parts, as explained by the list and formula below:

(1) an aromatic residue with an acidic group (lipophilic); (R_1 where R = radical);

(2) a connecting intermediate aliphatic chain (with ester or amide link), usually an amino-alcohol; (R_2);

(3) a terminal substituted amino group (hydrophilic); (R_3 and R_4).

Thus a general formula may be written as follows, the three parts being numbered
as in the preceding list:

$$R_1CO\text{---}R_2\text{---}N\!\!\begin{array}{l} \diagup R_3 \\ \diagdown R_4 \end{array}$$

$$(1) \qquad (2) \qquad (3)$$

Note that R_3 and R_4 may form part of a cyclic system as in mepivacaine and
bupivacaine, two of the agents included in Fig. 7.1, which shows the structure of
some common local anaesthetics according to the common plan described above.

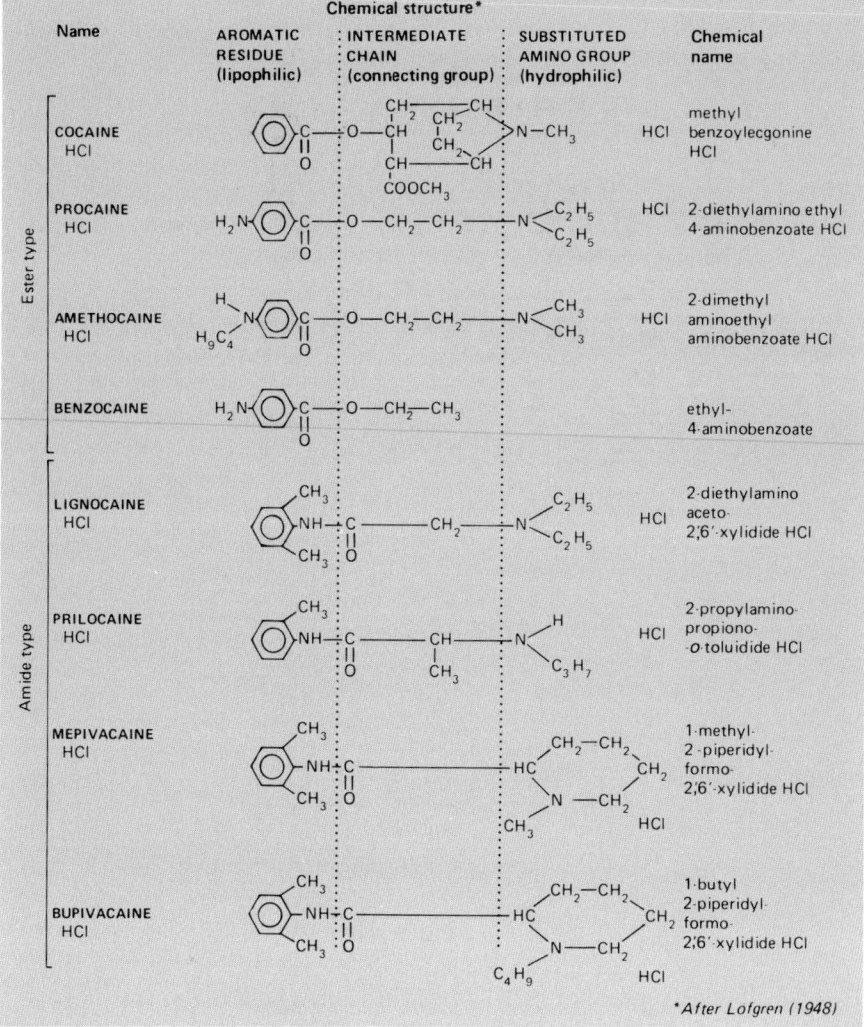

Fig. 7.1. Chemical structures of some local anaesthetics.

Physico-chemical properties

There are three that need to be considered, namely ionization, the partition coefficient, and protein binding.

Ionization

As local anaesthetics are weak bases, it follows that they will exist partly in an un-ionized form and partly in an ionized form, the proportion of each depending upon the pK_a or dissociation constant of the particular drug (i.e. the pH at which the ionized and non-ionized forms of the drug are present in equal amounts), and the pH of the surrounding medium (see Table 7.1 below and also Chapter 1). For example, procaine (as procaine hydrochloride) with a pK_a of 9.0 will ionize according to the following equation:

cation

$$H_2N\bigcirc C\!-\!O\!-\!CH_2\!-\!CH_2\!-\!N\!\!<^{C_2H_5}_{C_2H_5} \underset{acid}{\overset{alkaline}{\rightleftharpoons}} H_2N\bigcirc C\!-\!O\!-\!CH_2\!-\!CH_2\!-\!N^+\!\!<^{C_2H_5}_{C_2H_5}$$

$+H^+ + Cl^-$

$+Cl^-$

anion

un-ionized form   ionized form

The proportion of procaine that is un-ionized at the physiological pH of 7.4 can be calculated from the Henderson–Hasselbach equation (see Chapter 1):

$$\text{For procaine, } pK_a = 9.0$$

$$pH = 7.4$$

$$\text{For bases, } pH = pK_a - \log_{10}\frac{\text{ionized base}}{\text{un-ionized base}},$$

$$\text{so re-writing, } \log_{10}\frac{\text{ionized base}}{\text{un-ionized base}} = pK_a - pH$$

$$= 9.0 - 7.4$$

$$= 1.6.$$

Taking antilogs on both sides of the equation,

$$\frac{\text{ionized base}}{\text{un-ionized base}} = \frac{39.8}{1.0}$$

$$\text{i.e. approximately} = \frac{40.0}{1.0}.$$

Therefore, the percentage ratio of ionized/un-ionized molecules ($=40$) within a total of $40+1$ molecules ($=41$) is:

$$\frac{40}{41} \times 100 = 97.6\%.$$

Expressed the opposite way round, the ratio of un-ionized/ionized molecules is 1/41 (2.4 per cent). Thus, at pH 7.4 only a small proportion of a dose of injected procaine will be present in the un-ionized form that is lipid-soluble and readily crosses the lipid-containing sheaths of nerves. At one time it was believed that the un-ionized form of a local anaesthetic was responsible for producing the local anaesthetic effect, but the work of Ritchie and his colleagues (see Ritchie and Greengard 1966; Ritchie 1975) has indicated it is the *ionized* form that is able to block nerve conduction (see later). However, it is now clear that *both* the un-ionized and ionized forms are important if a local anaesthetic effect is to be achieved. Thus, the un-ionized form, being lipid-soluble, is able to cross the fatty sheath of nerves and gain ready access inside the nerve fibres; having gained entry to the cytoplasm of the nerve cell it is the ionized form that is able to block conduction (see later under 'Mechanism of action of local anaesthetics'). As these two forms of a local anaesthetic are in equilibrium it follows that as soon as some un-ionized molecules arrive inside the cell, some will become ionized, the proportion depending upon the pK_a of the drug and the intracellular pH, which is normally lower (e.g. pH 7 or less) than the extracellular pH of 7.4; see Fig. 7.3, p. 119).

   Table 7.1 lists the pK_a of those local anaesthetics commonly used in dentistry (together with some others), and also indicates the percentage of each drug in the un-ionized and ionized forms at pH 7.4. It can be seen that in general the amide types have a lower pK_a than the ester types (with the exception of benzocaine, which does not form soluble salts and can therefore only be used as a surface local anaesthetic). This means that the proportion of the lipid-soluble (i.e. un-ionized) form present in solution at physiological pH (7.4) is considerably greater with the amides (e.g. for lignocaine, 25 per cent) as compared with the ester type (e.g. for procaine, 2.4 per cent). This accounts for the faster onset of action of lignocaine (1–2 min) compared with procaine (2–5 min).

Partition coefficient

The partition coefficient measures lipid solubility or, to be more precise, the relative solubilities of an agent in fat and water—so that the more fat-soluble and the less water-soluble a compound is, the higher the numerical value (compare procaine = 0.6 with lignocaine = 3; see Table 7.1). All other things being equal, the greater the fat solubility, the greater the ease and rapidity with which a compound will cross a lipid barrier such as a nerve sheath.

Protein binding

Most drugs bind to plasma proteins in varying degrees (see Chapter 1) and local anesthetics are no exception (see Table 7.1). The two proteins chiefly involved are

Table 7.1. Pharmacokinetic data for certain local anaesthetics

	Drug[a] (MW)	pK_a[a]	% un-ionized[b] (pH 7.4)	% ionized[b] (pH 7.4)	Partition[c] coefficient	Plasma[d] protein binding %	Toxicity	Vol. of[d] distribution (litres)	Estimated[d] hepatic extraction ratio	Clearance[d] ($l\ min^{-1}$)	$T_{0.5}$[d]
Ester type	Cocaine (303)	8.6	6	94	?	?	V. high	118	?	0.71–3.08	0.7–1.5
	Procaine (236)	9.0	2.4	97.6	0.6	5.8	Low	?	?	?	<1
	Amethocaine (264)	8.5	7	93	80	75.6	High	?	?	?	?
	Benzocaine (165)	2.5	—	—	?	—	Low	—	—	—	—
Amide type	Lignocaine (234)	7.9	25	75	3	64	Medium	91	0.65	0.95	1.6
	Prilocaine (220)	7.9	25	75	1	50	Low/ medium	191	?	2.37	1.6
	Mepivacaine (283)	7.6	33	67	1	77	Medium	84	0.52	0.78	1.9
	Bupivacaine (302)	8.1	17	83	28	96	Medium	73	0.38	0.58	2.7

Abbreviations: pK_a = dissociation constant; ? = data not available; — = not applicable; MW = Molecular weight; $T_{0.5}$ = systemic; $T_{0.5}$ i.e. the time (hours) take for the amount of drug absorbed into the circulation to fall by one half.
Partition coefficient = lipid/water solubility ratio.
Vol. of distribution = effective volume (litres) into which, after absorption, the drug is finally distributed.
Clearance ($l\ min^{-1}$) = number of litres of plasma cleared of the drug per minute.
Hepatic extraction ratio = fraction of drug removed from the blood during a single passage through the liver (NB: high > 0.7).
(*Sources*: [a]Martindale (1982) [b]calculated from Henderson–Hasselbach equation (see text) [c]Wildsmith (1986) [d]Tucker and Mather (1979), and Arthur *et al.* (1979).)

α-1 acid glycoprotein, which has high affinity but low capacity, and albumin, which has low affinity but high capacity. The binding is a simple reversible one and tends to increase in proportion to the number of side chains of the molecule; for example, lignocaine 64 per cent binding compared with bupivacaine 96 per cent. In general the degree of protein binding is related to the duration of action of the local anaesthetic. This is because the bound portion acts as a reservoir from which free drug can be released in order to replace that which has left the site either due to diffusion or metabolism. Thus, we may compare the duration of action of lignocaine (plain), which is 15 to 45 minutes, with that of bupivacaine (plain), which is six hours. However, it should be noted that other factors may alter this relationship. Thus, prilocaine is less protein-bound (50 per cent) than lignocaine (64 per cent) and yet has a longer duration of action because it does not have the vasodilator action of lignocaine, and this more than compensates for its physico-chemical disadvantages (Wildsmith 1986).

Relevance of chemical structure to clinical use

Local anaesthetics form one of the most important groups of drugs used by the dental practitioner, who should therefore have some general awareness of their chemical structure. There are also at least four special categories in which some knowledge of this structure is relevant to clinical use; these are now detailed.

Local anaesthetic activity of amines

Figure 7.1 (above) shows that although the chemical structures of those local anaesthetics in clinical use have general features in common, there is considerable variation between the different formulae. Many drugs in other groups that are amines also possess local anaesthetic activity—for example, mepyramine (H_1-blocker), atropine (antimuscarinic), pethidine (opioid), and quinidine (anti-arrhythmic). However, this action is not made use of clinically because, of course, these drugs have other actions as well, and some are irritant on injection into the tissues. Knowledge of this action explains some of their side effects, such as the numbing effect on the tongue produced by some antihistamines (H_1-blockers). Similarly, it accounts for the fact that the inadvertent intravenous administration of a sufficiently large dose of an H_1-blocker may interfere with the normal conduction processes within the heart (see Chapter 15).

Biotransformation of local anaesthetics

The presence or absence of an esteratic link in the intermediate chain determines whether or not a compound is susceptible to attack by the cholinesterase group of enzymes. Thus, the ester link in procaine is susceptible to the ubiquitous pseudocholinesterase (plasma esterases), and this is an important reason why procaine is rapidly inactivated after injection (see later). By contrast, the amide link in lignocaine can only be broken by amidases located in the liver, so accounting in part for the longer systemic half-life of this drug (see Table 7.1 above).

Hypersensitivity

Drug allergy due to a local anaesthetic is obviously important, and the main features and underlying mechanism of it are dealt with in Chapter 21. In this context, a direct consequence of chemical structure is that if a patient is known to be hypersensitive to a certain local anaesthetic with a formula based on p-aminobenzoic acid (e.g. procaine) it is almost certain that they will show cross-hypersensitivity to any other local anaesthetic based on that acid (e.g. amethocaine). On the other hand, they might well not show cross-hypersensitivity to lignocaine or prilocaine because these compounds are not derivatives of p-aminobenzoic acid (see Fig. 7.1). Nevertheless, it would be unwise to make this assumption in the absence of specific tests for hypersensitivity to lignocaine or prilocaine, tests that are not without their own risks and should be carried out by a specialist in this field.

Drug interactions

Local anaesthetics that are derivatives of p-aminobenzoic acid (e.g. procaine and amethocaine) can under certain conditions interfere with the bacteriostatic action of sulphonamides (see Chapter 10). This is because sulphonamides act as competitive antagonists to p-aminobenzoic acid, which is normally an essential growth factor for micro-organisms sensitive to the sulphonamide group of drugs. The presence of these local anaesthetics during sulphonamide therapy would make available p-aminobenzoic acid and so redress the balance in favour of the bacteria. In practice, however, as Laurence and Bennett (1987) have pointed out: '. . . with wounds, or when local anaesthesia is being used for lumbar puncture or other exploration in sulphonamide-treated patients, local sulphonamide antagonism followed by infection is a theoretical risk.' It is noteworthy that local anaesthetics with no p-aminobenzoic acid moiety (e.g. lignocaine, prilocaine) do not antagnoize sulphonamides.

PHARMACOLOGICAL ACTIONS OF LOCAL ANAESTHETICS

These may be listed as follows:

(1) reversible block of conduction in nerve endings and nerve trunks;

(2) muscle: (i) direct relaxation of smooth muscle (e.g. vasodilatation via vascular smooth muscle; (ii) interference with neuromuscular transmission (i.e. in skeletal muscle)—usually not clinically significant;

(3) quinidine-like action on the heart (see Chapter 15);

(4) stimulation and/or depression of the CNS.

These apparently different actions of local anaesthetics are due largely, if not entirely, to a common mechanism of action on excitable cell membranes, as is now described.

Nerve conduction and the mechanism of action of local anaesthetics

The conduction of a nerve impulse along a nerve fibre depends critically upon the movement of certain ions across the nerve cell membrane. In the resting state (i.e. in the absence of a nerve impulse) this membrane is permeable to potassium ions but only very slightly permeable to sodium ions (Fig. 7.2); the result is a difference of electrical potential, such that the inside of the nerve cell is approximately 80 millivolts negative to the outside. The intracellular concentration of sodium ions is normally kept low by means of an active extrusion process known as the sodium pump. During conduction of a nerve impulse, sodium permeability transiently increases by several hundred times and, as the concentration of sodium ions outside the nerve cell is more than ten times that inside the fibre (i.e. there is a concentration gradient of sodium ions from outside to inside the cell), these ions diffuse rapidly into the cell. As a result, there is a temporary reversal of electrical polarity across the cell membrane (Fig. 7.2), and this permits an outflow of potassium ions down their concentration gradient (which is opposite to that of sodium, i.e. from within to without the cell). The outward movement of potassium ions brings about a repolarization during which a short-lived hyperpolarization (i.e. reversal or overshoot) occurs (Fig. 7.2b). The sodium pump, which is temporarily overwhelmed during the momentary inward rush of sodium ions, then extrudes the excess of sodium ions and this is accompanied by a re-entry of potassium ions with recovery of the membrane potential to the resting value (Fig. 7.2c). Those who elucidated these mechanisms (see, for example, Hodgkin and Huxley 1945) have shown that if these ionic movements are prevented, especially the inward entry of sodium ions, then nerve conduction no longer takes place.

There is much evidence to support the contention that local anaesthetics prevent the inward entry of sodium ions, which is essential for normal impulse transmission. As a result they prevent the generation and conduction of action potentials. Voltage clamp experiments, and other studies using radioactive neurotoxins and antibodies, have revealed the presence of sodium channels with several sites at which local anaesthetics could interfere with the normal changes in sodium permeability (Hille et al. 1975; Cahalan and Almers 1979). Thus blocking agents may act at specific receptor sites on the external or internal part of the sodium channels located in the nerve cell membrane. The biotoxins, tetrodotoxin and saxitoxin, are both potent local anaesthetics; they bind to a

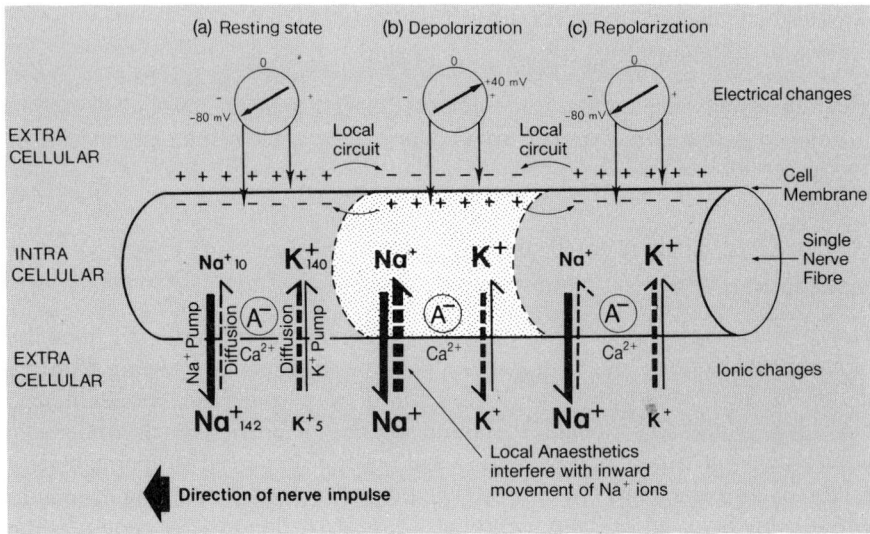

Fig. 7.2. Diagram of a single nerve fibre to illustrate the electrical (upper surface) and ionic (lower surface) changes that occur during the conduction of a nerve impulse (central shaded area) passing in the direction from right to left (i.e. (c) to (a). (a) Resting state: the extracellular concentration of sodium ions (Na$^+$) greatly exceeds the intracellular concentration, whilst the opposite is true for potassium ions (K$^+$). (Indicated by relative size of symbols; the actual amounts in mmol/l are also shown). Active transport of ions is indicated by continuous arrows ($\rightarrow$) and diffusion by broken arrows (--$\rightarrow$). The presence of intracellular indiffusible and negatively charged protein anions (A$^-$) and extracellular calcium ions (Ca^{2+}), which are essential components, is also shown. (b) Depolarization: the reversal of membrane polarity caused by the transient inward rush of Na$^+$ is followed by the outward movement of K$^+$. (c) Repolarization: the sodium pump extrudes the excess of intracellular Na$^+$ and this is rapidly followed by the inward movement of K$^+$. The presence of local electrical circuits at the junctions between normal and depolarized segments of nerve are indicated by semicircular arrows. Local anaesthetics are believed to block nerve conduction by interfering with the inward movement of Na$^+$ which is essential for normal transmission. (This diagram is an oversimplification of a complicated process; for further details see text.)

receptor on the external aspect of the sodium channel and thereby block the pore. Unfortunately they are unsuitable for clinical use. By contrast, local anaesthetics in common clinical use act at receptors situated on the internal or intracellular aspect of the sodium channel. It also seems likely that local anaesthetics can alter the membrane structure of the nerve to distort and close the sodium channels. Thus, local anaesthetics probably act by both mechanisms.

Sodium channels

The available evidence suggests that the sodium channel involves at least two 'gates'. One of these is a barrier and is named an 'activation' or 'm' gate, whereas the other is an 'inactivation' or 'h' gate (see Fig. 7.3). The depolarization that occurs with the arrival of a nerve impulse opens the 'm' gate and sodium ions are

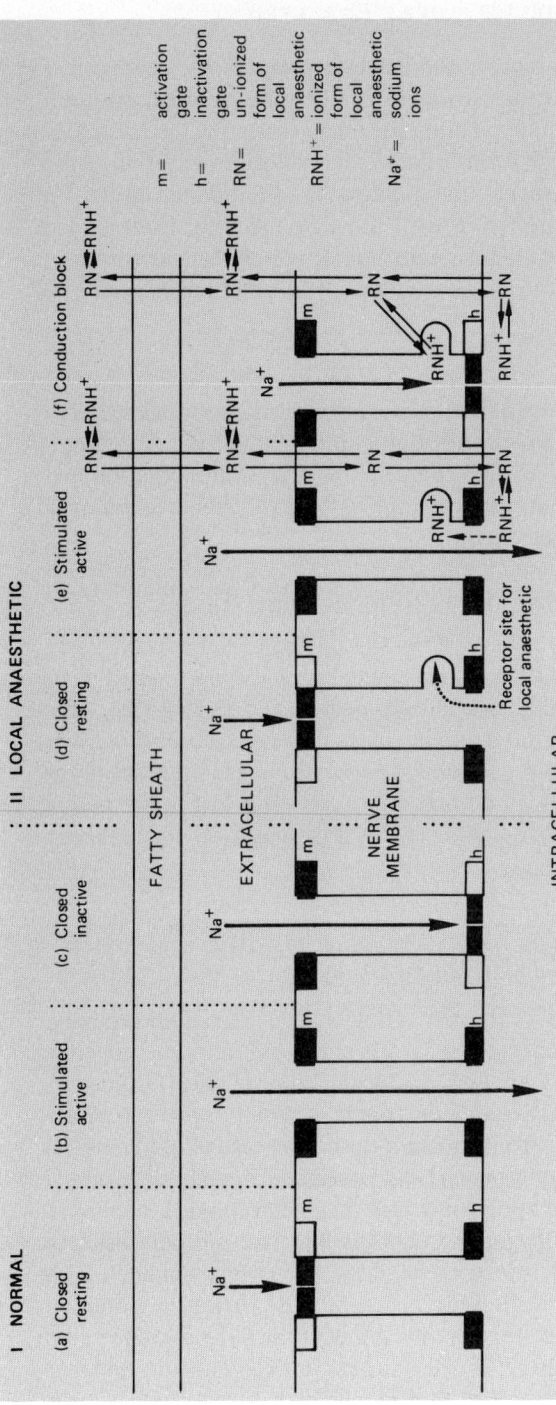

Fig. 7.3. Diagram to illustrate mechanism of action of a local anaesthetic. A section of nerve cell membrane is shown containing sodium channels with the m and h gates that control them. A length of accompanying fatty nerve sheath is also shown. I. NORMAL. The nerve cell membrane may be in one of three phases. (a) Closed resting: m closed, h open, sodium channel closed. (b) Stimulated active: m and h open, sodium channel open with inward movement of sodium ions. (c) Closed inactive: m open, h closed, sodium channel closed and remains so until full repolarization has taken place (thus accounting for refractory period). Note carefully that stages (a), (b), and (c) in this diagram correspond to stages (a), (b), and (c) in Fig. 7.2. II. LOCAL ANAESTHETIC. (d) Closed resting as in (a) but includes proposed receptor site for local anaesthetic which is linked to the h gate. (e) Local anesthetic has been applied outside the nerve sheath where it exists partly in the unionized (lipid soluble) form and partly in the ionized (lipid insoluble) form. The unionized form has diffused across the nerve sheath where it exists partly in the unionized (lipid soluble) form and partly in the ionized (lipid insoluble) form. The unionized form has diffused across the nerve sheath to the space beneath it and thence across the nerve membrane to the internal end of the sodium channel where it partially reionizes (according to the Henderson–Hasselbach equation: see text). The ionized moiety then enters the internal end of the sodium channel to occupy and activate the local anaesthetic receptor site which closes the h gate: the situation depicted in (e) is just prior to the closure of the h gate by the local anaesthetic. (f) The h gate has now been activated and the membrane is held in the closed inactive state as in (c). Note: it seems probable that when the h gate has been closed by the presence of local anaesthetic, the latter can continue to gain access to the receptor site by diffusing to it directly from within the nerve membrane, as indicated by the pair of diagonal arrows. RN represents unionized form of local anaesthetic, RNH$^+$ represents ionized form of local anaesthetic.)

able to move through the membranes, but this is soon stopped by the operation of the 'h' gate, which closes the channel. Once closed, it cannot re-open until full repolarization has taken place, thus explaining the phenomenon of the refractory period after excitation during which a nerve cannot be excited however large the stimulus. Local anaesthetics first traverse the sodium channel and then bind to an intracellular receptor, thereby interfering with the gate mechanism described above. They may also gain access by diffusing through the lipophilic membrane of the axon and then enter the intracellular opening of the sodium channel (see Fig. 7.3).

Role of calcium
An adequate extracellular concentration of calcium is essential for normal nerve transmission. Thus, reducing this concentration can potentiate the action of a local anaesthetic because both agents compete for the same phospholipid receptor. Nevertheless it seems clear that calcium is not involved in the primary nerve-blocking action of local anaesthetics.

Differential sensitivity of nerve fibres to local anaesthetics

As a general rule the susceptibility of nerve fibres to local anaesthetics is inversely proportional to their diameter, so that smaller nerve fibres are more sensitive to their blocking action than larger diameter fibres (Gasser and Erlanger 1929). This appears to be related to the greater susceptibility of smaller nerve fibres to sodium lack (Nathan and Sears 1962). As sensory information is carried by nerve fibres smaller than those that carry motor information, sensation is lost before motor activity is blocked. In general terms, pain is the first sensation to disappear followed by temperature, touch, and pressure.

Measurement of local anaesthetic activity

There are many different methods for the estimation of local anaesthetic activity, which include the measurement of variables such as minimal effective concentration, latency of onset of anaesthesia, or duration of effect. Unfortunately, there is no standard method available so that it is difficult or inappropriate to compare the results obtained from different tests. One particularly useful method by which the relative potency of two local anaesthetics can be determined in man is that devised by Mongar (1955). in which local anaesthetic is applied to an exposed area of dermis on the flexor aspect of the forearm. A modification of this method, using intradermal injections of drug or placebo (saline), also produces informative and useful results (see Fig. 7.4, p. 124). However, it must be appreciated that results obtained by this method are not directly applicable to the use of local anaesthetics in dentistry; in this context, an elegant and relevant method is that of Bjorn (1946), in which local anaesthetics are tested on teeth subjected to electrical stimulation.

FATE AND METABOLISM OF LOCAL ANAESTHETICS

Local anaesthetics are not absorbed from intact skin but many of them, when applied to mucous membranes (or *damaged* skin), or injected into tissues, are absorbed into the blood stream. The rate at which absorption takes place depends principally upon:

(1) the particular drug and its concentration;

(2) the vascularity of the tissues, the rate of absorption being faster the more vascular the part;

(3) whether or not a vasoconstrictor drug has been added in order to prolong the action of the local anaesthetic (discussed later).

All local anaesthetics undergo metabolism in the liver to inactive metabolites. In addition, as we have seen, those which contain an ester link in their chemical structure are also broken down by plasma cholinesterase (pseudocholinesterase) so that procaine is split into its constituents namely, *p*-aminobenzoic acid (sometimes abbrev. PABA) and diethylaminoethanol (see Fig. 7.1). Kalow (1952) and Brodie *et al.* (1948) have shown that procaine is broken down by this enzyme at about 20 mg per minute. Amethocaine, which also contains an ester linkage, is hydrolysed by plasma cholinesterase at about one quarter the rate of procaine. By contrast, lignocaine and prilocaine contain amide and not ester linkages and so are not susceptible to plasma cholinesterase; these molecules are split by amidases in the liver.

Thus, there are two ways in which the liver is of importance in the metabolism of local anaesthetics: (i) it is the major site of metabolism of many of them, and (ii) it is the source of plasma cholinesterase, which is important in the metabolism of those that contain an ester linkage. For these reasons, a normal dose of local anaesthetic given to a patient suffering from impaired liver function could result in relative overdosage (see Chapter 21).

THE PROPERTIES OF THE 'IDEAL' LOCAL ANAESTHETIC

Although no such compound exists, consideration of these properties is a convenient way to highlight the advantages and disadvantages of those local anaesthetics that are available for clinical use. It also leads us into the discussion of some of the important problems associated with the unwanted effects of this group of drugs.

The 'ideal' local anaesthetic should have the following properties:

1. The drug should exert a specific and fully reversible paralytic action on nerves and nerve endings in concentrations that do not injure or irritate the tissues. Surprisingly, there is no standard method to compare the potency of local

anaesthetics. As noted earlier, methods for undertaking this in man are those devised by Bjorn (1946) and Mongar (1955).

2. The drug should produce rapid onset of anaesthesia without preliminary excitation. One of the disadvantages of cinchocaine is that local anaesthesia takes from five to ten minutes to develop, whereas with lignocaine the onset of action is very rapid (see Table 7.2 below).

3. The drug should be soluble, chemically stable, and capable of sterilization by heat. Whereas cocaine is unstable when heated, lignocaine is very stable and can be sterilized by this means.

4. The drug should have penetrating properties so that it can be used for topical anaesthesia. In this respect, procaine is useless whereas lignocaine is effective.

5. The drug should have a high safety margin or therapeutic ratio. As discussed in Chapter 1, the therapeutic ratio is commonly expressed as:

$$\frac{LD_{50}}{ED_{50}}$$

where LD_{50} = dose that kills 50 per cent of a group of animals; ED_{50} = dose that produces a desired effect in 50 per cent of a group of animals.
The higher the value of this ratio, the greater the safety margin, i.e. the less toxic the drug. (The use of the term 'toxic(ity)' is in general undesirable; but in relation to testing the safety of a drug, particularly with reference to LD_{50} estimations in animals, the term 'toxicity' is established by long usage.)

Unfortunately, for local anaesthetics the problem of drug safety is more complex than hitherto realized and many of the data recorded in the literature are of doubtful clinical relevance. This is because most of the testing of local anaesthetics has been carried out by administering them to animals by the subcutaneous route. In *clinical practice*, the chief danger is inadvertent *intravenous* administration and, as Weatherby (1964) has pointed out, the '. . . maximal potential hazard associated with the use of an anaesthetic can therefore be expressed most accurately in terms of the LD_{50} obtained by *rapid intravenous injection*. With rapid intravenous injection, sufficient time is not available for the elimination of an appreciable fraction of the dose, and susceptible structures are exposed to the maximal concentration almost immediately.'

Ideally, estimates of potency should be performed on man although, at the present time, initial measurements must be done by means of animal tests. Purely objective tests on the isolated sciatic nerve of the frog can be carried out using complicated electronic stimulating and recording apparatus, as described by Rud (1961). On the other hand, available tests in man depend upon subjective assessment and utilize experimentally induced pain, which is vastly different from that of pathological origin. Thus, the measurement of therapeutic ratios for local anaesthetics is at present a compromise; in Table 7.2 below, these ratios for the drugs listed have been calculated using acute IV LD_{50} values in the rabbit and relative potencies obtained from isolated frog sciatic-nerve experiments (data from Truant and Takman 1965). On the basis of these calculations, procaine has the highest therapeutic ratio, followed (in descending order) by mepivacaine, prilocaine, lignocaine, cocaine, amethocaine, and bupivacaine.

6. When necessary, the drug should allow combination with a vasoconstrictor agent. The reasons usually given for the desirability of adding such an agent are threefold:

(i) in order to prolong the duration of local anaesthesia by delaying absorption of the drug into the general circulation;

(ii) in order to reduce the risk of an unwanted effect by reducing the rate of absorption of the drug into the general circulation;

(iii) in order to produce a relatively bloodless field to facilitate surgery.

It seems clear that the addition of a vasoconstrictor achieves number (i) of these listed objectives; Fig. 7.4 shows the results of a class experiment in which the time course of the local anaesthetic effect produced by procaine in the presence and absence of adrenaline was compared using Mongar's method (Mongar 1955). From common experience it is known that objective number (iii) is also attained, but the results of experiments in animals suggest that the objective number (ii) may not always be achieved with all local anaesthetics. Thus, when Avant and Weatherby (1960) compared the effect of the presence and absence of adrenaline on the LD_{50} values of five local anaesthetics, they found that only with amethocaine was the addition of a vasoconstrictor accompanied by a highly significant reduction in toxicity; with the four other compounds there was no appreciable difference, whilst procaine containing adrenaline 1:50 000 appeared more toxic than procaine alone. The trend toward a reduction in the amount of vasoconstrictor added without loss of effect (Gangarosa and Halik 1967), coupled with Avant and Weatherby's findings, make it important to ensure that the amount of vasoconstrictor added to any local anaesthetic is the minimum required.

In this context it should be noted, as pointed out by Cawson (1984), that mere psychological stress can raise plasma catecholamine levels by a factor of from five to ten (Dimsdale and Moss 1980), which is greater than that resulting from the use of a local anaesthetic with added vasoconstrictor.

UNWANTED EFFECTS OF LOCAL ANAESTHETICS

From time to time, the administration of a local anaesthetic is followed by some unfavourable response of the patient (see, for examples, Cawson et al. 1983). It appears that the majority of adverse reactions are due to inadvertent overdosage rather than to other causes (Moore and Bridenbaugh 1960). In such an event, it is important for the dental practitioner to have available a plan that will enable the possible causes and treatment of an adverse reaction to be considered quickly.

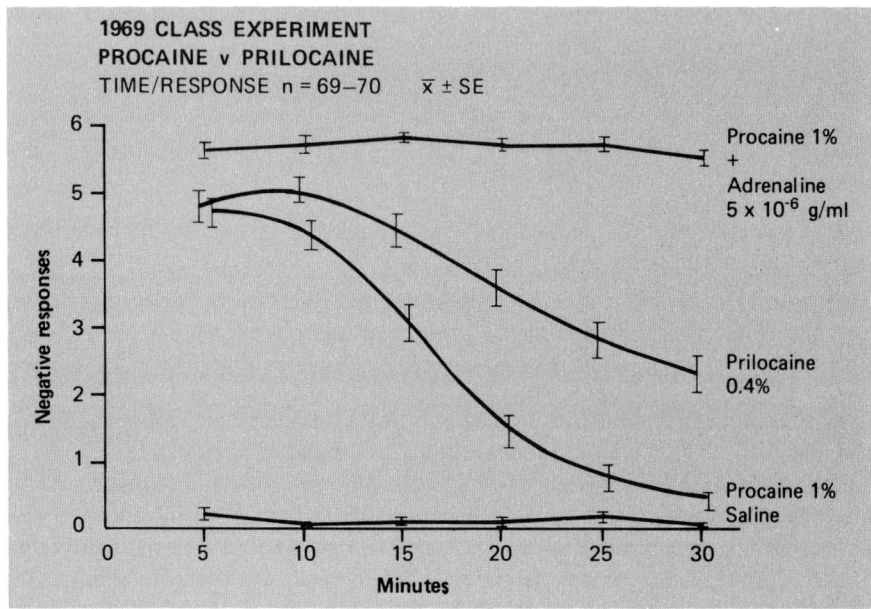

Fig. 7.4. Graph comparing the duration of local anaesthesia obtained with intradermal injections of procaine 1 per cent, procaine 1 per cent with adrenaline 5×10^{-6} g/ml ($= 1:200\,000$), prilocaine (Citanest) 0.4 per cent and physiological saline solution, using the method of Mongar (1955). The figures plotted are the mean results $\bar{x}$ ($\pm$ standard error) obtained by 69–70 medical students during a class experiment in pharmacology. The experiment was designed as a 'double-blind' trial and the intradermal weals containing the four different doses were made in a random order to allow for differences in sensitivity along the flexor surface of the forearm. Each weal was tested for anaesthesia by pricking with a pin six times in different parts of the weal, using a standardized stimulus. The test was repeated every five minutes for half an hour and the total number of pricks not felt gave a measure of anaesthetic activity. The highly significant potentiation of the duration of action of procaine by the addition of adrenaline is shown. The longer duration of action of prilocaine 0.4 per cent compared with procaine 1 per cent is also illustrated; the saline control produced a trivial effect.

The first important decision to be made is whether the unwanted effect is due to the local anaesthetic or to some other factor. The second decision concerns the institution of the correct treatment.

The following classification is based on that of Sadove *et al.* (1952); its correspondence with the Type A/B classification (Rawlins and Thompson 1985) is indicated.

I. Unwanted effects that are due to the local anaesthetic agent

    (1) In normal individuals (Type A reactions):

        A. *Central nervous system*

            (i) Stimulation   (a) Cerebral cortex

    (ii) Depression   (b) Medulla

          (i) respiratory centre;

          (ii) vasomotor centre;

         (iii) others.

B. *Cardiovascular system*

    (i) Direct action on the heart

   (ii) Action on the vascular bed

(2) In intolerant individuals: effects include those in (1) above that follow a standard (or even sub-standard) dose.

(3) In abnormal individuals (Type B reactions):

    (i) hypersensitivity (drug allergy);

   (ii) idiosyncrasy.

II. Unwanted effects that are *not* due to the local anaesthetic

    (i) psychomotor;

   (ii) vasopressor (Type A).

Each of these problems will now be discussed in the format given in the list above.

Unwanted effects that are due to the local anaesthetic

In normal individuals (Type A reactions)

Central nervous system

All local anaesthetics are potential central stimulants (possibly through interference with central inhibitory mechanisms) and may produce apprehension, confusion, excitement, or frank euphoria. The patient may complain of giddiness, tinnitus, a metallic taste in the mouth, headache, nausea, and sometimes a feeling of coldness (Horton 1966). This stage may be followed by muscle twitchings and convulsions, the latter severe enough to require intravenous thiopentone to control them, administered as increments of 50 mg in 2.5 per cent solution (Horton 1966). Alternatively, midazolam (2.5–7 mg) can be given intravenously or 5 mg intramuscularly; if necessary, a further dose can be given half to one hour later.

Initial central stimulation may be followed by central depression, which leads to a fall in blood pressure with consequent loss of consciousness and respiratory depression. If this occurs it will be necessary to start artificial respiration. Occasionally the excitatory onset is absent and the clinical picture begins with sudden collapse due to depression of the respiratory, vasomotor, and other centres in the brain. In any collapse, the patient should be laid flat (on the floor if necessary), ideally with the head down, and steps should be taken to ensure that artificial respiration and cardiac massage can be instituted if needed. As pointed out by Moore and Bridenbaugh (1960), oxygen is the most important factor in the treatment of this emergency.

Although large doses of local anaesthetics are contra-indicated in epileptics, the relatively small amounts used in most dental procedures would seem to carry little risk of provoking a fit (E. A. Cooper, personal communication).

Cardiovascular system

If a dose of local anaesthetic is administered intravenously by accident it may cause cardiac arrest due to the direct depressant action of the drug on the heart and, in particular. on its conduction system. If this occurs it is vital to give external cardiac massage combined with artificial respiration immediately. On the other hand, the quantity of local anaesthetic inadvertently injected into a vein may instead be distributed in the body so that its effects are exerted mainly on the peripheral vasculature. When this happens, the clinical picture will be one of peripheral vascular collapse, which may require the administration of vasopressor drugs to restore the blood pressure.

In abnormal individuals (Type B)

Hypersensitivity

In certain individuals, the administration of a local anaesthetic is followed rapidly by anaphylactic shock or, after a latency of minutes or hours, by asthma, rhinitis, angio(neurotic) oedema, or urticaria. These responses are due to hypersensitivity and are the result of an antigen–antibody reaction in which the offending local anaesthetic has acted as a hapten (for details see Chapter 21). The majority of hypersensitivity reactions to local anaesthetics have been produced by procaine, or by a drug chemically related to procaine in which the acidic group is p-aminobenzoic acid (Hanauer 1955). By contrast, lignocaine, which is widely used, appears to be remarkably safe; one case of an anaphylactic reaction to lignocaine has been reported by Holti and Hood (1965), whose paper contains three references to other cases of suspected hypersensitivity to this drug (Noble and Pierce 1961; Kirkler 1962; Gregg et al. 1963). (See also a reference quoted by Trimble 1962). An unusual hyperpigmentation caused by lignocaine has been reported by Curley et al. (1987).

As discussed above, if a patient is found to be sensitive to one local anaesthetic, for example procaine, it is highly probable that they will exhibit cross-hypersensitivity to others that are chemically related to the offending one. On the other hand, it is less likely that they will be hypersensitive to any chemically unrelated local anaesthetic, such as, in this example, lignocaine, although it will be necessary to arrange for special sensitivity tests to be performed (by an expert).

In spite of the foregoing comments it should be noted that with those local anaesthetics in common use in dentistry, the incidence of allergy as a cause of adverse effects is very low (Cawson et al. 1983). The subject of local anaesthetics and allergic reactions is reviewed by Giovannitti and Bennett (1979), and by Reynolds (1987), to whom the reader is referred for further details.

In dentists and others, contact dermatitis due to application of ointments containing local anaesthetics or due to constant handling of these drugs may occur. Contact dermatitis is an example of delayed-type hypersensitivity (see Chapter 21); the use of ointments and creams containing local anaesthetics always carries risk of this hazard and these preparations should therefore be avoided wherever possible (see later).

Intolerance

For any given drug the population contains a very small minority of individuals whose response to the standard dose is exaggerated (see Chapter 21). Thus, if a very small dose of local anaesthetic is followed by one (or more) of the central nervous-system and/or cardiovascular responses classified under IA or IB in the list above (and is clearly not due to hypersensitivity or idiosyncrasy), it is most probably due to intolerance.

Idiosyncrasy

This unwanted effect comprises very rare reactions of a bizarre nature that cannot be explained by any of the other known mechanisms. When such an event occurs with a local anaesthetic containing an ester link, it is worthwhile considering the possibility that the patient's plasma may contain an atypical pseudocholinesterase, such as would also be revealed by an idiosyncratic response to suxamethonium (Downs 1966; see also p. 413).

Unwanted effects *not* due to the local anaesthetic

Psychomotor

This group includes effects in patients who faint at the sight of a needle, or whose psychological reaction is abnormal and may take the form of hysterical behaviour. This situation calls for sympathetic but firm handling; difficult cases may require appropriate sedation (see Chapter 8).

Vasopressor

The addition of vasoconstrictor substances, such as adrenaline or other sympathomimetic amines, to local anaesthetic solutions may produce local or general unwanted effects (see also earlier).

Local adverse effects include a change from initial vasoconstriction with pallor to local cyanosis accompanied by a local reduction in oxygen tension (Klingenstrom and Westermark 1964). This state of affairs can be followed by a reactive hyperaemia, which may increase the risk of postoperative bleeding.

General adverse effects of adrenaline in the concentrations and amounts used in dentistry do not commonly occur, although it should be noted that entry of adrenaline from local anaesthetic solutions into the circulation is known to be rapid (Tolas *et al.* 1982). However, if the solution is injected inadvertently into a vein, or undergoes rapid absorption, adverse effects could include tachycardia (interpreted by the patient as palpitations), apprehension, and a rise of blood pressure that may be dangerous in subjects with cardiovascular disease; these effects may also occur with other sympathomimetic amines. It is thus essential that all local anaesthetic administration in dentistry should be with an aspirating technique. It is just conceivable that in an exceptional case of adverse reaction to adrenaline, specific therapy in the form of an adrenergic α-receptor blocking drug, e.g. phentolamine, might be needed (see Chapters 13 to 15); under these circumstances medical aid should be sought immediately.

Recently it has been shown that adrenaline in amounts commonly injected with local anaesthetic during dental anaesthesia reduces plasma potassium concentrations within 10 minutes (Meechan and Rawlins 1987). Although this is unlikely to be a hazard in healthy individuals, it might predispose to cardiac arrhythmias in patients with incipient hypokalaemia caused by prolonged medication with potassium-losing diuretics (see Chapter 15).

SPECIFIC LOCAL ANAESTHETICS: 1. ESTER TYPE

(Throughout see Fig. 7.1 above for chemistry; see Table 7.2 for details of preparations including doses.)

Cocaine

In addition to being a local anaesthetic, this alkaloid, which is obtained from the leaves of the coca plant (*Coca erythroxolon*), has sympathomimetic properties, and also powerful stimulant actions on the central nervous system including the ability to induce psychic dependence. Consequently, cocaine is too dangerous to use by injection but, in special circumstances, can be employed topically, for example in dental apicectomies. Its sympathomimetic properties, at one time thought to be due to inhibition of amine oxidase, are now known to be due to its ability to block the uptake by the amine pump of noradrenaline released from adrenergic nerve endings (see Chapter 13). The use of cocaine is now restricted to topical application. The smallest effective dose should be used and never in higher concentration than 10 per cent. It is metabolized in the liver and also by plasma esterases, the plasma route being probably the more important in man (Van Dyke *et al.* 1976).

Procaine

Until the advent of lignocaine, procaine was for 50 years the nearest to the 'ideal' local anaesthetic. The fact that it is rapidly metabolized by the readily available plasma esterases is no doubt an important factor in its safety. However, this drug is useless topically and, as it is an active vasodilator, it is essential to add vasoconstrictor agents to solutions for injection. Although it is certainly one of the safest local anaesthetics, it may produce adverse reactions, including death, in patients hypersensitive to it (Criep and Ribeiro 1953). An additional hazard for the dental practitioner is contact dermatitis (see above). These disadvantages, coupled with the availability of better agents, mean that procaine is now used rarely in dentistry, and only occasionally for very special reasons in medicine.

Amethocaine

This local anaesthetic was first synthesized by O. Eisleb in Germany in 1928. It is the most potent (9.5 times the potency of lignocaine) of the ester type to be used clinically. It is rather unstable to heat and inactivated by alkalis. Amethocaine is an excellent topical anaesthetic although its onset of action is slow. As better and safer local anaesthetics (of the amide type; see below) are available, it is rarely used in dentistry and then only by topical application, such as to anaesthetize the gum prior to injection of another local anaesthetic.

Pharmacokinetics

Amethocaine is hydrolysed by plasma cholinesterase but about four times more slowly than procaine (see earlier 'Fate and metabolism of local anaesthetics'). Although its rate of onset is slow it is rapidly absorbed from mucous membrane because of its very high lipid solubility, as shown by a partition coefficient of 80 (see Table 7.1).

Unwanted effects

Amethocaine is particularly liable to produce the unwanted effects that characterize local anaesthetics as a group, including hypersensitivity. For this reason it is only occasionally used in dentistry (see above).

Benzocaine

Unlike all other local anaesthetics used in dentistry, benzocaine does not contain the hydrophilic amine group common to the others (see Fig. 7.1). It is therefore unable to ionize (at a physiological pH) and, as a consequence, can neither form water soluble salts nor be used for injection. It is thus restricted to topical use. Its inability to ionize raises the question as to how it acts as a local anaesthetic. The answer is that it diffuses directly across the nerve cell membrane and gains access to the gating mechanism of the sodium channel via the lipid component (i.e. without passing through the sodium channel as do the ionized anaesthetics; see Fig. 7.3). It has limited use in dentistry (see Table 7.2).

Table 7.2. Some local anaesthetics used in dentistry

Chemical class	Chemical Name (and synonyms)	(a) Relative potency (isolated nerve)	(b) Relative toxicity IV LD$_{50}$ rabbit	(a/b) Therapeutic ratio	Preparations type	Preparations Description	Contents Local anaesthetic	vasoconstrictor (if present)	Onset of action min	Duration of action	Maximum 'safe' dose mg	Indications	Comments (stability refers to plain local anaesthetic unless stated otherwise)
Ester type	Cocaine HCl	2.5	1.5	0.6	Topical only	Cocaine hydrochloride 10%	Cocaine HC1 10%	—	rapid	1 h	100	Applied to floor of nose to facilitate supraperiosteal injections in maxillary incisor region.	Decomposes on boiling. Stimulates CNS and causes vasoconstriction and mydriasis. Dependence. Restricted to topical use due to toxicity.
	Procaine HCl	0.26	0.47	1.8	Injection only	Procaine and adrenaline injection	Procaine HCl 2%	Adrenaline acid tartrate 1:50,000	2-5	1 h	500	Seldom used now, but may be useful for patient hypersensitive to anilide derivatives, e.g. lignocaine.	Moderately heat stable. Active vasodilator therefore added vasoconstrictor essential. Useless topically. Sulphonamide antagonism a theoretical risk.
	Benzocaine		insoluble		Topical only	Benzocaine lozenges DPF / Benzocaine compound lozenges BPC	Benzocaine 10 mg / Benzocaine 100 mg + menthol 3 mg	— / —	rapid	duration of contact	—	To help patients otherwise unable to tolerate an impression or new dentures. Occasionally to relieve pain of severe ulceration.	Insoluble. Stable, but protect from light.
Amide type	Lignocaine HCl (lidocaine)	1.0	1.0	1.0	Injection	Xylocaine 2% plain	Lignocaine HCl 2%	—	1-2	15-45 min	200	Indicated when use of adrenaline dangerous, e.g. patients with severe cardiovascular disease or uncontrolled hyperthyroidism. More usual alternative prilocaine with felypressin (see below).	
						Xylocaine 2% with adrenaline	ditto	Adrenaline Acid tartrate 1:80,000	1-2 infiltration	2-4 h	500	Most commonly used local anaesthetic solutions	WARNING (see below)
						Xylocaine 2% with noradrenaline (all three preparations available in 2 ml cartridges)	ditto	l-noradrenaline* 1:- 80,000	4-5 nerve block	2-4 hr	500		
						Xylocaine spray	lignocaine 10 mg per spray dose	—	0.25	25-30 min	200 (=20 spray-doses)	Useful topical preparations.	
					Topical	Xylodase (a cream)	lignocaine 5% hyaluronidase 0.015%	—	1-2	25-30 min	200 (=4 g cream)		

Drug				Form	Preparation	Local anaesthetic	Vasoconstrictor	No.	Duration	Max dose	Indications	Comments
Prilocaine hydrochloride (Citanest)	0.65	0.77	1.18	Injection	Citanest 4% plain (2 ml cartridge)	Prilocaine	—	1	30 min	400	For use when adrenaline or noradrenaline contra-indicated, e.g. patients with cardiovascular disease, hyperthyroidism. Note: In doses higher than those recommended, prilocaine causes cyanosis due to methaemoglobinaemia. In a healthy patient this is usually of little account, but in one unable to compensate for reduced oxygen-carrying capacity, e.g. anaemia, it would be prudent to choose an alternative drug.	Stable and heat-resistant. Solutions with vasoconstrictors are stable for 2 years if stored away from light and at a temperature not exceeding 15°C (to preserve vasoconstrictor). Methaemoglobinaemia due to prilocaine can be prevented or reversed with the aid of the reducing agent, methylene blue, 1 mg/kg IV
					Citanest 3% + Octapressin 0.03 I.U./ml (2 ml cartridge)	Prilocaine HCl 3%	felypressin 0.03 I.U./ml = 0.54 µg/ml (1 I.U. = 0.018 mg)	2–5	2.5 hr	600	For use when longer acting preparation required and when adrenaline contra-indicated, e.g. patients with cardiovascular disease, hyperthyroidism.	
Mepivacaine HCl	0.55	0.81	1.47	Injection	3% (1.8 ml cartridge)	Mepivacaine HCl 3%	—	1–2	Upper jaw 15–30 min lower jaw 30–40 min	400	Short-acting local anaesthetic	Stable and heat-resistant
Bupivacaine hydrochloride (Marcain)	4	7.8†	1.95	Injection	Marcain 0.25% 0.5%	Bupivacaine HCl 0.25% 0.5%	—	4	6 hr	2 mg/kg	Situations where there is likely to be immediate severe postoperative pain; reduces postoperative analgesic requirements.	Prolonged anaesthesia increases risk of trauma due to biting or hot drinks; some patients find prolonged dental anaesthesia unpleasant.
					0.25% 0.5%	Adrenaline acid tartrate 1:200,000 1:200,000 (=5 µg/ml)			6+ hr	2 mg/kg		

*The use of noradrenaline as an added vasoconstrictor to local anaesthetics is not advised because:
1. It is a very potent pressor agent and is potentially dangerous, especially in patients with cardiovascular disease
2. Adrenaline is normally satisfactory as an added vasoconstrictor and is much less potentially hazardous.
3. If it is essential to AVOID the administration of adrenaline then either
(i) a local anaesthetic without any added vasoconstrictor can be used or, alternatively
(ii) felypressin (Octapressin), a polypeptide vasoconstrictor (a derivative of vasopressin) can be used; a suitable preparation is Citanest 3% + Octapressin 0.03 i.u./ml.

†IV LD$_{50}$ mice (Reynolds 1987)

N.B. Measurement of strength of solutions: It is traditional, although illogical, to employ one system of units to measure the strength of a solution of local anaesthetic and another system to measure the strength of vasoconstrictor contained within the same solution! Nevertheless it is obviously important for every dental practitioner to be thoroughly familiar with this dual system.

1. The strength of a local anaesthetic solution is usually expressed as a *percentage concentration* so that, for example, a 2 per cent solution is one that contains 2 g of the particular local anaesthetic per 100 ml of solution.
2. The amount of vasoconstrictor added to a solution of local anaesthetic is expressed as a *dilution*. Thus a solution labelled 1:200 000 indicates that it contains 1 g of the particular vasoconstrictor dissolved in 200 000 ml of local anaesthetic solution. As this system indicates dilution it follows that a dilution of 1:400 000 is twice as dilute (half as concentrated) as a dilution of 1:200 000. Dilution values can be converted to concentration values (and vice versa) by using the following relationship:

$$\text{a dilution of } 1{:}y = \text{a concentration of } \frac{100}{y} \text{ mg/ml};$$

$$\text{conversely, a concentration of } x \text{ mg/ml} = \text{dilution of 1 g in } \frac{1000}{x}$$

In this Table the strength of vasoconstrictor has been expressed in both systems.

Pharmacokinetics

Benzocaine is hydrolysed very rapidly by plasma esterases to para-aminobenzoic acid, and this presumably accounts for its low toxicity.

Unwanted effects

The metabolite, para-aminobenzoic acid, is liable to act as a hapten and to cause allergic responses. Thus, of 887 patients with dermatitis or eczema patch tested with 5 per cent benzocaine in yellow soft paraffin, nearly 6 per cent gave a positive reaction (Rudzki and Kleniewska 1970). It is therefore particularly important for dentists to exercise great care so as not to come into skin contact with benzocaine (or any other local anaesthetic for that matter).

SPECIFIC LOCAL ANAESTHETICS: 2. AMIDE TYPE

Lignocaine (Xylocaine, Lidocaine)

Lignocaine (Löfgren 1948) was introduced in the early 1950s and soon replaced procaine, being more potent than it and also effective topically. According to which method of comparison is used, lignocaine is between one to four times as active as procaine for infiltration anaesthesia, and two to four times as active as procaine in nerve block (Wiedling 1964). Although lignocaine can be used without the addition of vasoconstrictor (plain), this is generally not very successful in producing dental anaesthesia. It may be used for minor surgical procedures but, again, adequate anaesthesia is unpredictable and it is better to use prilocaine with felypressin (see later) if adrenaline is thought to be contraindicated.

Lignocaine 2 per cent *with* adrenaline 1:80 000 ($=12.5$ μg/ml) is certainly the most useful local anaesthetic available for dentistry at the present time. In dental outpatients injected with lignocaine 2 per cent plus 1:100 000 adrenaline, the outcome was effective infiltration anaesthesia in 91 to 100 per cent of injections (Cowan 1968; Brown and Ward 1969; Epstein 1969; Chilton 1971). Other important properties of lignocaine are: (i) rapidity of onset of analgesia; (ii) useful duration of action when combined with adrenaline 1:80 000 (2–4 hours); and (iii) very low incidence of toxic effects.

Pharmacokinetics

Lignocaine is highly lipophilic (partition coefficient $= 3$; see Table 7.1) and so is rapidly absorbed. It undergoes virtually complete biotransformation in the liver and has a systemic $T_{0.5}$ of approximately 100 minutes. Figure 7.5 shows that lignocaine is subject to three metabolic transformations, namely oxidative-N-dealkylation, hydrolysis, and hydroxylation. Thus, it is first dealkylated to the monoethyl derivative, after which the amide link is broken by hydrolysis yielding

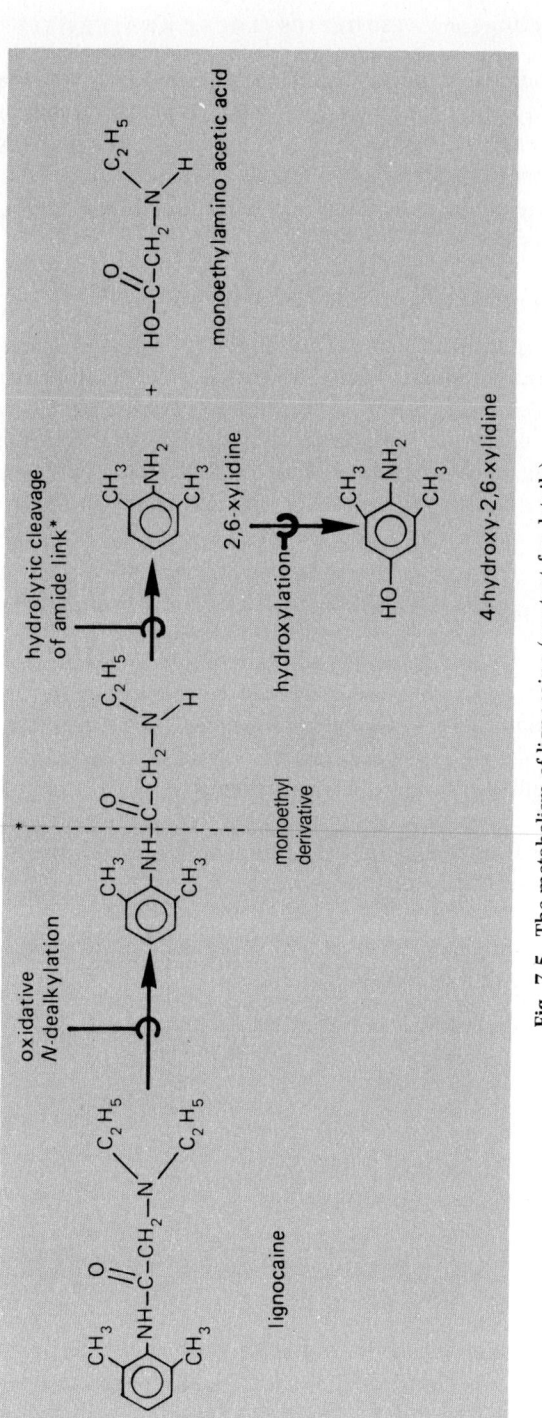

Fig. 7.5. The metabolism of lignocaine (see text for details).

2,6-dimethylxylidine and monoethyl aminoacetic acid. Finally, the dimethylxylidine undergoes hydroxylation to 4-hydroxy-2,6-dimethylxylidine. It seems that only the first metabolite (monoethyl aminoacetyl-2,6-xylidide) possesses local anaesthetic properties, and all of the metabolites have longer half-lives and are less toxic than the parent drug. Only negligible amounts of unchanged drug are excreted in the urine.

Unwanted effects

When used in the correct dosage and in the correct way, the toxicity of lignocaine is low. Nevertheless, adverse reactions involving the central nervous system or cardiovascular system can occur, as have been described earlier in this chapter. Allergy to lignocaine is also rare (Rood 1973; Cawson *et al.* 1983); it is most likely to occur following repeated application to the skin either in the form of a cream or ointment (allergy in the patient), or during recurrent careless handling by an operator (allergy in the dentist, doctor, etc.).

Prilocaine (Citanest, propitocaine)

This is a more recent and important addition to the range of local anaesthetics. It is equipotent with lignocaine and has the lowest toxicity of the amide drugs (see Table 7.2). A comparison made between prilocaine 3 per cent with adrenaline 1:300 000 and lignocaine 2 per cent with 1:80 000 adrenaline has shown that the drugs are similar although, two hours after injection, a higher proportion of the soft tissues had recovered from prilocaine anaesthesia (Goldman and Gray 1963). Thus, the shorter duration of action combined with the reduced amount of adrenaline required is a distinct advantage of prilocaine during the average dental session.

The following compares the duration of anaesthesia in soft tissue and dental pulp for lignocaine and prilocaine:

Preparation	Duration of anaesthesia (hours)	
	Soft tissue	Pulp
Lignocaine 2% + adrenaline 1:50 000	3 +	3/4
Prilocaine 3% + adrenaline 1:300 000	2 +	1/3
Prilocaine 3% + felypressin 0.03 IU/ml	2	1/2–3/4

Pharmacokinetics

Prilocaine has a similar profile to that of lignocaine, although it differs from it in several important ways that account for its lower toxicity. Thus it does not produce any vasodilatation (or vasoconstriction); it is distributed more rapidly and has a larger volume of distribution (see Chapter 1) than lignocaine; and its rate of clearance ($2.37 \, l \, min^{-1}$) is higher than that of all other amide local anaesthetics, suggesting (Tucker 1986) that it may undergo extensive extrahepatic metabolism (see Table 7.1), so resulting in relatively low blood concentrations. These reasons account for the maximum 'safe' dose of prilocaine (400 mg) being twice that of lignocaine.

In the liver, prilocaine is acted on by amidases (Geddes 1965), which cause hydrolytic cleavage of the molecule into α-propyl-aminopropionic acid and o-toluidine (Fig. 7.6), the latter then undergoing oxidation to nitrosotoluidine. The metabolite o-toluidine is capable of causing methaemoglobinaemia but this is only likely to be significant when more than 600 mg of prilocaine have been administered. It must be remembered that under normal circumstances methaemoglobin is being formed continuously during red cell metabolism but does not exceed about 1 per cent of the total haemoglobin. Cyanosis does not occur until more than 1.5 per cent of haemoglobin is present as methaemoglobin. If a dose of prilocaine sufficient to cause cyanosis is given, the condition is likely to disappear spontaneously within 24 hours and is not likely to be clinically significant, except in a patient who already suffers from anaemia or an impaired circulation (see next section; unwanted effects).

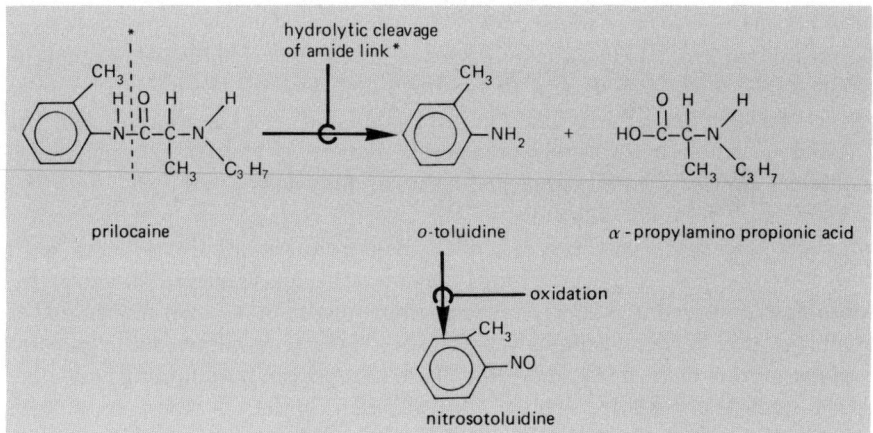

Fig. 7.6. The metabolism of prilocaine (see text for details).

Unwanted effects

Since its introduction, prilocaine appears to have been remarkably free from such effects, apart from occasional cyanosis (described above) due to mild methaemoglobinaemia, which usually occurs only with dosage above that recommended. This form of systemic toxicity is unique to prilocaine, is dosage-related and, as has been explained, is not directly due to the parent substance but to its metabolite, o-toluidine. Although cyanosis will occur in the presence of small amounts of methaemoglobinaemia. It seldom causes any embarrassment to the patient unless the oxygen-carrying capacity and/or the oxygen requirements are already compromised. When necessary the methaemoglobinaemia may be rapidly reversed by intravenous injection of methylene blue 1 mg/kg, the normal haemoglobin levels being restored in 15 to 20 minutes.

Problems associated with the use of adrenaline in local anaesthetic solutions

In the past, the need to add adrenaline to prilocaine, or indeed to any other local anaesthetic used in dentistry, was considered to be a disadvantage in treating patients already taking tricyclic antidepressants (see Chapter 14). There are theoretical reasons why an interaction might occur between adrenaline and tricyclic antidepressant but, in practice, this interaction has not occurred and it would therefore seem that the anticipated risk has been overestimated (Cawson *et al.* 1983). Nevertheless, it was not unreasonable to anticipate the possibility of such an interaction, particularly in view of the evidence obtained from experimental studies (Boakes *et al.* 1973). In passing, it should be said that it has been better to err on the side of caution rather than to ignore such evidence, as was the case for the dangerous interaction that can occur between monoamine oxidase inhibitors (MAOI) and the indirect-acting sympathomimetic amines, particularly tyramine, found in fermented foods, e.g. cheese (see Chapter 22). The MAOI interaction was entirely predictable and could have been prevented if available knowledge in this area had been carefully considered at the time.

The use of adrenaline in local anaesthetic solutions has been discussed above, where it was seen that there is little risk from its use in patients with cardiovascular problems if aspirating injection techniques are used. However, for those dental surgeons who have reservations about its use, an alternative is available; this is the synthetic vasopressor polypeptide known as felypressin (Octapressin), which is related chemically to vasopressin (antidiuretic hormone, ADH) from the posterior lobe of the pituitary gland. It differs only from vasopressin in that phenylalanine replaces the molecule of tyrosine normally located at position 2. When present in a final concentration of 0.03 IU/ml (1 IU = 0.018 mg), this vasoconstrictor, which is less potent than adrenaline, nevertheless resulted in a marginal increase in the duration of anaesthesia produced by prilocaine 3 per cent compared with the same strength of local anaesthetic combined with adrenaline 1:300 000 (Goldman and Evers 1969). These authors also observed that 0.03 IU/ml felypressin appeared to be an optimal concentration; lower and higher concentrations decreased the duration of pulpal analgesia, suggesting that vasoconstriction may not be the only factor in the prolongation of analgesic effect by this substance.

It should be noted that felypressin does not necessarily limit the level of prilocaine in the plasma (Cannell and Whelpton, 1986), and that it causes prolonged coronary vasoconstriction *in animals*, although the evidence for this in patients is controversial (see Cannel, 1983).

Mepivacaine (Carbocaine)

This drug resembles lignocaine pharmacologically but is distinguished from it chemically in that the hydrophilic end of the molecule consists of a ring structure (an N-methylated pyridine) instead of a diethyl amino group as in lignocaine (see Fig. 7.1). It is chemically stable, being resistant to acid and alkaline hydrolysis. It is not a vasodilator. It is a short-acting anaesthetic and is only available as a 3 per cent solution without vasoconstrictor. It does not appear to be widely used, and the interested reader should consult Mumford and Geddes (1961), and Goebel *et al.* (1980) for further information.

Pharmacokinetics

Mepivacaine, like lignocaine, is metabolized in the liver where the amide link is cleaved to yield pipecolylxylidine and monoethylamino acetic acid, with some unchanged drug excreted in the urine. However, unlike lignocaine, in neonates it is not metabolized but eliminated by the kidneys. In adults the maximum dose is 5 mg/kg or 400 mg.

Unwanted effects

It is claimed that mepivacaine is a little less toxic than lignocaine. One case of an acute anaphylactic reaction has been reported (Seskin 1978) following a mandibular block with mepivacaine 3 per cent without vasoconstrictor. As mepivacaine has a chemical structure similar to the other amide local anaesthetics, cross-hypersensitivity may be expected to occur.

Bupivacaine

Bupivacaine (0.25–0.5 per cent with or without adrenaline) is a long-acting local anaesthetic, similar in chemical structure to mepivacaine (see Fig. 7.1). It was introduced for use where prolonged local anaesthesia is required, such as in orthopaedic and accident work, and including epidural administration and intravenous regional analgesia. Thus, it was not originally designed for dental use but it has found a use in dentistry where there is likely to be immediate and severe postoperative pain, such as in patients undergoing removal of impacted third molars (Moore and Dunsky 1983; Wilson *et al.* 1986). Under these conditions it has been found valuable and, as a consequence of the prolonged analgesia, it reduces the need for postoperative analgesic medication. However, the disadvantage of such prolonged dental analgesia (six to eight hrs) is the risk of trauma, which occurs as a result of self-biting or the ingestion of hot drinks.

Furthermore, some patients find prolonged dental analgesia an unpleasant experience.

Pharmacokinetics

The major part of a dose of bupivacaine is metabolized in the liver where, after dealkylation and cleavage of the amide link, the metabolite, pipecolylxylidine, is excreted in the urine. Bupivacaine is absorbed into the systemic circulation from the site of injection more slowly than the shorter-acting amide local anaesthetics (lignocaine, prilocaine, and mepivacaine). An important factor here is the greater binding of this drug to plasma and tissue proteins (Tucker 1986).

Unwanted effects

The risk of an adverse reaction with bupivacaine does not appear to be any greater than with lignocaine, provided that it is given in the correct dosage and inadvertent intravenous injection is carefully avoided. The main experience with this drug is outside dentistry, where it has been found to have a wide therapeutic margin when used correctly (Reynolds 1987). Thus, primary ventricular fibrillation has developed after the injection of excessive amounts of bupivacaine into the general circulation (Covino 1984). As bupivacaine is chemically similar to lignocaine, prilocaine, and mepivacaine, there is likely to be cross-hypersensitivity between these agents.

INTRALIGAMENTARY INJECTION OF A LOCAL ANAESTHETIC SOLUTION

The periodontal ligament provides the attachment between the root surface and alveolar bone, and comprises a series of well-organized collagen bundles and a rich blood supply. The width of the ligament in health is 0.1 to 0.25 mm. The nerve supply to teeth must traverse the ligament to reach the apical foramen, and thus an injection of local anaesthetic solution into the ligament will anaesthetize the nerve supply to that tooth. This technique is known as intraligamentary anaesthesia and has been practiced by dental surgeons for many years. The recent introduction of high-pressure syringes with ultra-fine needles (Ligmaject and Peri-press) has renewed interest in this method of administering a local anaesthetic. The advantages and disadvantages of this technique are listed below:

Advantages

1. Rapid onset of anaesthesia (15–45 seconds).

2. Less of the local anaesthetic solution is administered when compared with conventional local anaesthesia. This reduces the risk of unwanted effects.

3. Lower teeth are anaesthetized without the need of an inferior dental nerve block, thereby reducing the risk of tongue and lip trauma. Hence, intraligamen-

tary anaesthesia may be especially useful in children. The technique also allows for bilateral anaesthesia of mandibular teeth, thus avoiding bilateral inferior-dental nerve block.

Disadvantages

1. The technique is destructive to the periodontal ligament and can cause resorption of the crestal bone (Walton and Garnick 1982). It is not advisable to use this technique in patients with periodontal disease.

2. Postoperative discomfort: the incidence of this is uncertain, and depends upon whether the injection was given for restorative procedures or tooth extraction (Jones 1981; Faulkner 1983). If intraligamentary anaesthesia is used for restorative procedures, the tooth may be tender to bite on for up to 24 hours. The injection may introduce infection into the periodontal ligament but the incidence of this can be reduced by swabbing the gingiva with 0.2 per cent chlorhexidine solution prior to injection.

3. It is reported that there is a higher incidence of dry socket (alveolar osteitis) after teeth have been extracted with intraligamentary anaesthesia than after conventional anaesthesia (J. G. Meechan, personal communication). This may be attributable to the direct action of the vasoconstrictor in inhibiting haemorrhage and thus the formation of the necessary blood clot in the socket.

Evidence now suggests that intraligamentary anaesthesia may be useful as an adjunct to conventional anaesthesia for restorative procedures. Its use in routine extractions is yet to be evaluated.

THE USE AND ABUSE OF TOPICALLY APPLIED LOCAL ANAESTHETICS

In dental practice, local anaesthetics can be applied topically in the form of solutions, aerosols, ointments, or lozenges (see Table 7.2). Thus, the use of a topical preparation to facilitate a subsequent injection of local anaesthetic is an example of a reasonable use of topical anaesthesia. However, this use should be restricted to a minimum because of the risks involved. These may be listed as follows:

1. Absorption of local anaesthetics from mucous membranes can be rapid and substantial. Adriani and Campbell (1956) measured blood levels of amethocaine in dogs: they found that a quantity of drug, which when injected subcutaneously failed to produce detectable blood levels, if applied topically produced blood levels similar to those achieved by one-third to one-half the same dose given intravenously. Thus the risk of producing unwanted effects due to overdosage may be considerable when local anaesthetics are applied topically.

2. Excessive use of topical preparations, particularly lozenges, may lead to a

dangerous degree of anaesthesia in the oropharynx with consequent inhalation of food into the respiratory tract during eating.

3. Prolonged use of topical preparations carries the risk of inducing hypersensitivity, with the development of severe swelling of the mouth. Subsequent exposure of the patient to the same or a chemically related local anaesthetic could lead to renewed hypersensitivity responses, including the possibility of anaphylactic shock.

4. The dental practitioner should take great care in handling topical preparations because of the risk of becoming hypersensitive to them, as described earlier.

REFERENCES

Adriani, J. and Campbell, D. (1956). Fatalities following topical application of local anaesthetics to mucous membranes. *Journal of the American Medical Association*, **162**, 1527–30.

Arthur, G. R., Scott, D. H. T., Boyes, R. N., and Scott, D. B. (1979). Pharmacokinetic and clinical pharmacological studies with mepivacaine and prilocaine. *British Journal of Anaesthesia*, **51**, 481–5.

Avant, W. E. and Weatherby, J. H. (1960). Effects of epinephrine on toxicities of several local anaesthetic agents. *Proceedings of the Society for Experimental Biology (N.Y.)*, **102**, 353–6.

Bjorn, H. (1946). Electrical excitation of teeth. *Svensk tandlakaretidskrift*, **39**, suppl.

Boakes, A. J., Laurence, D. R., Teoh, P. C., Barer, F. S. K., Benedikter, L. T., and Prichard, B. N. C. (1973). Interactions between sympathomimetic amines and antidepressant agents in man. *British Medical Journal*, i, 311–15.

Brodie, B. B., Lief, P. A., and Poet, R. (1948). Fate of procaine in man following its intravenous administration and methods for estimation of procaine and diethylaminoethanol. *J. Pharmacology and Experimental Therapeutics*, **94**, 359–66.

Brown, G. and Ward, N. L. (1969). Prilocaine and lignocaine plus adrenaline. A clinical comparison. *British Dental Journal*, **126**, 557–62.

Cahalan, M. D. and Almers, W. (1979). Interactions between quaternary lidocaine, the sodium channel gates and tetrodotoxin. *Biophysical Journal*, **27**, 39–56.

Cannell, H. (1983). The hazards of dental local anaesthetics. *British Dental Journal*, **155**, 6.

Cannell, H. and Whelpton, R. (1986). Systemic uptake of prilocaine after injection of various formulations of the drug. *British Dental Journal*, **160**, 47–9.

Cawson, R. A. (1984). Vasoconstrictor preference (letter). *Journal of the American Dental Association*, **109**, 542–3.

Cawson, R. A., Curson, I., and Whittington, D. R. (1983). The hazards of dental local anaesthetics. *British Dental Journal*, **154**, 253–8.

Chilton, N. W. (1971). Clinical evaluation of prilocaine hydrochloride 4 per cent solution with and without epinephrine. *Journal of the American Dental Association*, **83**, 149–54.

Covino, B. G. (1984). Current controversies in local anaesthetics. In *Regional anaesthesia 1884–1984*. (ed. D. B. Scott, J. H. McClure, and J. A. W. Wildsmith), pp. 74–81. ICM, Södertälje.

Cowan, A. (1968). Further clinical evaluation of prilocaine (Citanest) with and without epinephrine. *Oral Surgery*, **26**, 304–11.

Criep, L. H. and Ribeiro, C. de C. (1953). Allergy to procaine hydrochloride with 3 fatalities. *Journal of the American Medical Association*, **151**, 1185–7.

Curley, R. K., Baxter, P. W., and Tyldesley, W. R. (1987). An unusual cutaneous reaction to lignocaine. *British Dental Journal*, **162**, 113–14.

Dimsdale, J. E. and Moss, J. (1980). Short-term catecholamine response to psychological stress. *Psychosomatic Medicine*, **42**, 493–7.

Downs, J. R. (1966). Atypical cholinesterase activity: its importance in dentistry. *Journal of Oral Surgery*, **24**, 256–7.

Epstein, S. (1969). Clinical study of prilocaine with varying concentrations of epinephrine. *Journal of the American Dental Association*, **78**, 85–90.

Faulkner, R. K. (1983). The high pressure periodontal ligament injection. *British Dental Journal*, **154**, 103–5.

Gangarosa, L. P. and Halik, F. J. (1967). A clinical evaluation of local anaesthetic solutions containing graded epinephrine concentrations. *Archives of Oral Biology*, **12**, 611–21.

Gasser, H. S. and Erlanger, J. (1929). The role of fiber size in the establishment of a nerve block by pressure or cocaine. *American Journal of Physiology*, **88**, 581–92.

Geddes, I. C. (1965). Studies of the metabolism of Citanest C114. *Acta Anaesthesia Scandinavica*, (suppl.) **16**, 37–41.

Giovannitti, J. A. and Bennett, C. R. (1979). Assessment of allergy to local anaesthetics. *Journal of the American Dental Association*, **98**, 701–6.

Goebel, W. M., Allen, G., and Randall, F. (1980). Comparative circulatory serum levels of 2 per cent mepivacaine and 2 per cent lignocaine. *British Dental Journal*, **148**, 261–4.

Goldman, V. and Evers, H. (1969). Prilocaine felypressin: a new combination for dental analgesia. *Dental Practitioner*, **19**, 225–31.

Goldman, V. and Gray, W. (1963). A clinical trial of a new local anaesthetic agent. *British Dental Journal*, **115**, 59–65.

Gregg, J. B., Barnett, G. L., and Ensberg, D. L. (1963). Mucosal slough reactions to topical anesthetic agent, lidocaine. *Archives of Otolaryngology*, **77**, 1–2.

Hanauer, A. (1955). Gruppensensibilisierung gegenuber anasthetika chemotherapeutika under antibiotika. *Deutsche Medizinische Wochenschrift*, **80**, 1175.

Hille, B., Courtney, K., and Dunn, R. (1975). Rate and site of action of local anesthetics in myelinated nerve. In *Molecular mechanisms of anesthesia*, (ed. B. R. Fink), pp. 13–20. Raven Press, New York.

Hodgkin, A. L. and Huxley, A. F. (1945). Resting and action potentials in single nerve fibres. *Journal of Physiology*, **104**, 176–95.

Holti, G. and Hood, F. J. C. (1965). An anaphylactoid reaction to lignocaine. *Dental Practitioner*, **15**, 294–6.

Horton, J. A. G. (1966) The complications of local anaesthetics. *Newcastle Medical Journal*, **29**, 125–30.

Jones, P. C. (1981). *Dental Advertiser*, (August), 26–9.

Kalow, W. (1952). Hydrolysis of local anaesthetics by human serum cholinesterase. *Journal of Pharmacology and Experimental Therapeutics*, **104**, 122–34.

Kirkler, D. M. (1962). Allergy to lignocaine. *Lancet*, **i**, 159.

Klingenstrom, P. and Westermark, L. (1964). Local tissue-oxygen tension after adrenaline, noradrenaline & octapressin in local anaesthesia. *Acta Anaesthesia Scandinavica*, **8**, 261–6.

Koller, C. (1928). Historical notes on the beginning of local anaesthesia. *Journal of the American Medical Association*, 90, 1742–3.

Laurence, D. R. and Bennett, P. (1987). *Clinical pharmacology*, (6th edn.), p. 451. Churchill Livingstone, Edinburgh.

Löfgren, N. (1948). *Studies on local anaesthetics—Xylocaine*. Hoegstroms, Stockholm.

Martindale: The Extra Pharmacopoeia (1982) 28th edn. (ed. J. E. F. Reynolds and A. B. Prasad). The Pharmaceutical Press, London.

Meechan, J. G. and Rawlins, M. D. (1987). A comparison of the effect of two different dental local anaesthetic solutions on plasma potassium concentration. *British Dental Journal*, 163, 191–3.

Mongar, J. L. (1955). Study of 2 methods for testing local anaesthetics in man. *British Journal of Pharmacology*, 10, 240–6.

Moore, D. C. and Bridenbaugh, L. D. (1960). Oxygen: the antidote for systemic toxic reactions from local anaesthetic drugs. *Journal of the American Medical Association*, 174, 842–7.

Moore, P. A. and Dunsky, J. L. (1983). Bupivacaine anesthesia—a clinical trial for endodontic therapy. *Oral Surgery*, 55, 176–9.

Mumford, J. M. and Geddes, I. C. (1961). Trial of carbamazepine in conservative dentistry. *British Dental Journal*, 110, 92–4.

Nathan, P. W. and Sears, T. A. (1962). Differential nerve block by sodium-free and sodium-deficient solutions. *Journal of Physiology. (Lond.)*, 164, 375–94.

Noble, D. S. and Pierce, G. F. M. (1961). Allergy to lignocaine: a case history. *Lancet*, ii, 1436.

Rawlins, M. D. and Thompson, J. W. (1985). Mechanisms of adverse drug reactions. In *Textbook of adverse drug reactions*, (ed. D. M. Davies), pp. 12–38. Oxford University Press.

Reynolds, F. (1987). Adverse effects of local anaesthetics. *British Journal of Anaesthesia*, 59, 78–95.

Ritchie, J. M. (1975). Mechanism of action of local anesthetic agents and biotoxins. *British Journal of Anaesthesia*, 47, 191.

Ritchie, J. M. and Greengard, P. (1966). On the mode of action of local anaesthetics. *Annual Review of Pharmacology*, 6, 405.

Rood, J. P. (1973). A case of lignocaine hypersensitivity. *British Dental Journal*, 135, 411–12.

Rud, J. (1961). Local anaesthetics. An electrophysiological investigation of local anaesthesia of peripheral nerves with special reference to xylocaine. *Acta Physiologica Scandinavica*, 51 (suppl. 178), 1–171.

Rudzki, E. and Kleniewska, D. (1970). The epidemiology of contact dermatitis in Poland. *British Journal of Dermatology*, 83, 543–5.

Sadove, M. S., Wyant, G. M., Gittelson, L. A., and Kretchmer, H. E. (1952). Classification and management of reactions to local anaesthetic agents. *Journal of the American Medical Association*, 148, 17–22.

Seskin, L. (1978). Anaphylaxis due to local anaesthesia hypersensitivity: report of case. *Journal of the American Dental Association*, 96, 841–3.

Tolas, A. G., Pflug, A. E., and Halter, J. B. (1982). Arterial plasma epinephrine concentrations and haemodynamic responses after dental injection of local anaesthetic with epinephrine. *Journal of the American Dental Association*, 104, 41–3.

Trimble, G. (1962). Allergy to lignocaine. *Lancet*, i, 435, quotes *U.S. Armed Forces Medical Journal* (1957) 8, 740.

Truant, A. P. and Takman, B. (1965). Local anaesthetics. In *Drill's pharmacology in medicine*, (3rd edn), pp. 133–56. McGraw-Hill, New York.

Tucker, G. T. (1986). Pharmacokinetics of local anaesthetics. *British Journal of Anaesthesia*, **58**, 717–31.

Tucker, G. T. and Mather, L. E. (1979). Clinical pharmacokinetics of local anaesthetics. *Clinical Pharmacokinetics*, **4**, 241–78.

Van Dyke, C., Barash, B. G., Tatlow, P., and Byck, R. (1976). Cocaine: plasma concentration after intranasal application in man. *Science*, **191**, 859–61.

Walton, R. E. and Garnick, J. J. (1982). The periodontal ligament injection. Histologic effects on the periodontium in monkeys. *Journal of Endodontics*, **8**, 22–6.

Weatherby, J. H. (1964). Local anaesthetics. In *Evaluation of drug activities: pharmacometrics*, Vol. 1. (ed. D. R. Laurence and A. L. Bacharach), pp. 205–14. Academic Press, London.

Wiedling, S. (1964). *Xylocaine*, (2nd edn.). Almqvist and Wiksell, Stockholm.

Wildsmith, J. A. W. (1986). Peripheral nerve and local anaesthetic drugs. *British Journal of Anaesthesia*, **58**, 692–700.

Wilson, I. H., Richmond, M. N., and Strike, P. W. (1986). Regional analgesia with bupivacaine in dental anaesthesia. *British Journal of Anaesthesia*, **58**, 401–5.

8

General anaesthesia and sedation

INTRODUCTION

GENERAL anaesthesia is the drug-induced absence of the perception of all sensation thus allowing surgery or other painful procedures to be carried out. This state is usually achieved by inhalation agents. Several other drugs are used in conjunction with general anaesthetic agents to ensure a safe, smooth, and uneventful operative procedure. These include drugs used to premedicate the patient, neuromuscular blocking agents, induction agents, and inhalation anaesthetic agents.

PREMEDICATION AGENTS

Premedication may be defined as the administration of drugs before an anaesthetic with a view to facilitating the operation and anaesthetic. Drugs used for this purpose are divided into (a) those used for their sedative effects, and (b) those used for their anticholinergic effects. The features required of premedication agents are as follows:

(1) to alleviate pre-operative anxiety;

(2) to provide some degree of postoperative amnesia, especially in children; so that a possible unpleasant experience is not remembered;

(3) to make the induction and maintenance of anaesthesia easier;

(4) to reduce the amount of anaesthetic agents required by enhancing their effects;

(5) to provide additional analgesia during surgery and in the postoperative period;

(6) to reduce salivary and bronchial secretions;

(7) to reduce activity in the parasympathetic nervous system, especially in the vagal plexus.

Opioids, anxiolytics, neuroleptics, and anticholinergic drugs are used as premedication agents.

Opioids

Morphine, pethidine, and papaveretum (a mixture of opium alkaloids) are the main opioids used in this way. Their pharmacological properties and mode of action have been discussed in Chapter 6. Their analgesic, sedative, and euphoriant properties make them popular as premedication agents. The dose regimes are shown in Table 8.1. Morphine does produce certain unwanted effects, in particular, nausea and vomiting. The incidence of postoperative vomiting with morphine is about 20 per cent, but this increases if the patient is ambulatory. Postoperative vomiting and nausea can be reduced by use of an anti-emetic such as cyclizine or prochlorperazine. The incidence of these effects is less after papaveretum. Pethidine is a less powerful analgesic than either morphine or papaveretum, but has a lower incidence of unwanted effects.

All the opioids produce a degree of respiratory depression and suppression of the cough reflex, which is important after abdominal and chest surgery where coughing is essential to clear the lungs of excessive secretions, thus reducing the risk of pneumonia.

Table 8.1. Dosage and routes of administration of opioids used as premedication agents

Drug	Route	Adult Dose	Child Dose	Times of administration
Pethidine hydrochloride	IM	50–100 mg	1–2 mg/kg	1 hour before operation
Morphine sulphate	IM	10 mg	150 μg/kg	1–1.5 hours before operation
Papaveretum	IM	10–20 mg	1–5 years: 2.5–5 mg 6–12 years: 5–10 mg	45–60 mins before operation

Anxiolytics

The benzodiazepines (diazepam, lorazepam, midazolam, and temazepam) may be used orally to provide pre-operative sedation. Their use is discussed below in the section 'Oral sedation' (p. 165).

Antipsychotics (neuroleptics)

Phenothiazine derivatives, such as promethazine and trimeprazine, are sometimes used as premedication agents. These drugs are effective as pre-anaesthetic sedatives and they have a powerful potentiating effect on general anaesthetics. Phenothiazine derivatives also have important anti-emetic properties and are valuable in patients who fear or who have a predisposition to postoperative

Table 8.2. Dosages and routes of administration of neuroleptic drugs used as premedication agents

Drug	Route	Adult Dose	Child Dose	Time of administration
Promethazine hydrochloride	Oral	—	6–12 months: 10 mg 1–5 years: 15–20 mg 6–10 years: 20–25 mg	1–2 hours before operation
"	IM	25–50 mg	6.25–12.5 mg	1 hour before operation
Trimeprazine tartrate	IM	3–4.5 mg/kg	2–4 mg/kg	1–2 hours before operation
Chlorpromazine hydrochloride	IM	20–50 mg	—	1 hour before operation

vomiting. They also depress respiration and cause a varying amount of hypotension. Dose regimes are shown in Table 8.2.

Anticholinergic premedication agents

Most gaseous anaesthetic agents cause an increase in salivary and bronchial secretions during induction and light anaesthesia. This excessive production of saliva and mucus may cause respiratory obstruction, which will interfere with the smooth course of the anaesthetic but, more seriously, may put the patient's life at risk. The need to depress salivary secretion during anaesthesia is even more important in children than in adults: the larynx and trachea are so small that a minimal quantity of secretion may seriously impair respiration. It is thus essential that every patient, except those having the briefest of anaesthetics, should receive a drug that reduces these secretions. Anticholinergic drugs also prevent overactivity of the parasympathetic nervous system especially in the vagus nerve. Drugs used to reduce salivary and bronchial secretions are atropine sulphate, hyoscine, and glycopyrolate.

Atropine sulphate

Atropine is commonly used to reduce salivary and bronchial secretions during anaesthesia. It produces these effects by antagonizing the actions of acetylcholine at muscarinic receptors (see Chapter 13). Atropine can be given intravenously immediately before anaesthesia, the adult dose being 300 to 600 micrograms (μg). The same dose can be given intramuscularly 30 to 60 minutes before induction.

Hyoscine

Like atropine, this antagonizes the effect of endogenous acetylcholine at muscarinic receptors. In order to dry up salivary and bronchial secretions, the adult dose of hyoscine is 200 to 600 μg given subcutaneously 30 to 60 minutes before induction of anaesthesia. Unlike atropine, hyoscine is a central nervous-system depressant, and causes a varying amount of drowsiness and depression of the vomiting centre; hence it is anti-emetic. Atropine, at high doses, may act as a stimulant of the central nervous system. Elderly people are sometimes confused by hyoscine and it is therefore best avoided in their premedication.

Both atropine and hyoscine depress vagal nerve endings in the heart. This gives some protection against the vagal stimulation that occurs with anaesthetic agents like trichlorethylene.

Glycopyrolate

This is a quaternary ammonium anticholinergic agent. It is highly ionized at physiological pH and thus penetrates poorly the blood–brain barrier and the placenta. Glycopyrolate produces prolonged and good control of salivary and pharyngeal secretions at doses that do not produce marked changes in heart rate. It has less effect on the cardiovascular system than atropine.

Glycopyrolate is also used as a preoperative or intra-operative antimuscarinic to attenuate or prevent the intra-operative bradycardia sometimes associated with the use of suxamethonium, or due to cardiac vagal reflexes. The usual adult does of glycopyrolate is 0.2 to 0.4 mg intravenously or intramuscularly before the induction of anaesthesia. For children, the dose is 0.004 to 0.008 mg/kg up to a maximum of 0.2 mg.

NEUROMUSCULAR BLOCKING AGENTS

These are widely used in anaesthetic practice because, by specific blockage of the neuromuscular junction, they enable light levels of anaesthesia to be achieved yet with adequate relaxation of the muscles of the abdomen and diaphragm. Neuromuscular blocking agents produce relaxation of abdominal muscles and paralysis of respiratory muscles. Prior to their introduction into anaesthetic practice, anaesthesia had to be very deep indeed to achieve the same degree of relaxation. They also relax the vocal cords, so allowing the passage of a tracheal tube.

There are two types of neuromuscular blocking agents depending on their mechanisms of action: (1) non-depolarizing (competitive) muscle relaxants, and (2) depolarizing muscle relaxants. These are detailed below, but to understand their action it is necessary to review the events of muscle contraction.

Muscle contraction

Acetylcholine bridges the gap between a motor nerve terminal and the motor/muscle end-plate or postsynaptic membrane. The sequence of events leading up to muscle contraction is as follows:

1. An action potential travels down the motor nerve and causes release of packets or 'quanta' of acetylcholine. Each quantum consists of many millions of acetylcholine molecules.

2. The released acetylcholine crosses the synaptic cleft and interacts with cholinergic receptors on the end-plate of a muscle fibre.

3. In the resting phase the muscle cell membrane is polarized, the interior being electronegative to the exterior. The surge of released acetylcholine impinging upon the end-plate receptor of the muscle brings about a massive increase in the permeability of the postsynaptic membrane to sodium ions and, to a lesser extent, potassium ions. Sodium ions enter and generate a local end-plate potential. When this depolarization of the end-plate potential reaches a critical threshold, this triggers off a muscle action potential that is propagated along the muscle fibre, so that a wave of depolarization is also propagated along the fibre, causing it to contract.

4. Acetylcholine is very rapidly broken down by cholinesterases in the neuromuscular junction; the motor end-plate repolarizes and is then ready to be stimulated again.

Non-depolarizing muscle relaxants

Tubocurarine

At one time natives of South America used to smear their arrows with curare to paralyse their victims. The active principle of curare is D-tubocurarine.

Tubocurarine is highly ionized and ineffective by mouth, so it is therefore given intravenously. In man it produces paralysis of all voluntary muscles, including those of respiration, so patients should always have their respiration controlled until the drug has been inactivated. Its action commences about 3 to 4 minutes after injection and lasts up to 40 minutes.

Tubocurarine produces its action by occupying acetylcholine receptors on a muscle end-plate, so preventing the occurrence of an end-plate potential. It competes with acetylcholine for the motor-end-plate and prevents the access of acetylcholine to the receptor so that the depolarization necessary for muscular contraction does not occur. Tubocurarine is therefore a competitive neuromuscular blocking agent.

Tubocurarine is largely used as an adjunct to general anaesthesia. To produce deep muscular relaxation by means of a general anaesthetic substance the depth of anaesthesia has to be profound, and this may cause serious depression of the medullary centres of respiration and circulation. Tubocurarine will produce a profound muscular relaxation of about 30 to 45 minutes duration and, at the same time, only a minimal amount of the general anaesthetic agent will be required. It does not in itself affect consciousness.

The actions of tubocurarine can be reversed by the administration of neostigmine, which is an anticholinesterase. The competitive antagonism between acetylcholine and tubocurarine for the same receptor sites is a quantitative phenomenon. Neostigmine prevents the destruction of acetylcholine by cholinesterases and so prolongs its effects with the result that the activity of tubocurarine is overcome. When tubocurarine has been used as an adjunct to general anaesthetic agents it is customary to assist recovery by the intravenous injection of neostigmine. However, before giving neostigmine, it is essential to administer atropine sulphate intravenously to prevent the muscarinic actions of accumulated acetylcholine (e.g. slowing of the heart).

In addition to producing neuromuscular blockade, tubocurarine is a weak ganglion blocker, and it also causes the release of histamine. Peripheral vaso-dilatation caused by the histamine release, together with the sympathetic ganglia blockade, will lower the blood pressure. In fact, if tubocurarine is rapidly injected intravenously, there is likely to be a severe drop in blood pressure. The release of histamine may also cause flushing of the skin and bronchospasm.

Tubucurarine does not cross the blood–brain barrier or the placenta.

Pancuronium

This is more potent than tubocurarine but has a shorter period of action. It acts in the same way by competitive block but, unlike tubocurarine, it does not normally block transmission in autonomic ganglia and so does not significantly alter the blood pressure. However, if rapidly injected intravenously, the drug may actually cause ganglionic stimulation with a rise in blood pressure. Pancuronium does not cause histamine to be released from mast cells and so is unlikely to induce bronchospasm. It thus has obvious advantages and is widely used to produce relaxation in clinical anaesthesia.

In addition to producing muscular relaxation during anaesthesia, such agents may be used to produce relaxation in a number of pathological conditions, e.g. tetanus.

Atracuronium and vecuronium

These are the neuromuscular blocking agents most likely to be used at the present time. They have little effect on the cardiovascular system and so there is relatively little change in blood pressure. Atracuronium (but not vecuronium) may produce histamine release but this is much less marked that with tubocurarine. Neither drug produces sympathetic blockade.

Depolarizing muscle relaxants

Suxamethonium

This depolarizes the postsynaptic membrane and maintains this state so that the adjacent muscle fibres are electrically inexcitable. Although suxamethonium is fairly quickly hydrolysed by pseudocholinesterase its action is long enough (5 minutes) to be clinically useful. It is the ideal agent for use when passing an endotracheal tube. The drug is injected intravenously and within half a minute it produces complete muscular relaxation. Its rather short duration of action makes it useful in preventing muscular movements during electroconvulsive therapy. If longer procedures are required then the drug can be used in repeated dosage.

The action of suxamethonium may be prolonged in patients with low pseudocholinesterase levels due to liver disease. On the other hand, the prolonged apnoea that may occasionally follow the administration of suxamethonium could prove to be due to the presence of an abnormal cholinesterase. It has been estimated that about 1 to 2 800 persons have this atypical esterase, which hydrolyses suxamethonium more slowly than pseudocholinesterase so that the duration of neuromuscular block is prolonged (this is an example of an unwanted effect—idiosyncrasy).

Suxamethonium promotes release of intracellular potassium and this may be important in patients taking digoxin and/or diuretics, because digoxin may itself promote intracellular depletion of potassium, and many diuretics increase the excretion of potassium. The drug has a number of muscarinic actions, which include increased salivary secretion. Muscle injury may occasionally occur with suxamethonium; this may be due to a direct action of the drug on muscle or follow on potassium depletion from muscles. Occasionally, malignant hyperpyrexia has followed the use of halothane with suxamethonium; it is fairly certain that this condition is genetically based, and it is a very serious one, as the mortality rate is in the region of 60 to 70 per cent.

INDUCTION AGENTS
(INTRAVENOUS ANAESTHETIC AGENTS)

These are widely used to induce anaesthesia. They are very potent drugs and, once injected, little can be done to terminate their action. Some can be used for short, painful operations such as reduction of a dislocation. The most widely used intravenous anaesthetic agents are sodium thiopentone, methohexitone, etomidate, and propofol. Ketamine is sometimes used for intravenous induction.

Sodium thiopentone

Sodium thiopentone is an ultrashort-acting barbiturate (ethyl thiobarbiturate). The sodium salt is water-soluble and the anaesthetic dose is 4 mg/kg of body weight.

Pharmacokinetics

Sodium thiopentone is given intravenously and produces loss of consciousness in 10 to 20 seconds. The maximum depth of anaesthesia occurs at 40 seconds after dosage and the patient becomes conscious some 2 to 3 minutes after dosage. The drug rapidly enters the brain because of its high lipid solubility. Its short action is attributable to the rapid fall in plasma concentration that is due to distribution into the tissues (especially into muscles, followed by adipose tissue). About 85 per cent of sodium thiopentone is bound to plasma protein, and the drug is metabolized in the liver, the metabolites being excreted via the kidney.

Pharmacological properties

Sodium thiopentone depresses many of the functions of the CNS (see Chapter 14), resulting in sedation, anaesthesia, and a dose-related respiratory depression. Like other barbiturates, it has no analgesic properties and low doses may even increase sensitivity to pain (Dundee 1960). It is also an anticonvulsant and can be used in emergency for status epilepticus.

Anaesthetic doses of sodium thiopentone produce a reduction in cardiac output and force of cardiac contraction. There is also a transient drop in blood pressure. Administration of thiopentone is often associated with laryngospasm and even bronchospasm, but the mechanism of these reactions is unknown. It has no effect on the uterus, but it does cross the placenta and can depress the fetal cardiovascular system.

Uses

Sodium thiopentone is used to induce unconsciousness prior to inhalation anaesthesia, and to provide anaesthesia for short operative procedures, such as reduction of a dislocation, and in electroconvulsive therapy.

Unwanted effects

Cough, laryngospasm, and bronchospasm are the more common of these. Because of the high incidence of laryngospasm and bronchospasm, thiopentone should not be used in asthmatics. An extravascular injection of sodium thiopentone will cause pain and, if the concentration of the solution is greater than 2.5 per cent, then tissue necrosis may occur. If it is inadvertently injected into an artery, the endothelial and deeper layers are immediately damaged, followed by an endarteritis and sometimes thrombosis. This damage is caused by the drug crystallizing out of solution due to reduced dilution in blood. If untreated, ischaemia and even gangrene may result. Damage to the arterial wall is instantaneous and treatment should be rapid. The needle should be left *in situ* and the artery infused with 5 to 10 ml of 1 per cent procaine, which will reduce the pain and arteriospasm. Heparin should then be administered to inhibit thrombus formation, and a regional block of the sympathetic nerves performed, to cause arterial dilatation. The damage from intra-arterial injections of sodium thiopentone is greatly reduced if the concentration of the solution does not exceed 2.5 per cent.

Sodium thiopentone, together with other barbiturates, must not be given to patients with porphyria, a condition which has a high incidence in South Africans of Afrikaaner descent. If a porphyria sufferer is given barbiturates, they will cause widespread demyelination of the peripheral and cranial nerves and disseminated lesions throughout the central nervous system, resulting in pain, weakness, and paralysis; these may be life-threatening.

Methohexitone

Like sodium thiopentone, this is also a short-acting barbiturate (sodium oxybarbiturate), and consequently both drugs have similar pharmacological properties. Anaesthesia is induced with a dose of 1 mg/kg of body weight, and recovery is rapid. Intra-arterial injection of methohexitone is very dangerous. The drug is not an anticonvulsant and can possible induce fits during anaesthesia.

Etomidate

This is a relatively new intravenous anaesthetic agent; chemically it is a carboxylated imidazole derivative. For induction purposes it is used at a dose of 0.3 mg/kg of body weight. Its main advantage over the short-acting barbiturates is the rapid recovery with no 'hangover' effect. Both these properties may be due to the short plasma half-life (approx. one hour). Intravenous injections of etomidate are painful and cause extraneous muscle movements. It does not cause histamine release, and so it can be used as an induction agent in asthmatics and in patients with a history of drug hypersensitivity. Etomidate has little or no effect on the cardiovascular system and is therefore mainly used for patients with cardiac disease.

Ketamine

This soluble anaesthetic agent is usually given intravenously, but can be given intramuscularly. It is used as either a 1, 5, or 10 per cent solution. Ketamine has high lipid solubility and rapidly passes the blood-brain barrier. An intravenous dose of 12 mg/kg of body weight produces anaesthesia within 30 seconds that lasts for 5 to 10 minutes. Unlike the short-acting barbiturates, ketamine administration is associated with profound sedation and analgesia. The main unwanted effect of ketamine is vivid hallucinations and nightmares. The drug also raises blood pressure and pulse rate, and so should not be used in hypertensive patients. Ketamine, an anaesthetic induction agent, is particularly useful in the management of mass casualties, especially for anaesthesia of trapped patients to carry out amputations or the like.

Propofol

This is a new phenolic (diisopropylphenol) intravenous anaesthetic induction agent. The drug is also licensed for use in maintenance of anaesthesia, provided the surgical procedure does not exceed one hour. The dose needed for induction is 2 to 2.5 mg/kg of body weight. Light general anaesthesia can be maintained by repeated bolus injections of between 25 to 50 mg. Recovery from such an anaesthesia is usually rapid and uneventful.

Pharmacokinetics

Propofol is highly lipophilic and, following an intravenous dose, there is a rapid decline in blood concentrations, indicating a swift distribution into the tissues. The pharmacokinetic profile is best described as a three-phase sequence:

(1) a very rapid distribution from blood ($T_{0.5}$ about 2 to 4 minutes);

(2) a rapid intermediate phase reflecting metabolic clearance ($T_{0.5}$, 35 to 45 minutes).

(3) a slower final phase, representing the slow return of drug to the blood from a poorly perfused deep compartment, probably body fat ($T_{0.5}$, 200 to 300 minutes).

The drug is mainly metabolized in the liver, and the metabolites are excreted via the kidney.

Unwanted effects

Cardio-respiratory depression is the main one of these; apnoea occurs on induction and the drug has a marked hypotensive effect. Another frequent unwanted effect is pain on injection, and this is particularly marked when propofol is injected into a small vein. Accidental extravasation does not produce any tissue damage.

Propofol is more expensive than existing intravenous induction agents, but its recovery characteristics make it particularly suitable for day-case procedures.

INHALATION ANAESTHESIA

This is the most widely used form of anaesthesia in the UK.

The various stages of anaesthesia were first described by Guedel (1937) with reference to ether. Hence the guidelines listed below must be subject to careful interpretation, and are clearly modified by modern anaesthetic techniques and agents. Many of the widely used anaesthetic agents bring the patient to Stage III very rapidly, and the subtle differences between the stages of anaesthesia may not be distinguishable. Furthermore, the depth of anaesthesia cannot be judged by the degree of muscular relaxation if a neuromuscular blocking agent has been used.

In the classical description, inhalation anaesthesia occurs in four stages, as listed next.

Stage I—analgesia stage

During this stage, the patient is still conscious and can talk, but feels giddy and sleepy. There is a progressive decrease in reaction to painful stimuli, and an increase in respiratory and pulse rate. The eyelash reflex is gradually lost.

Stage II—excitement stage

Although the patient is unconscious, this stage is known as the excitement stage because during it they may be agitated and struggle. Alternatively, they may be quiet, and much of this variable response may depend on the type of patient, the presence or absence of stimuli, and the skill of the anaesthetist. During the excitement stage, conscious control is removed, and the patient may struggle from a fear that has been concealed during Stage I or because they are being subjected to some stimulus, such as a premature attempt to extract teeth. In stage II, the pupils dilate, the pulse is rapid and strong, but respiration is irregular.

Stage III—surgical anaesthesia

The characteristic features of surgical anaesthesia concern eye signs and the muscles of respiration. There is a decrease in the range and activity of the movements of the eyeballs until eventually the eye comes to rest in the central position and remains there. In the early phase of surgical anaesthesia there is complete functioning of the intercostal muscles and diaphragm.

Stage IV—respiratory paralysis

At the stage of respiratory paralysis, the heart still beats and the patient may be kept alive if adequately oxygenated by artificial means. If such support is not given, the pulse will be rapid, there will be a drop in blood pressure, and the pupils will dilate. This will be followed by complete respiratory and circulatory collapse, and the patient will die.

The depth of anaesthesia will depend upon the type of operation. Most dental procedures can be carried out during the early phases of Stage III.

INHALATION ANAESTHETIC AGENTS

The properties of an ideal inhalation anaesthetic agent are:

(1) a rapid and pleasant induction of, and recovery from anaesthesia;

(2) the ability to produce rapid changes in the depth of anaesthesia;

(3) the ability to produce adequate relaxation of skeletal muscles;

(4) a wide margin of safety;

(5) no unwanted effects or other adverse properties in normal use.

Inhalation anaesthetic agents can be classified into two groups, gaseous agents (nitrous oxide and cyclopropane) and volatile liquids (halothane, enflurane, isoflurane, trichlorethylene, and ether).

Nitrous oxide

This colourless, odourless gas was the first agent to be used as an anaesthetic. It is stored as a liquid under pressure in metal cylinders, and evaporates when released. The gas is not flammable but supports combustion. Nitrous oxide has a very low solubility in blood (but not as low as nitrogen), and a state of equilibrium between alveolar and arterial tension is quickly reached. It is excreted unchanged in the expired gases.

Pharmacological properties

Nitrous oxide is a weak anaesthetic agent, mainly used as an adjunct to other agents (e.g. halothane). Surgical anaesthesia can be obtained in a minority of patients with nitrous oxide alone at concentrations in excess of 80 per cent. However, at these concentrations there is every danger of hypoxia. The mechanism for nitrous oxide-induced anaesthesia remains uncertain. It is an excellent analgesic agent, and may exert its analgesic properties by initiating the release of the endogenous opioids (see Chapter 6 and Berkowitz et al. 1977). When nitrous oxide is mixed with an adequate amount of oxygen (30 per cent), the mixture has little or no significant effect on the cardiovascular or respiratory system. However, it is a direct myocardial depressant, and also stimulates the sympathetic nervous system. As a result of these two actions, cardiac output remains unchanged.

Unwanted effects

The incidence of nausea and vomiting after administration of nitrous oxide alone is approximately 15 per cent, which compares unfavourably with halothane. *In vitro* studies have shown that nitrous oxide interrupts cell division in the presynthetic (G-1) phase of the DNA-synthesis cycle (Brinkley and Rao 1973; see also Chapter 17). Excessive use of nitrous oxide may suppress spermatogenesis and the production of white and red blood cells in the bone marrow (Kripke et al. 1976). However, this problem does not appear to arise in normal clinical use (Ames et al. 1978).

In experimental animals, nitrous oxide can cause megaloblastic anaemia and neuropathy through oxidation of the cobalt ion of vitamin B_{12}. This finding may be significant to personnel repeatedly exposed to nitrous oxide, such as anaesthetic and operating-theatre staff. Scavenger systems should be fitted to all systems where nitrous oxide is used to ensure that the atmosphere does not contain more than 50 p.p.m. A neuropathy similar to that of vitamin B_{12} deficiency has been observed in dental surgeons who regularly use nitrous oxide (Layzer 1978). Nitrous oxide may have a deleterious effect if used in patients who have an air-containing closed space in their bodies as the gas diffuses into such a space with a resulting build-up of pressure. This effect may be dangerous in cases of pneumothorax, which lesion may enlarge and so compromise respiration.

Uses

Nitrous oxide is used as an adjunct to other inhalation anaesthetic agents such as halothane or enflurane. Low doses are used in sedation and are discussed later. 'Entonox' is a commercially available mixture of 50 per cent nitrous oxide and 50 per cent oxygen; it is widely used to produce analgesia without loss of consciousness, and is especially useful in obstetric practice, for changing painful dressings, as an aid to postoperative physiotherapy, and in emergency ambulances. In ambulance emergencies, the mixture is very efficacious at reducing the pain of myocardial infarction. Cylinders containing 'Entonox' must always be stored in a warm room because, at low temperatures, the gaseous mixture separates out and the less dense nitrous oxide rises to the top of the cylinder. When such separation has occurred, the next patient will be exposed to 100 per cent nitrous oxide.

Halothane

This halogenated hydrocarbon is the most widely used anaesthetic agent. At room temperature, it is a colourless liquid that decomposes on contact with light. The liquid has a pleasant smell and readily vapourizes with a boiling point of 50°C. It is not inflammable and is non-explosive. Halothane can be used to induce anaesthesia at a concentration of 2 to 4 per cent, and anaesthesia can be maintained with a concentration of 1 to 2 per cent. Although intraveous anaesthetic agents are commonly used to induce anaesthesia (see p. 150), induction can be achieved with halothane. The vapour does not irritate the larynx so induction is smooth and a rapid depth of anaesthesia can readily be achieved.

Pharmacokinetics

Sixty to eighty per cent of halothane is eliminated unchanged in the expired gases. That portion absorbed is biotransformed in the liver, and the metabolites excreted via the kidney.

Pharmacological properties

Halothane has a marked effect on the cardiovascular system causing a dose-related reduction in blood pressure. The hypotension is due to a reduction both in cardiac output and in the baroreceptor response. Halothane also causes a slowing of the heart rate mediated by the vagus nerve and, more importantly, sensitizes the myocardium to catecholamine, which can provoke severe dysrhythmia. Such sensitization can be a problem in certain dental surgical procedures where injections of a local anaesthetic solution containing adrenaline may be used to maintain a relatively bloodless field. It is recommended that the amount of adrenaline should not exceed 0.1 mg in 10 minutes or 0.3 mg in 1 hour (Katz *et al.* 1962).

Halothane depresses respiration causing a reduction in gaseous exchange. However, it also produces bronchodilatation, thus making it a suitable agent for use in asthmatics and bronchitics. Halothane does not have any analgesic properties but does produce a degree of muscle relaxation, although rarely enough for most types of surgery.

Unwanted effects

Hepatic necrosis has been associated with halothane anaesthesia at an incidence of 1:10 000 anaesthetic administrations. However, the incidence increases with repeated halothane anaesthesia (Summary of the National Halothane Study 1966). Clinical signs and symptoms of a halothane-induced hepatic necrosis usually arise 2 to 5 days after administration. The patient becomes pyrexic, and complains of nausea and vomiting. Death occurs in 50 per cent of these patients. The mechanism of hepatic necrosis is uncertain: any residual halothane that is not expired is likely to be metabolized in the liver; however, a metabolite may induce an immune response resulting in hepatitis. Although halothane hepatitis is serious, other complications of general anaesthesia occur with much greater frequency.

A rare, unwanted effect of halothane is the syndrome of malignant hyperpyrexia, characterized by a rapid rise in body temperature, and a massive increase in both oxygen consumption and production of carbon dioxide. This condition can be fatal unless treated.

Enflurane

This is a halogenated ether; at room temperature it is a colourless, non-inflammable liquid with a mild, sweet odour. Anaesthesia can be smoothly induced with enflurane 4 per cent, and maintained with concentrations of 1.5 to 3 per cent. Induction is associated with mild stimulation of salivary flow and tracheobronchial secretions, but these are not usually troublesome. Enflurane also alters certain types of electrical activity in the brain that may be epileptogenic. Therefore, this agent should not be used in patients with a history of epilepsy.

Pharmacokinetics

About 80 per cent of enflurane is excreted unchanged in the expired gases. Of the remainder, only 2 to 5 per cent is metabolized in the liver; metabolites are excreted via the kidney.

Pharmacological properties

Enflurane produces a dose-dependent reduction in blood pressure in a manner similar to halothane. Its effect on the heart is also similar to that produced by halothane, but there is a smaller incidence of arrhythmias. Adrenaline-containing local anaesthetic solutions can be used safely with it.

Enflurane causes respiratory depression, and patients are usually ventilated when this agent is being used. Deep anaesthesia with enflurane is associated with muscle twitching of the limbs, jaw, face, and neck. These muscular movements are usually self-limiting, and are prevented by reducing the depth of anaesthesia. Because of this unwanted effect, enflurane should be avoided in epileptic patients. It has no significant effect on the liver and is often used in preference to halothane when repeated anaesthesia is required.

Isoflurane

This is an isomer of enflurane; chemically, it is a halogenated methyl ethyl ether. Its physical properties are similar to those of enflurane. Induction of anaesthesia with isoflurane is smooth and rapid, and can be achieved with a concentration of 3 per cent; maintenance is achieved with 1.5 to 2.5 per cent.

Pharmacological properties

Like the other halogenated volatile liquids, isoflurane causes a reduction in blood pressure, but has little or no effect on cardiac output. Administration is associated with an increase in heart rate but no arrhythmias. It does not sensitize the heart to catecholamines so adrenaline-containing local anaesthetic solutions can be used safely with this agent. Respiration is depressed with isoflurane, which may also stimulate airway reflexes, causing increased secretion, coughing, and laryngospasm. The incidence of nausea and vomiting is similar to that produced by the other halogenated compounds, and hepatotoxicity does not appear to be a problem

Trichlorethylene

This is a weak anaesthetic agent and a poor muscle relaxant, but a potent analgesic. It is rarely used as an anaesthetic agent because of slow induction and long recovery, due to its poor solubility.

Ether (diethyl ether)

This was one of the earliest and safest volatile liquids to be used in anaesthetic practice. Liquid ether is very pungent, irritating to the mucous membrane, inflammable, and explosive. Induction with ether was slow and unpleasant, and recovery was often associated with nausea and vomiting. Because of these unwanted effects, ether is now rarely used.

ASSESSMENT, AND ANAESTHETIC PROBLEMS OF THE MEDICALLY COMPROMISED PATIENT

Before any general anaesthetic is administered it is essential to check that the patient has had nothing to eat or drink for a period of six hours before induction. If possible, the patient's bladder should be empty. Where anaesthetics are being administered to out-patients, the patient must be accompanied by a responsible adult.

The medical conditions listed below can cause complications during anaesthesia and, where possible, such patients should be treated under local anaesthesia. If a general anaesthetic has to be used then they should be referred to hospital, and the anaesthetic should always be administered by an experienced anaesthetist.

Pregnancy

During the first trimester, drugs employed in anaesthetic practice could impair the development of the fetus and placenta. The middle trimester is probably the optimal time for a general anaesthetic if this is definitely required. In the final trimester, the bulky uterus will cause a reduction in gastric emptying, and it may impair venous return from the lower extremities, which will also cause a reduction in cardiac output.

Cardiovascular problems

Any disorders of this, the body's main transport system, will have serious implications during general anaesthesia.

Patients with angina pectoris should have a percutaneous preparation of glyceryl trinitrate (Transiderm-Nitro) applied to their skin before an anaesthetic. Those with ischaemic heart disease are already suffering from some degree of oxygen deprivation and any additional deprivation may produce an infarct.

All antihypertensive drugs are potentiated by general anaesthetic agents, especially the barbiturates and halothane, and a severe hypotensive attack could result from this interaction. Halothane may have some ganglion-blocking activity, and could also enhance the antihypertensive effects of other drugs.

Respiratory disorders

General anaesthesia should be postponed in patients with acute diseases of the upper respiratory tract (i.e. the common cold). Those with disease of the lower respiratory tract are prone to excessive mucus production, and such patients should be referred for a medical opinion before a general anaesthetic is administered.

Haematological disorders

All types of anaemia can affect the course of a general anaesthetic, but the two most serious forms are sickle cell disease and thalassaemia.

Sickle cell disease is an inherited disease found in about 10 per cent of people of African or West Indian origin. There are two types, a homozygous form (sickle cell disease) and a heterozygous form (sickle cell trait). In homozygous sickle cell disease, the red blood cells contain an abnormal haemoglobin (Hb_S). When such cells are exposed to a reduced oxygen tension, or a rise in blood pH, they become sickle-shaped (sickling) and haemolysis occurs. Dehydration, stasis of the circulation, and pyrexia also predispose to sickling. Patients with the heterozygous sickle cell trait may have some Hb_S in their red blood cells and the amount needs to be determined before a general anaesthetic is administered.

Thalassaemia is a rare inherited anaemia that occurs mainly in mid- and southern Europeans. The red blood cells in thalassaemia have a short life-span and contain fetal haemoglobin. Sufferers usually have a severe hypochronic anaemia.

Endocrine disorders

The problem of administering a general anaesthetic to patients suffering from diabetes or who have adrenocortical suppression is discussed in Chapter 18.

Hyperthyroidism causes tachycardia, and disturbances such as arrhythmias or even cardiac failure. Therefore the hyperthyroid patient is at risk when a general anaesthetic is administered because of the possible precipitation of dangerous arrhythmias.

Neurological disorders

Methohexitone should not be used as an intravenous anaesthetic agent in patients with a history of epilepsy (see p. 152). In such a patient, methohexitone could result in status epilepticus under general anaesthesia.

Patients with a history of spasticity, myasthenia gravis, and multiple sclerosis are a special anaesthetic risk and should be be anaesthetized in hospital.

Drug therapy

Patients taking mono-amine oxidase inhibitors should not be given pethidine as a premedication, as severe and life-threatening interactions occur between them (see Chapter 22).

ANAESTHETIC EMERGENCIES

The two emergencies to be discussed in this section are respiratory obstruction and hypersensitivity reactions. Other emergencies can occur at any phase of general anaesthesia, i.e. cardiac arrest, syncope, etc., and these are discussed in Chapter 24.

Respiratory obstruction

Obstruction of the airway during anaesthesia can be caused by the several factors listed below:

(1) *Anatomical:* large tongue, retrognathic mandible, enlarged adenoids and tonsils;

(2) *Operative problems:* obstructing the airway by applying too much back pressure during extraction, or too much flexion of the head;

(3) *Pathological problems:* upper respiratory tract infection, blocked nasal airway;

(4) *Laryngeal spasm:* caused by blood, saliva, mucus, pus, vomit, or foreign bodies touching the vocal cords;

(5) *Obstruction below vocal cords:* caused by inhaled foreign body, or broncho-spasm.

Signs and symptoms

If respiratory sounds can still be heard, this is an indication of only *partial* blockage of the airway; no respiratory sounds means *total obstruction*. With complete obstruction there is alternate indentation of the intercostal spaces and jerking movements of the abdominal wall because of the efforts of the diaphragm, which is the most powerful muscle of respiration. Respiratory obstruction, if not urgently treated, will lead to circulatory collapse.

Treatment

In the first instance, try and find the cause of the obstruction: the cervical spine should be extended to open the pharynx and the mandible lifted forward. With a laryngoscope, inspect the larynx for foreign material such as blood, saliva, and mucus; remove with suction. This, however, can be an extremely difficult procedure even for an experienced anaesthetist. Foreign bodies, such as tooth fragments, should be removed with McGill's forceps. Respiratory obstruction in small children can usually be cleared by holding them upside down and thumping their back.

If the condition does not improve with these measures, then a cricothyrotomy should be carried out. For this technique, the neck is extended and a cricothyroid cannula inserted through the cricothyroid membrane. If a cricothyroid needle is not available, then a large venepuncture needle could allow sufficient air (200 ml) to pass into the lungs. Oxygen should be administered through the cannula. If circulatory collapse has occurred, resuscitation techniques described in Chapter 24 should be employed.

Hypersensitivity reactions

Any of the drugs used in general anaesthesia are capable of causing a hypersensitivity reaction. However, such reactions are more likely to occur with the intravenous anaesthetic agents, and this was especially true of Althesin and propanidid, which contain the solvent, cremophor E-L. These two drugs are no longer used, but other compounds may still cause a problem. The signs, symptoms, and treatment of hypersensitivity reactions are discussed in Chapter 21.

SEDATION

Introduction

Fear of dental treatment is a common reason for failure to seek regular dental care; all dentists encounter apprehensive patients and are aware of the problems of managing their anxiety so that treatment can be carried out. Sedation is one of the most widely used methods for reducing such axiety. The Wylie Report (1978) defines sedation as '. . . a technique in which the use of a drug or drugs produces a state of depression of the central nervous system enabling treatment to be carried out, but during which verbal contact with the patient is maintained throughout the period of sedation. The drugs and techniques used should carry a margin of safety wide enough to render unintended loss of consciousness unlikely.'

Hill and Morris (1983) list the ideal properties of a sedation agent as follows:

(1) alleviation of fear and anxiety;

(2) production of a degree of amnesia and analgesia;

(3) suppression of vomiting reflexes, but not of protective reflexes;

(4) prolongation of potential operating time;

(5) readily effective;

(6) having a sufficiently long effect but which then quickly wears off;

(7) no side effects;

(8) safety and easily administered by the operator;

(9) not requiring special procedures or precautions before or after use;

(10) the associated techniques and equipment should be simple and the drugs inexpensive.

Sedation techniques used in dentistry can be categorized into three types depending on the route of administration—these being inhalation, oral, and intravenous. Whatever sedation technique is used, local anaesthesia must be also employed. Sedation techniques on their own are not sufficient to reduce painful impulses arising from dental procedures.

Inhalation methods of producing sedation

Nitrous oxide is the main inhalation agent used to provide sedation in dentistry, although the efficacy of low concentrations of enflurane and isoflurane is also being evaluated. After its introduction as an anaesthetic agent, it was soon recognized that low concentrations (20 to 25 per cent) of nitrous oxide could produce sedation. This property has been incorporated into two sedation techniques, inhalation sedation and relative analgesia.

Nitrous oxide, in the concentrations required for sedation, is a very safe drug producing very little systemic disturbance. The gaseous mixture (see below) can be rapidly cleared from the blood stream in the lungs within five minutes of breathing normal air. There are a few patients who are very sensitive to nitrous oxide and these may become anaesthetized with the concentrations used for sedation.

Inhalation sedation

This method involves the administration of a fixed concentration of 25 per cent nitrous oxide in an oxygen-enriched (25 per cent) air mixture at a flow rate in excess of the patient's anticipated minute volume. With the concentration of nitrous oxide fixed at 25 per cent, loss of consciousness cannot occur; thus this technique is safe for single operators. The gaseous mixture is administered via a nasal mask, and the level of sedation is determined by the amount of nose or mouth breathing, with nose breathing producing deeper sedation and mouth breathing recovery, whereby the level of sedation is controlled by the patient.

The mixture of nitrous oxide and oxygen-enriched air, when supplied at a flow rate above the normal minute volume, causes a small positive pressure in the breathing circuit. This minimizes the problem of dilution of the inspired gas mixture by air in a leaky breathing circuit.

Relative analgesia

In this method of sedation, the gas flow from the machine is below the minute-volume requirements and, to compensate, the air dilution valve on the nosepiece is partially opened to admit additional volumes of air. This results in a variable and unpredictable dilution of the inspired gases according to changes in the partial pressure in the system. Such changes result from the inspiratory effort, which can vary from breath to breath. Consequently, the level of sedation must be monitored by the operator by altering the flow rate of the gases.

Patient preparation and administration of inhalation sedation

The patient does not need to starve before inhalation sedation. Patients must be accompanied, and should not be permitted to drive or to place themselves in a situation where they might be a hazard either to themselves or others. Lingering, subtle effects on judgement or co-ordination cannot be completely excluded in the aftermath of sedation. Furthermore, one who is approaching a dental appointment in a state of anxiety and fear is not fully rational at the time and is at a greater hazard than the normal population. The euphoria commonly experienced after sedation may also interfere with judgement and responses; this is apart from any possible effects of the drug.

Prior to the appointment, the patient should be given details of the sedative technique and its likely effects. At the appointment, they should be placed in the supine position and allowed to familiarize themselves with the nosepiece, making adjustments for comfort. When the nosepiece is in position, the gaseous mixture is turned on and the patient instructed to breath slowly and regularly. During induction, quiet and reassuring verbal contact should be maintained between operator and patient, which produces a state of semi-hypnosis.

Signs of sedation

The signs and symptoms of inhalation sedation produced by nitrous oxide are listed by Edmunds and Rosen (1983), and categorized as either objective or subjective.

Objective signs

The patient remains awake, follows instructions, and responds to questions. There is a reduced response to painful stimuli, and the patient appears drowsy and relaxed. The respiratory rate is normal and smooth with little or no gagging or coughing. There is no excessive movement of the limbs; the pupil size, eye reactions, pulse, and blood pressure are normal.

Subjective signs
These are:

(1) mental and physical relaxation, and relief of anxiety;

(2) euphoria, headiness, and a feeling of floating;

(3) an indifference to surroundings and to the passage of time;

(4) feelings of warmth and tingling of extremities;

(5) buzzing or ringing in ears;

(6) sounds seeming distant.

Once the patient is sedated, the local anaesthetic can be injected and the operative procedure carried out. On completion of treatment, the patient breathes 100 per cent oxygen for 2 minutes, and within 10 minutes they should be fit to leave the surgery.

Contra-indications to inhalation sedation

This technique should not be used during pregnancy. In the early stages of pregnancy there is the possibility of teratogenicity from nitrous oxide and, in the later stages, there is the risk of relaxation of the uterus, although this is most unlikely if the concentration of nitrous oxide stays below 25 per cent. Inhalation sedation techniques are not suitable for patients with acute or chronic nasal obstruction: these include upper respiratory tract infections, chronic bronchitis, or an attack of hay fever. The obese may be intolerant of the supine position because of difficulties in breathing due to diaphragm compression. Psychiatrically disturbed patients are best treated in hospital after consultation with their psychiatrist.

Summary

Inhalation sedation techniques are safe and usually well-tolerated by most anxious patients. The administration of nitrous oxide by the inhalation sedation method has the advantage over relative analgesia by allowing a fixed dose of the gas to be given. Thus the operator is not distracted by having to adjust the nitrous-oxide level, being left free to concentrate on the dental procedure. Inhalation sedation techniques also appear to 'cure' dental anxiety, and it is then possible to 'wean' patients off sedation onto conventional treatment under local anaesthesia.

Oral sedation

The oral administration of drugs to produce sedation has the advantage of relative safety and acceptability. Oral sedation is particularly useful in children. The disadvantages of the oral route are the delayed onset of action, unreliable drug absorption, inability to regulate easily the intensity of the drug effect, and often a prolonged duration of action. For these reasons, oral sedative agents are mainly used to ensure that patients have a restful night before a dental procedure and to provide some degree of sedation in the period before the appointment. Drugs used for this purpose include the benzodiazepines, antihistamines, and triclofos.

Benzodiazepines

Diazepam, temazepam, lorazepam, and midazolam are the main benzodiazepines used for oral sedation. The general pharmocology of these drugs is dealt with in Chapter 14, and dose regimes are shown in Table 8.3. Elderly patients are unusually sensitive to diazepam and, if this drug is to be used in them, then the normal adult dose should be halved. Conversely, children show a degree of resistance to diazepam and should be prescribed a dose regime of 0.2 to 0.5 mg/kg of body weight (Trapp 1981). Unwanted effects of diazepam include dizziness, an

Table 8.3. Dose regimes of drugs used for oral sedation.

Drug	Adult Dose	Child Dose	Time of administration
Diazepam	5 mg	5–10 mg	5 mg at night 5 mg on wakening 5 mg 2 hours before dental procedure
Temazepam	10–30 mg	—	40–60 minutes prior to dental procedure
Lorazepam	1–5 mg	—	1–3 mg at night 1–5 mg, 2–6 hours before dental procedure
Trimeprazine tartrate	3–4.5 mg/kg	2–4 mg/kg	1–2 hours before dental procedure
Promethazine hydrochloride	—	6–12 months: 10 mg 1–5 years: 15–20 mg	1–2 hours prior to dental procedure
Triclofos sodium	1–2 g	1 year: 100–250 mg 1–5 years: 250–500 mg 6–12 years: 0.5–1 g	30 minutes before retiring to bed

increased awareness of painful stimuli, ataxia, and prolonged postoperative drowsiness.

Temazepam and lorazepam are both classified as sedative-hypnotics. They are especially useful in the anxious patient for ensuring undisturbed sleep before a dental appointment. Both drugs have a short half-life and there is little hangover effect.

Antihistamines

Some antihistamines (H$_1$-antagonists; see Chapter 4) cause drowsiness and sedation as unwanted effects, but they can also be used therapeutically for this purpose. Trimeprazine and promethazine are widely used as sedative agents especially in children; dosages are shown in Table 8.2. Both drugs also have anti-emetic properties. Trimeprazine is especially useful for out-patient sedation, but unwanted effects include persistent drowsiness, disturbed dreams, nasal stuffiness, and headache. Promethazine is less effective than trimeprazine as a sedative agent and may produce restlessness, irritability, and hallucinations.

Triclofos sodium

This is chemically related to chloral hydrate, both of which are discussed in Chapter 14. It is mainly used as a sedative/hypnotic in children, and dosages are shown in Table 8.2. Unwanted effects from triclofos sodium include drowsiness, dizziness, headache, and gastro-intestinal disturbances.

Intravenous sedation agents

The administration of sedative agents via the intravenous route is probably the most reliable and effective method of producing sedation. Furthermore, this route provides a rapid onset of action, and the dose of agent used can be titrated to each patient's needs. The disadvantage of intravenous sedation is the inability to reverse the actions of the drug once administerd. The technique also requires a certain amount of patient co-operation to allow venepuncture, hence this method is not suitable for young children. Intravenous sedation is particularly useful for the moderate to very anxious patient, and the physically and mentally handicapped.

Early pioneers of intravenous sedation were Jorgenson (see Jorgenson 1976) and Drummond-Jackson (see Drummond-Jackson 1967). Jorgenson's technique involved the intravenous administration of an incremental dose of pentobarbitone, followed by pethidine and hyoscine. Not only did the patients become sedated, but many fell asleep. This technique is rarely used now because it is slow and requires skilled training. When patients are asleep their protective reflexes may be reduced. Recovery from this sedation technique is very slow and so it is not suitable for out-patients.

Drummond-Jackson advocated the intravenous administration of incremental doses of methohexitone producing ultra-light anaesthesia. Much controversy surrounded the safety and efficacy of this technique, especially the use of the same person acting as operator/anaesthetist. This technique is condemned by anaesthetists as dangerous; it has been replaced with the advent of the benzodiazepines. Diazepam and midazolam are the most widely used intravenous sedation agents used in dentistry. As well as producing sedation, both drugs produce amnesia, which is especially useful for certain dental procedures (Greg *et al.* 1974).

Diazepam

Diazepam is available as a 5 mg/ml viscous solution, and as an emulsion preparation (Diazemuls[R]) for intravenous sedation. The drug is administered into a vein usually in the antecubital fossa. The solution should be injected slowly (5 mg/min) until the required level of sedation is achieved. During the period of injection, the patient's speech becomes slurred and there is ptosis of the upper eyelid (Verril's sign). Apnoea may occur during the onset of sedation and oxygen must always be available in case this problem presents. Normal adults usually require 5 to 20 mg; the duration of sedation is usually 45 to 60 minutes. Most patients can usually leave the dental surgery about 1 to 1.5 hrs after administration, but there is a rebound effect, where the patient may feel drowsy, which occurs 6 to 8 hours after dosage. This is probably due to the release of an active metabolite, desmethyl diazepam. Consequently, patients should always be accompanied and escorted home. They should not be allowed to drive or operate machinery during the 24 hours after intravenous diazepam.

Other unwanted effects arising from intravenous diazepam are pain at the site of injection, and sometimes thrombosis (Olesen and Huttel 1980) because the solution is irritant to the vein. This problem can be overcome by preparing the drug in an emulsified oil solvent (Diazemuls[R]; Rosenbaum 1982).

Midazolam

This is a new benzodiazepine that is water-soluble and may well replace diazepam as an intravenous sedation agent. The water solubility means there is less tendency for pain on injection and thrombophlebitis. In comparison to diazepam, midazolam has a shorter half-life (1.7 hours) and a shorter duration of action. Midazolam is 50 per cent more potent that diazepam and has a superior amnesic effect (Maisel 1980; see Chapter 14).

Combined intravenous preparations for sedation in dentistry

Over the years, it has become the practice of some operators to supplement intravenous sedation with benzodiazepines by adding a centrally acting analgesic such as pentazocine or pethidine. The rationale for this procedure is two-fold. Firstly, the opioids will potentiate the sedative properties of the benzodiazepines and the patient will therefore require a reduced dose of the latter. Secondly, when this sedation mixture is used for dental surgical procedures, the opioids may provide some degree of postoperative pain relief.

Opioids and benzodiazepines produce respiratory depression and deaths have occurred following the use of this sedation technique. It should also be noted that the efficacy of the opioids in postoperative dental pain is uncertain (Seymour and Walton 1982; 1984), and their use for this purpose is very questionable. With the new generation of benzodiazepines, there seems little point in supplementing sedation with other drugs that could be life-threatening.

Conclusions

Sedation techniques have had a tremendous impact on the practice of dentistry and patients' perception of dental treatment. There are some practitioners who never attempt sedation techniques and others who employ them all the time, whether they are required or not. It is important to realize that all sedation techniques have potential problems, and the drugs, if misused, can be life-threatening. A practitioner may consider him or herself competent at administering various sedation techniques, but must always have respect for the agents used. In all instances, emergency resuscitation equipment and drugs must be available to treat any unforeseen problem.

REFERENCES

Ames, J. A. L., Burman, J. F., Rees, G. M., Nancekievill, D. G., and Mollin, D. L. (1978). Megablastic hemopoiesis in patients receiving nitrous oxide. *Lancet*, **2**, 339–41.

Berkowitz, B. A., Fink, A. D., and Nga, S. H. (1977). Nitrous oxide analgesia: reversal by naloxone and development of tolerance. *Journal of Pharmacology and Experimental Therapeutics*, **203**, 539–47.

Brinkley, B. R. and Rao, P. N. (1973). Nitrous oxide: effects on the mitotic apparatus and chromosome movement in Hela cells. *Journal of Cell Biology*, **58**, 96–106.

Drummond-Jackson, S. L. (1967). Minimal incremental methohexitone in intravenous anaesthesia. In *Society for the Advancement of Anaesthesia in Dentistry* (3rd edn), p. 143. London.

Dundee, J. W. (1960). Alterations in response to somatic pain associated with anaesthesia. II. The effect of thiopentone and pentobarbitone. *British Journal of Anaesthesia*, **32**, 407–14.

Edmunds, D. H. and Rosen, M. (1983). Inhalation sedation. *Dental Update*, **10**, 469–76.

Greg, J. M., Ryan, D. E., and Levin, K. H. (1974). The amnesic actions of diazepam. *Journal of Oral Surgery*, **32**, 651–64.

Guedel, A. E. (1937). *Inhalation anaesthesia: a fundamental guide.* Macmillan, New York.

Hill, C. M. and Morris, P. J. (1983). *General anaesthesia and sedation in dentistry.* Wright, Bristol.

Jorgensen, N. B. (1976). Local anaesthesia and intravenous pre-medication. *Anaesthesia Progress*, **13**, 168–76.

Katz, R. L., Matteo, R. S., and Papper, E. M. (1962). The injection of epinephrine during general anaesthesia. II. Halothane. *Anaesthesiology*, **23**, 597–600.

Kripke, B. J., Kelman, A. D., Shah, N. K., Balogh, K., and Handler, A. H. (1976). Testicular reaction to prolonged exposure to nitrous oxide. *Anaesthesiology*, **44**, 104–13.

Layzer, R. B. (1978). Myeloneuropathy after prolonged exposure to nitrous oxide. *Lancet*, **ii**, 1222–30.

Maisel, G. M. (1980). Midazolam: second generation of benzodiazepines. *Anaesthesia Progress*, **27**, 159–60.

Olesen, A. S. and Huttel, M. S. (1980). Local reactions to I.V. diazepam in different formulations. *British Journal of Anaesthesia*, **52**, 609–11.

Rosenbaum, N. L. (1982). A new formulation of diazepam for intravenous sedation in dentistry: a clinical evaluation. *British Dental Journal*, **153**, 192–3.

Seymour, R. A. and Walton, J. G. (1982). Analgesic efficacy in dental pain. *British Dental Journal*, **153**, 291–7.

Seymour, R. A. and Walton, J. G. (1984). Pain control after third molar surgery. *International Journal of Oral Surgery*, **13**, 457–85.

Summary of the National Halothane Study. (1966). *Journal of the American Medical Association*, **197**, 775–88.

Trapp, L. D. (1981). Pharmacological management of pain and anxiety. In *Pediatric Dentistry* (ed. R. E. Stewart, T. K. Barber, K. C. Troutman and S. H. Y. Wei). Mosby. St. Louis.

The Wylie Report (1978). Report of the working party on training of dental anaesthetists. *British Dental Journal*, **151**, 385–7.

9

Antiseptics and disinfectants

AT one time antiseptics and disinfectants formed a major part of the dental students' teaching in dental pharmacology. Today they play a lesser role, but nevertheless an important one. Some of these substances are of great use in medicine and dentistry; the dental surgeon should be able to choose, from all those available, those with real advantages and, at the same time, appreciate their limitations. The prevention of cross-infection, and the use of antiseptics for this purpose, are referred to later in this chapter.

Many chemical substances kill bacteria. The use of phenol in operating theatres, associated historically with the name of Lister, introduced a new era into antisepsis. The trouble with most chemical agents is that in concentrations destructive to micro-organisms, they are also destructive to other living tissue.

TERMINOLOGY

Antiseptics are substances that kill or prevent the growth of micro-organisms; the term is generally applied to substances used on living tissues. In contrast, the term disinfectant is usually applied to substances used on inanimate objects. Disinfectants prevent infection by the destruction of pathogenic organisms, and are generally regarded as being bactericidal. The distinction between antiseptics and disinfectants is not so much that one group is bacteriostatic and the other bactericidal, but that the distinction is implicit in the way they are used. For instance, antiseptics are applied to living surfaces and, by preventing the growth and multiplication of organisms, they assist the natural defence mechanisms of the body. If the vitality of the micro-organisms can be reduced below a certain level, then these natural mechanisms will have a chance to repel the microbial invasion. Usually disinfectants are too toxic to be applied to living tissues; they not only kill off bacteria but also they kill healthy living tissue. Disinfectants are therefore used on objects, e.g. instruments—when, for instance, heat sterilization is not possible.

INDIVIDUAL ANTISEPTICS AND DISINFECTANTS

These will be considered under separate headings, those with similar chemical structures being grouped together.

Alcohols

Alcohol is a protoplasmic poison; it acts by precipitating the proteins of the protoplasm.

Ethyl alcohol and isopropyl alcohol are effective antibacterial agents and are used for disinfection of the skin, but alcohol is ineffective when applied to the oral mucosa. The curious thing is that alcohols are effective in concentrations of 50 to 70 per cent by weight, but higher concentrations are useless. The activity of other antiseptics, e.g. chlorhexidine, iodine (see later), is increased in the presence of alcohol.

Surgical spirit, which is a mixture of ethyl and methyl alcohols, is used for cleaning surgical surfaces.

Aldehydes

Formaldehyde

This has bactericidal activity against bacteria, fungi, and viruses. However, its action is very slow—in 0.5 per cent concentrations it would take about 12 hours to kill bacteria. Formaldehyde is usually used in 2 to 8 per cent concentrations as a means of disinfecting inanimate objects.

Glutaraldehyde

This aldehyde is much superior to formaldehyde as a sterilizing agent and acts against all micro-organisms, including viruses. It is much less volatile than formaldehyde and causes less odour. It is marketed as a useful preparation in a 2 per cent concentration. This is used for 'cold sterilization' of instruments. It is recommended for the treatment of articles that have been contaminated by hepatitis B virus (see below), and that cannot be heat sterilized. Exposure should be for at least 1 hour, but preferably for a longer period, e.g. up to 12 hours.

Chlorhexidine

Chlorhexidine (Hibitane) finds extensive use in medicine and in dentistry as an antiseptic and disinfectant. Many preparations are available, and a few are now listed:

1. *Hibiscrub ICI*—chlorhexidine gluconate 4 per cent in non-ionic detergent base. The solution is used for pre-operative preparation of skin, and for hand disinfection.

2. *Hibisol ICI*—chlorhexidine gluconate 0.5 per cent in isopropyl alcohol. This solution is used for disinfection of the skin and hands. It should be applied to clean dry skin/hands and rubbed briskly until dry.

3. *Corsodyl ICI*—chlorhexidine gluconate 1 per cent: dental gel (red). There is

also a Corsodyl Mouthwash, which is a chlorhexidine gluconate 0.2 per cent solution.

4. *Hibitane ICI*—chlorhexidine gluconate 1 per cent cream. Pre-operative preparation of hands and skin.

5. *Hibitane Concentrate*—chlorhexidine gluconate 5 per cent; used as a general purpose antiseptic.

Chlorhexidine is a highly effective agent against a wide variety of organisms, both Gram-positive and Gram-negative, but more particularly Gram-positive. It is especially effective when in alcoholic solution. It is non-irritant to the tissues in the recommended concentration, and is non-toxic. Chlorhexidine 0.5 per cent in 70 per cent alcohol is a useful solution for pre-operative skin preparation of both surgeons and patients. 'Hibiscrub' is also used for the same purposes. Chlorhexidine may also be used for storing sterile instruments.

A particular use for chlorhexidine has been found in dentistry (see Chapter 11). In 0.5 per cent solution in 70 per cent alcohol it is useful for sterilizing the mucosa prior to local anaesthetic injection. More importantly, the aqueous solution has been found to inhibit dental plaque formation. Daily mouth rinsing with a 0.2 per cent solution has been shown to inhibit the deposition of plaque, and this leads to a reduction in the amount of gingival inflammation. Unwanted effects, seemingly few, include some disturbance of taste, perhaps due to the unpleasant taste of the mouthwash. It also produces a staining of the teeth that is not all that easy to remove. Occasionally it is said to have induced swellings of the parotid glands. Although the long-term use of chlorhexidine does not seem to be accompanied by problems of a serious nature, perhaps its use would best be limited to short courses associated with current periodontal treatment. The reader is referred to modern textbooks on preventive dentistry for further information.

Dyes

These are complex organic substances, which are all derived in some way from coal tar, and they include the aniline dyes, gentian violet, and brilliant green. Also included are the acridine dyes, acriflavin and proflavine.

Gentian violet and brilliant green are effective against some Gram-positive organisms, but Gram-negative organisms are very resistant. Their effectiveness is decreased by the presence of pus and serum. Gentian violet is a fungicide and, prior to the introduction of the antifungal antimicrobials, was used in the treatment of oral thrush (acute candidiasis). It stains the tissues blue and is messy; with newer agents now available, it is no longer used.

Acriflavine and proflavine differ considerably from the aniline dyes in that they are active against Gram-negative as well as Gram-positive organisms, and they are not inactivated to any extent by organic matter. They may be used for application to superficial wounds.

Halogens

These substances are effective because they unite with proteins of bacteria and this chemical action is toxic.

Chlorine

This halogen is bactericidal, used in the disinfection of water and for disinfecting drains. In practice it is the hypochlorites that find particular use, and they exert their effect by liberating chlorine. Chlorine is inactivated by organic matter: it combines with the proteins of the tissues as well as with those of bacteria, with consequent rapid loss of its activity. In dentistry, a 2.5 per cent solution of sodium hypochlorite is used as an antiseptic irrigant of root canals, and is an effective solvent of necrotic tissues, e.g. the dead pulp. At one time this syringing was alternated with 5 to 10 volumes hydrogen peroxide and the final syringing done with saline solution. Care must be exercised to ensure that neither the hypochlorite solution nor the hydrogen peroxide get through the root apex where they would cause irritation, and hydrogen peroxide must not be sealed into a canal. Today, irrigation is generally by sodium hypochlorite alone.

Iodine

This acts as an antiseptic in much the same way as chlorine; it is bactericidal and is also a fungicide, but one difference is that it is not readily inactivated by organic matter. It is an effective agent in sterilization of the skin prior to surgery, when it is used in the form of weak iodine solution, 2.5 per cent iodine in potassium iodine, water, and alcohol. When painted on the skin this solution is said to produce a sterile area, in about five minutes, that lasts some time. Unfortunately, it does discolour the skin and just very occasionally causes hypersensitivity reactions. Weak solution of iodine was sometimes painted on inflamed gums when, supposedly, it acted as a counter-irritant.

Iodoform

This is mildly antiseptic due to slow liberation of iodine when applied to tissues. A number of preparations containing iodoform have been, or are still, used in dentistry; all have a strong, persistent, and characteristic smell. One such preparation is Whitehead's Varnish, which contains 10 per cent iodoform with benzoin, storax, and balsam of tolu in solvent ether. Whitehead's Varnish, usually incorporated into ribbon gauge, is used to treat infected sockets, and as a dressing after surgical removal of third molars and cysts. Another iodoform preparation, once very popular in dentistry, is Kri-Paste, which consists of Kri Liquid (40 per cent) and iodoform (60 per cent). Kri Liquid contains (approx.) parachlorphenol, 45 parts; camphor, 49 parts; and methanol, 6 parts. It was frequently used as a medicament to sterilize root canals, and the paste as a root-canal filler.

Iodophors

Are combinations of iodine and surface-active detergents, e.g. povidone–iodine. Povidone is a water-soluble polymer that seems to prolong the activity of many drugs, and does so with iodine by liberating it slowly from the complex. Such combinations are probably effective against most Gram-positive and Gram-negative organisms after about 15 seconds contact. They do not irritate or stain the skin. Povidone–iodine mouthwash (povidone–iodine, 1 per cent) is available, and may be used either undiluted or diluted with an equal volume of warm water as a mouthwash for mucosal infections.

Oxidizing agents

These act by liberating oxygen, which unites with proteins of bacteria, and also with tissue proteins. All the available oxygen is soon used up and the antiseptic action quickly exhausted.

Hydrogen peroxide

This oxidizing agent is a weak antiseptic; when brought into contact with living tissue it is decomposed into water and oxygen but it gives off its oxygen rapidly and so its germicidal action is limited. It has been used as a mild antiseptic mouthwash in the treatment of acute ulcerative gingivitis (15 ml of the 20 volume solution (approx 6 per cent) to a half tumbler full of warm water). Its use in this form of gingivitis was advocated because of the anaerobic nature of the infection. Apart from its antiseptic properties, hydrogen peroxide exerts a mechanical cleansing action through the effervescence produced by the liberation of the oxygen. A stronger solution of hydrogen peroxide (30 per cent aqueous solution) is used to bleach discoloured root-filled teeth.

Sodium perborate

In solution this may also be used in the treatment of acute ulcerative gingivitis, for it too liberates oxygen when in contact with organic matter. 'Bocasan' (buffered sodium peroxyborate monohydrate) is said by the manufacturers to release far more effervescent oxygen than ordinary sodium perborate.

Phenols, cresols, and their derivatives

Phenol

As mentioned in the Introduction to this chapter, phenol is associated with the pioneering work of Lister in the field of antiseptics. As an antiseptic it has now been largely superseded by less toxic chemicals. It was often used as liquified phenol, which is phenol 80 per cent in water. Its action on micro-organisms is largely due to the fact that it is more soluble in lipids and proteins than in water.

Consequently it leaves a watery medium and concentrates on the microbial bodies. There is significance in this differential solubility, for oily phenolic preparations are virtually valueless as antiseptics. When applied to the skin or mucous membranes in weak or moderately weak solutions, phenol produces some feeling of anaesthesia as it does have a depolarizing local anaesthetic action. It is this 'anaesthetic' property that made it popular as an ingredient of mouthwashes. If a strong solution is applied to the skin it is irritant and caustic, producing a burning pain. The area of skin will show a white slough if the application of the strong phenol is prolonged; this local action is due to the precipitation of proteins. Phenol is not firmly held in the protein precipitate and is thus capable of quite deep percutaneous penetration.

Camphorated paramonochlorphenol (CMCP)

This is a 35 per cent solution of parachlorphenol in camphor and has been widely used as a medicament in root canals. The pronounced disinfectant property of this preparation depends on the liberation of chlorine in the presence of phenol, the chlorine replacing one of the hydrogen atoms in phenol. It is comparatively non-irritant. A commonly used antiseptic today is a 1 per cent aqueous parachlorphenol solution.

Cresol

This has about three times the bactericidal potency of phenol and is about as toxic. However, metacresyl acetate (Cresatin) is a cresol that is used as a chemical antiseptic for the irrigation of root canals. It is not irritant to the periapical tissues and has an anodyne effect on residual pulp tissue.

Chloroxylenols

These are less effective against microbes than other phenolic agents and what activity they do have is considerably reduced in the presence of organic matter. Dettol (about 5 per cent chloroxylenol) is a well-known preparation. Solutions of chloroxylenol are often so ineffective that they are liable to be contaminated by one pathogen, namely *Pseudomonas pyocyanea*; indeed the growth of this organism may be encouraged by such solutions.

Hexachlorophane

This is very effective against Gram-positive cocci and is an excellent surface disinfectant. Preparations containing hexachlorophane are used on the skin prior to surgery, and as a pre-surgical hand cream. Hexachlorophane is not very irritant to the tissues but neurotoxic effects have been reported as a result of absorption following its application to babies in dusting powders. This problem may have related to the widespread application of the powder, particularly on raw skin surfaces.

Surface-acting agents

These alter surface tension; they have both fat- and water-soluble groups in the same molecule. They are variously classified, the classification depending on the electric charge on the water-soluble group—cationic, positive charge; anionic, negative charge; amphoteric, positive and negative charges; and non-ionic, that is un-ionized. Non-ionic forms have little activity, but the others all have some degree of antibacterial activity, the cationic agents being the most effective. These substances are very active detergents, but are really only weak antiseptics.

Some cationic surface-active agents have attracted interest; these are the quaternary ammonium compounds, a few examples of which include:

(1) *cetrimide (Cetavlon)*—used as an aqueous or as an alcoholic solution for skin disinfection and cleansing of wounds;

(2) *Benzalkonium chloride (Roccal)*—1 per cent solution used as pre-operative skin preparation.

The quaternary ammonium compounds are incompatible with soaps and are inhibited by organic matter. Sometimes these agents are combined with other substances: for instance, chlorhexidine gluconate 1.5 per cent and cetrimide 15 per cent in a solution called Savlon Concentrate, which is used for general antisepsis. They are poor antiseptics, but are used as anti-plaque agents in dentistry (see Chapter 11).

THE DENTAL USES OF ANTISEPTICS

These can be summarized as follows:

(1) skin preparation before surgery or injection;

(2) pre-operative preparation of the oral mucosa;

(3) sometimes as an ingredient of dentifrices;

(4) inhibition of dental plaque;

(5) cleaning of operating areas;

(6) the 'cold' sterilization of instruments and equipment (where 'heat' sterilization is impractical);

(7) storage of sterilized surgical equipment;

(8) preparation of the surgeon's hands;

(9) irrigation of root canals in endodontics.

ASTRINGENTS

These are substances that are said to precipitate proteins in superficial cells and thereby form a protective layer against irritants and bacterial invasion. This layer is also supposed to inhibit exudation of leucocytes and serum. There is much doubt about the efficacy of astringents; their effect is mainly subjective, merely causing the mucous membranes to feel shrunken and shrivelled.

Astringents are classified into two groups:

(1) the soluble salts of heavy metals, e.g. iron, lead, zinc, copper, aluminium, silver, and mercury;

(2) the vegetable astringents.

Metallic astringents

The zinc salts are the main components of this group; for example, zinc sulphate and zinc chloride mouthwash. It has been suggested that although the so-called astringent action of zinc mouthwashes may have little or no value, perhaps zinc salts themselves are helpful in promoting healing. Although such mouthwashes have been used in the healing of ulcers, their value is doubtful.

Silver nitrate is an astringent antiseptic that found much favour in dentistry at one time. Its astringent action is powerful but superficial, so concentrated solutions are caustic but not penetrating. A 10 per cent solution of silver nitrate has been used to reduce the sensitivity of dentine exposed at the necks of teeth. The solution is burnished into the exposed tissue by means of a plastic instrument. Even if this is effective, the solution stains and is not suitable for anterior teeth.

Vegetable astringents

Tannic acid is the example of a vegetable astringent. At one time it was used in dentistry in powder form as a haemostatic, the powder being applied to the bleeding tooth socket and covered with a gauze pack. It was also a constituent of some mouthwashes, but this substances no longer finds favour in dentistry as it is ineffective.

CAUSTICS

A number of substances, when concentrated, act as caustics, e.g. zinc chloride, zinc sulphate, silver nitrate, phenol, chromic acid. Trichloracetic acid is perhaps still of some interest in dentistry as a caustic. Sometimes a small amount placed beneath a gum flap with college tweezers will relieve the discomfort of a mild pericoronitis. It does so by simply destroying sensory nerve endings.

HEPATITIS AND AIDS

It seems appropriate to discuss these two diseases together and within this Chapter on antiseptics because the use of certain antiseptics is recommended in precautionary procedures when treating such patients.

Hepatitis B (serium hepatitis)

The hepatitis B virus (HBV) produces a number of serological markers; for instances the Dane particle is composed of, amongst other things, a surface antigen designated as HBsAG. This is detectable in patients with acute hepatitis and has usually disappeared from the serum in about six weeks from the onset of clinical jaundice. However, in some 4 to 5 per cent of patients, the HBsAG antigen can be detected many months after the onset of the illness, and these patients become chronic carriers. Another antigen from hepatitis B is the e antigen designated as HBeAG, and this is only found in HBsAG-positive serum.

Another group infected with the virus do not develop overt symptoms and the subclinical picture is not associated with jaundice; the majority so infected fall into this group. The carrier state is more likely to develop in those with a subclinical infection rather than in those who have had an acute infection.

Most patients with acute hepatitis B recover within a few weeks without ill consequences, but some may develop cirrhosis of the liver and a small percentage may eventually develop hepatocellular carcinoma.

Certain patients (and staff) are predisposed to become carriers of this disease and form a 'risk' group; these include:

(1) those frequently receiving blood products, e.g. haemophiliacs;

(2) those who, for whatever reason, have a defective immune response, e.g. on immunosuppressive drugs (including transplant patients) or who are immunodeficient;

(3) intravenous drug abusers;

(4) patients or staff in long-stay institutions, especially for the mentally handicapped;

(5) those undergoing haemodialysis;

(6) staff in renal dialysis units;

(7) the sexually promiscuous, particularly male homosexuals;

(8) patients from certain parts of the world where there is a high incidence of the disease, e.g. Asia and Africa;

(9) the tattooed individual.

Serum hepatitis is more likely to occur in those constantly exposed to blood or blood products, a category which must include dental surgeons. The disease is transmitted by blood and saliva. Most carriers of the virus will be unaware that they are carriers. The British Dental Association (BDA) suggests that all dental clinical staff should be immunized against hepatitis B, as an effective vaccine is available, which can be provided by a General Medical Practitioner under the National Health Service.

AIDS (acquired immunodeficiency syndrome)

A great deal of attention has been given to this disease, and to those who are infected with the human immunodeficiency virus (HIV). The public are alarmed about AIDS and, considering the likely mortality produced by the infection, this is understandable. AIDS is the name given to a group of disorders in which there is a serious cell-mediated immunodeficiency. Because of this deficiency, it is not surprising that sufferers tend to acquire various opportunistic infections, such as candidosis(-iasis) and, particularly, the otherwise rare *Pneumocystis carinii* pneumonia.

A characteristic of the disease is the long incubation period, varying from a few months to perhaps years. The full-blown picture of AIDS is often preceded by various syndromes, the most common being a persistent generalized lympha-denopathy accompanied by malaise, low-grade pyrexia, and weight loss. Oral candidosis may be an early feature, and the dental surgeon must recognize that this may be a pointer to the presence of the disease. Once AIDS is fully manifest, then opportunistic infections and/or malignant neoplasms are characteristic. A high percentage of patients have *Pneumocystis* pneumonia and Kaposi's sarcoma, a rare, usually cutaneous, tumour which may also be an early oral manifestation of AIDS, forming a red patch or nodule, often on the hard palate. Herpes simplex infections are often present, and are persistent and severe. The AIDS virus infects the brain and this may well lead to dementia.

The risk groups for AIDS are not dissimilar to those for hepatitis B. Throughout Britain, at the time of writing, the main risk groups are promiscuous homosexual or bisexual men, intravenous drug abusers, and haemophiliacs. The risk of transmitting AIDS appears to be low, the disease being less readily acquired than hepatitis B. Although the virus is present in saliva, transmission of the disease from this source is uncertain. Transmission is essentially through receptive anal intercourse, and by the administration of infected blood or blood products.

For both hepatitus B and AIDS, the practical aim in dentistry is to avoid cross-infection in the surgery, and to provide a safe environment for both patient and dental personnel. 'The Problems of Cross-infection in Dentistry' were considered by a BDA workshop convened on 27 November 1985 to look at the whole problem. The recommendations of the working party were considered under two headings: Appendix 1—Control of Cross Infection in Routine Dental Practice; and Appendix 2—Dental Treatment of Patients Carrying Blood-borne Viruses including Hepatitis B and HTLV III (AIDS). These BDA workshop recommenda-tions are stated below. (Published by kind permission of the Editor of the British Dental Journal).

Control of cross-infection in routine dental practice (Appendix 1)

Every member of the dental team has a duty to ensure that all necessary steps are taken to prevent cross-infection to protect both their patients and themselves.

While special precautions are recommended when treating patients known to be carrying blood-borne diseases such as hepatitis B and HTLV III, many patients will not have been identified and the only safe approach is to assume that any patient may be a carrier. It is necessary to strike a balance between cumbersome 'perfect' procedures and a reasonable approach which is practical while minimizing the hazards to a point where they present a negligible risk.

The following recommendations for procedures in routine dental practice are made in the light of current knowledge and may be subject to alteration and updating as further information becomes available.

1. Medical history

A thorough medical history should be taken for all patients and up-dated at subsequent examinations. The use of medical history sheets and questionnaires is recommended but they must be supported by direct questioning and discussion with the patient.

2. Cleaning of instruments

All instruments should be cleaned thoroughly before sterilization and all visible deposits must be removed. Ultrasonic cleaners are recommended for small instruments.

Gloves of the heavy duty ('kitchen') type should be worn. Great care should be taken when handling sharp instruments.

3. Sterilization of instruments

Sterilization procedures must be effective against all known pathogens. The method of choice for all instruments is an autoclave which reaches a temperature of 134°C for a minimum of 3 min. Hot air ovens may also be used at a temperature of 160°C for a minimum of 60 min. Hot air ovens should be of the type which ensures an uninterrupted timed cycle with an automatic locking device on the door. Boiling water is *not* an effective method for sterilizing instruments in dental practice. Its use should be discontinued.

Cold sterilizing solutions are not suitable for routine use and should only be employed when the instrument cannot be exposed to heat. The instrument must be scrupulously clean and the manufacturer's instructions followed precisely.

All instruments and equipment likely to be contaminated with blood should be sterilized, including aspirator tips and beakers where these are not disposable.

Some dental instruments, including handpieces, have been difficult to sterilize. Handpieces which can be autoclaved are now available and should be used.

4. Disposables

The general use of disposables, including aspirator tips, impression trays and beakers, is recommended whenever possible.

Disposable needles should always be used. They must *never* be re-used for another patient. Similarly, part-used local anaesthetic cartridges may contain blood from the patient and they must *never* be used for a second patient. Towels for hand drying should be disposable or of the roller type which presents a fresh section of towel each time it is used.

5. Surgery surfaces

The bracket table or similar working surface may accumulate infective material. The best solution is to use a system of sterilizable trays or, failing that, a disposable covering. Work surfaces should be cleaned and dried with a solution of 70 per cent isopropyl alcohol. If there is visible blood or pus, the surface should be cleaned with a disposable cloth and disinfected with hypochlorite solution containing 1 per cent available chlorine or, if the surface is metal, with 2 per cent glutaraldehyde. The solution should be left for a minimum of 3 minutes and the surface rinsed and dried. This routine should be followed at the end of each working session even in the absence of a spillage of blood. Equipment should be chosen which is easy to clean.

6. Personal protection

The dental profession has been unique in not taking precautions to prevent contact between patients' blood and unprotected skin. There is much to recommend the routine use of operating gloves for all dentists and close-support dental surgery assistants. They should certainly be worn whenever there is any likelihood of the hands coming into contact with blood. The gloved hands may be washed between patients using a proprietary handwash.

Cuts and abrasions should be kept covered with waterproof dressings at all times even if gloves are worn.

Protective glasses should be worn by operators, close-support dental surgery assistants and patients to protect the eyes against the splatter which may occur during cavity preparation, scaling and the cleaning of instruments.

It is recommended that a well-fitting face mask is worn during high-speed cavity preparation, when using an ultrasonic scaler or undertaking surgical procedures.

Particular care should be taken to avoid needlestick injuries, especially if local anaesthetic needles are resheathed.

Vaccination gives safe and effective protection against hepatitis B and it is recommended for all dental staff.

7. Aspiration and ventilation

The use of efficient high-speed aspirators which exhaust externally will reduce the risk of cross-infection from aerosols. This risk is further reduced by good ventilation. Aspirators should be cleaned regularly in accordance with the manufacturers instructions.

8. Disposal of waste

Sharp items, including needles and scalpels, and local anaesthetic cartridges should be placed in a rigid 'safe' container. Great care should be taken to avoid needlestick injuries. Other items, such as napkins and cotton wool rolls, should be consigned to stout plastic bags which are sealed before disposal.

Heavy duty gloves should be worn.

The collection and incineration of surgical waste should be arranged locally.

Needles, local anaesthetic cartridges and other surgical waste must *never* be dumped on a normal refuse tip.

9. Laboratory items

Impressions and appliances should be rinsed thoroughly before sending to the laboratory. Disposable impression trays are recommended. Technicians should be encouraged to wear gloves when handling impressions and pouring models.

10. Training

All dental staff should be trained thoroughly and should understand the policies adopted in the practice for the prevention of cross-infection. Particular attention should be given to the training of new members of staff. All procedures should be reviewed from time to time to ensure that they are being carried out correctly.

Dental treatment for patients carrying blood-borne viruses including Hepatitis B and HTLV III (Appendix 2)

Patients who are ill with hepatitis B or AIDS should normally receive dental treatment under hospital conditions.

Patients who are known, or may be presumed, to be infectious but are otherwise well may be treated in normal dental practice. The majority of carriers of these and other blood-borne viral diseases are not identified and many receive routine dental treatment each day. The treatment of known carriers would not add materially to the hazards of practice, and they should therefore be treated by general dental practitioners as a matter of course. It should be remembered that the transmissibility of HTLV III is low and there is little risk to health-care workers. It is not necessary to make any special arrangements for waiting rooms or other non-clinical areas.

It is unlikely to be possible for dentists to be informed of the names of all patients who may be carriers, and in some cases the passage of this information is further constrained by the need for confidentiality which is a legal requirement in the case of sexually transmitted diseases. It is therefore essential that a careful history is taken and that the approach to patients enables them to disclose sensitive information. Known carriers are counselled to inform their dentist and the response they receive will determine whether or not they continue to disclose their carrier state. A dentist should regard it as a privilege to be informed and should express gratitude for the information. Any unsympathetic response or a failure to provide treatment is likely to lead to concealment in the future. Confidentiality must be preserved and the information restricted to those members of staff who need to know.

Clinical procedures that minimize exposure to actually or potentially infectious material, including blood, must be employed routinely and all dentists should follow the guidelines in Appendix 1. The following additional precautions are recommended when treating patients known to be carriers of hepatitis B and HTLV III.

1. The appointment should normally be arranged at the end of the day. All the procedures for the control of cross-infection and for personal protection listed in Appendix 1 *must* be used. Protective eyewear, masks and gloves are essential

during treatment and when handling contaminated instruments and materials. Gowns, preferably disposable, should be worn.

2. All instruments, including handpieces, must be sterilizable or disposable. Freshly prepared 2% glutaraldehyde can be used, if necessary, for instruments which cannot be autoclaved. They should be soaked in glutaraldehyde for 1 hour before thorough cleaning and then left in fresh glutaraldehyde for a further period of 3 hours.

3. Aerosols should be minimized by the use of a high-volume aspirator which vents externally. Ultrasonic scalers should be avoided.

High-speed drills should not be used for patients known to be HBeAG positive unless the staff involved in providing treatment have been vaccinated. There is no evidence to suggest an infection risk from the use of high-speed drills when treating carriers of HTLV III.

4. Contaminated working surfaces or blood splashes elsewhere should be physically cleaned and swabbed with hypochlorite solution (1% available chlorine) left in contact for 30 minutes or, if metal, with 2% glutaraldehyde which is left in contact with the surface for 3 hours. The surface should then be rinsed and dried.

5. Aspirators should be flushed with 2% glutaraldehyde and the solution left in the system collector for 3 hours.

6. Impressions should be taken in a silicone-based material. These and any appliances should be placed in 2% glutaraldehyde for 1 hour. They should be rinsed and soaked in fresh solution for at least 3 hours before being sent to the laboratory.

7. Great care must be taken to avoid needlestick injuries. In the event of accidental innoculation or contamination of the eyes or mouth, the affected part should be washed with running water. The accident should be reported immediately and medical advice sought. The District Medical or Dental Officer will be able to provide information on the appropriate local contacts.

8. All disposable materials must be placed in plastic bags (sharp items in rigid 'safe' containers), labelled in accordance with local practice and incinerated.

9. Non-disposable laundry items such as towels may be safely washed in a washing machine with a cycle which holds the temperature at 90°C for a period of 10 minutes.

10. General anaesthetics should be avoided if at all possible. If general anaesthesia is essential, reference should be made to the guidance to anaesthetists provided by the Department of Health.

11. *Further information* The British Dental Journal book *Viral Hepatitis, AIDS and Dental Treatment* by R. C. W. Dinsdale is recommended as a source of more detailed information and advice. It contains many references to other published reports on the subject and may be obtained from Professional and Scientific Publications at BMA House, Tavistock Square, London WC1H 9JR, price £2.50.

Further advice is contained in:

1. Report of the Expert Group on Hepatitis in Dentistry London, HMSO, 1979.

2. Acquired Immune Deficiency Syndrome. London: DHSS

 (i) General Information for Doctors, 1985;

 (ii) Information for Doctors concerning the Introduction of the HTLV III Antibody Test, 1985;

 (iii) Guidance for Surgeons, Anaesthetists and Dentists, 1986.

The real point at issue is that many patients who are carriers of the blood-borne infections discussed above will not be identified as carriers. The recommendations of the working party as contained under Appendix 1 are aimed at making routine treatments in dental practice as safe as possible, without creating too burdensome surgery procedures.

FURTHER READING

Babajews, A., Poswillo, D. E., and Griffin, G. E. (1985). Acquired immune deficiency syndrome presenting as recalcitrant Candida. *British Dental Journal*, **159**, 106–8.

BDA Dental Health and Science Committee Workshop (1986). The problems of cross-infection in dentistry. *British Dental Journal*, **160**, 131–4.

Bystrom, A. and Sundqvist, G. (1985). The antibacterial action of sodium hypochlorite and EDTA in 60 cases of endodontic therapy. *International Endodontic Journal*, **18**, 35–40.

Field, A. E. and Martin, M. V. (1986). Handwashing: soap or disinfectant. *British Dental Journal*, **160**, 278–80.

Greenspan, D., Greenspan, J. S., Pindborg, J. J., and Schiodt, M. (1986). *AIDS and the Dental Team*, (1st edn). Munksgaard, Copenhagen.

Howell, R. A. (1980). Bleaching discoloured root-filled teeth. *British Dental Journal*, **148**, 159–62.

Leading article (1985). AIDS: safeguards, not Panic. *British Dental Journal*, **158**, 195.

Leading article (1986). Infection Control—changes Needed. *British Dental Journal*, **160**, 109.

MacFarlane, T. W. and Follett, E. A. C. (1986). Serum hepatitis: a significant risk in the dental care of the mentally handicapped. *British Dental Journal*, **160**, 386–8.

Matthews, R. (1987). Cross-infection—the phoney war? *Dental Practice*, **25**, 1–3.

Matthews, R. W., Hislop, W. S., and Scully, C. (1986). The prevalence of hepatitis B markers in high-risk dental out-patients. *British Dental Journal*, **161**, 294–6.

Matthews, R. W., Scully, C., and Dowell, T. B. (1986). Acceptance of hepatitis B vaccine by dental practitioners in the United Kingdom. *British Dental Journal*, **161**, 371–3.

Mentz, T. C. F. (1982). The use of sodium hypochlorite as a general endodontic medicament. *International Endodontic Journal*, **15**, 132–6.

Richards, J. M. (1985). Notes on AIDS. *British Dental Journal*, **158**, 199–201.

Samaranayake, L. P. and Lewis, M. A. O. (1985). AIDS and the dental practitioner. *Dental Update*, **12**, 551–62.

Scully, C. (1985). Hepatitis B: an update in relation to dentistry. *British Dental Journal*, **159**, 321–8.

Scully, C., Cawson, R. A., and Porter, S. R. (1986). Acquired immune deficiency syndrome: a review. *British Dental Journal*, **161**, 53–60.

Wray, D., Moody, G. H., and McMillan, A. (1986). Oral 'Hairy' Leukoplakia in a male homosexual with persistent lymphadenopathy syndrome: report of two cases. *British Dental Journal*, **161**, 338–9.

10

Antimicrobials

INTRODUCTION

CHEMOTHERAPEUTIC agents are substances that are used to kill micro-organisms or neoplastic cells. This chapter will be concerned with antimicrobial drugs, which are agents used against micro-organisms, and with the principles underlying their use. The term antibiotic refers to substances produced by micro-organisms that, in high dilution, will prevent the growth of, or kill, other micro-organisms. As many antibiotics are now synthesized, this restricted meaning may be somewhat academic.

Until the advent of the sulphonamides in 1935, the search for systemic chemotherapeutic agents to treat infection had met with little success. The sulphonamides heralded an era that has been prolific in the discovery of new substances capable of acting against infective organisms. Great successes can be claimed for the use of penicillin in the treatment of infections with haemolytic streptococci. On the other hand, the number of substances available for use against viral agents is somewhat limited.

The object of chemotherapy is to kill or to prevent the multiplication of invading organisms, with minimal damage to the host. Valuable though powerful chemotherapeutic agents are, they can also produce unwanted effects in the individual and the community. It is clearly important that they be used with discrimination. Although it is impossible to make definitive rules for the prescribing of chemotherapeutic agents, there are certain guiding principles.

GENERAL PRINCIPLES OF TREATMENT

Diagnosis

There must be some clear indication that chemotherapy is necessary. It is indefensible to prescribe antimicrobials for conditions not due to infection; nor indeed should trivial and self-limiting infections be treated with antimicrobial drugs.

Choice of drug

Ideally this should depend on bacteriological identification of the causative organisms, and sensitivity tests to establish the susceptibility of the particular organism to the antimicrobial of obvious choice. In dental practice, such specialist services are not usually available and are mostly unnecessary. Clinical experience has shown that most acute infections in dentistry respond to a limited range of antimicrobial agents, e.g. penicillin, and so the choice is dictated through clinical experience. Exceptions to this general statement will be discussed later. It should be kept in mind that severe infections should not be treated without bacteriological assistance, a position that has been well summed up by O'Grady (1973) in the following words:

Blind treatment of severe infections without bacteriological assistance, and delay of treatment while the wheels of the bacteriological machine slowly turn, are both wrong. Adequate specimens should always be obtained before therapy of dangerous infections begins. However, treatment should then be instituted with what appears to be the most appropriate agent.

Dosage and route of administration

The object of treatment is to maintain a sufficiently high concentration of the drug in the infected tissues for as long as is required to overcome the infection. The actual concentration in the blood may not be so directly important except in the case of septicaemia, endocarditis, or osteomyelitis, when blood levels need to be high. In order to achieve effective tissue levels it may be necessary, when a drug is excreted rapidly, to administer it frequently so that tissue levels can equilibrate with blood levels. A good example of this is the use of benzylpenicillin, which has a half-life of less than one hour. On the other hand, some antimicrobials, e.g. gentamicin, may accumulate and dose intervals should be altered appropriately.

The duration of therapy depends on several factors, not least being the precise nature of the infection and the response to treatment. Patients should be impressed with the importance of adhering to the therapeutic regime advocated and of not discontinuing treatment at their own discretion. Treatment should be continued until the infection is overcome, and the early response should be monitored. In general terms, in dentistry, if there is no response to treatment within 48 to 72 hours, the antibacterial substance is unlikely to prove effective. This would suggest wrong diagnosis or the choice of the wrong antimicrobial.

In dentistry, systemic antimicrobials are usually given orally or by intramuscular injection. In hospitals, antimicrobials are often administered by the intravenous route, either by slow injection or infusion. Where there is a choice, administration by injection is to be preferred in severe infections as absorption is likely to be more certain and it produces a more immediate effect. Sometimes treatment, or prophylaxis, is started by injection and followed up by oral administration.

Use of antimicrobial agents in renal failure

When it is essential to prescribe an antimicrobial agent in the presence of renal disease, it is mandatory to consider what effect any impairment of renal function may have on the dose regime to be employed. For those drugs that are excreted predominantly by the kidney it may be necessary to modify therapy under these circumstances. If such a problem is encountered by the dental surgeon the matter should be discussed with the medical practitioner. Some antimicrobials should be avoided altogether in the presence of renal impairment.

Antimicrobials to be avoided wherever possible, or where their dosage should be monitored carefully, include cephaloridine, chloramphenicol, neomycin, nalidixic acid, nitrofurantoin, sulphadiazine, tetracyclines (except doxycycline and minocycline), and parenterally administered vancomycin.

Antimicrobials (detailed later) where dosage should be reduced include cephalosporins, cotrimoxazole, amoxycillin, ampicillin, trimethoprim, and others. Examples where a major dosage adjustment (reduction) will be required, and where serum concentrations need to be monitored, include gentamicin, kanamycin, streptomycin, and amphotericin B (if used systemically).

Antimicrobials (detailed below) listed in the *Dental Practitioners' Formulary 1986–88* should be modified as follows:

Acyclovir	—reduce dosage
Amoxycillin	—reduce dosage
Ampicillin	—reduce dosage
Benzylpenicillin	—max. 6 g daily when GFR < 10
Cephalexin	—max. 500 mg daily when GFR < 10
Cephadrine	—reduce dosage
Co-trimoxazole	—max. 960 mg daily when GFR < 10
Lincomycin	—use clindamycin instead
Tetracyclines (except doxycycline and minocycline)	—avoid

GFR = Glomerular filtration rate; this indicates the degree of renal impairment.

Published by kind permission of The Pharmaceutical Society of Great Britain.

The reason why the plasma levels of some drugs should be monitored is simply to keep them within safe limits, especially when there is a very serious risk of ototoxicity, as may occur with streptomycin, for example.

Use of antimicrobial agents in liver disease

As many drugs are metabolized in the liver, prescribing of drugs in general should be kept to a minimum in the presence of liver disease. Clindamycin is the only antimicrobial listed in the *Dental Practitioners' Formulary* where the dose should be reduced. This is not to imply that other antimicrobials outside of that Formulary would not similarly require modification. For instance, the use of a particular preparation of erythromycin (see below), namely the estolate, is liable to cause idiosyncratic hepatotoxicity, and may cause jaundice in the absence of liver disease when used for a long period.

Accompanying treatment

Antimicrobials are not a substitute for necessary surgery; where pus is present, drainage should be established. It is unjustifiable to rely on antibiotics alone when drainage is obviously required; to do so may cause the formation of a tumour-like cold abscess surrounded by fibrous tissue. In many instances, drainage of an infected area will suffice in itself without recourse to antimicrobials.

Combination of drugs

Antimicrobial drugs are basically classified as bacteriostatic or bactericidal: bacteriostatic drugs inhibit the multiplication of organisms, and bactericidal drugs kill them. Some bacteriostatic drugs exhibit bactericidal activity when used in high concentrations, e.g. erythromycin. Drug combinations can sometimes reduce the development of resistant strains of organisms, a well-known example being the use of streptomycin and isoniazid together in the treatment of tuberculosis. Used alone, resistance quickly develops to either of these drugs, but is much reduced when they are combined. However, combined drug therapy is not always beneficial, and may indeed be harmful. For example, many bactericidal drugs only kill rapidly multiplying cells and, in the presence of a bacteriostatic agent, their killing effect is antagonized (e.g. penicillin in the presence of tetracyclines). Such combinations should be avoided.

Topical administration

The principal arguments against the topical use of antibiotics are:

(1) the risk of sensitizing the patient;
(2) the risk of development of resistant strains.

It is generally agreed that antimicrobials for topical use should be selected from those that are unlikely to be used systemically, possibly because they are not absorbed or because they are liable to produce unwanted effects. Common examples are neomycin and polymyxin B. Nevertheless, the topical use of antifungal agents (e.g. nystatin) has proved most valuable in dentistry; their usage will be considered later.

Previous hypersensitivity

If a patient gives a history of hypersensitivity to any particular antimicrobial agent, then drugs of similar structure should not be administered because of the likelihood of cross-allergenicity. Some patients provide doubtful evidence of previous reactions, but it would be unwise to ignore the history however seemingly improbable. Drug hypersensitivity reactions are more likely to occur in patients with an allergic diathesis.

INDICATIONS FOR THE USE OF SYSTEMIC CHEMOTHERAPEUTIC AGENTS IN DENTISTRY

Treatment of infections

Chemotherapeutic agents should not be used in the normally healthy patient for minor infections that are likely to respond to treatment by other means, or are self-limiting. Needless to say, if local measures appear to be inadequate, or in the presence of severe infection, antimicrobial therapy should be instituted. A number of indications for the use of antimicrobials in dental practice are indicated below:

(1) In severe acute ulcerative gingivitis, especially if there are signs of systemic involvement (e.g. pyrexia and lymphadenopathy). In less severe cases, but where systemic chemotherapy is deemed necessary, metronidazole is the drug of choice.

(2) In severe infections of dental origin, e.g. cellulitis, acute osteomyelitis, severe pericoronitis, and deep infections implanted by local anaesthesia.

(3) In sinus infection complicating oro-antral fistula.

General prophylaxis

Antimicrobials may be used prophylactically in an attempt to prevent infection following surgery. There is no overwhelming evidence to suggest that such prophylaxis will prevent postoperative infection, although there are circumstances where it is generally agreed that such chemoprophylaxis should be provided. Of course, the situation is different when the patient has some underlying medical condition, but even then the exact position of chemoprophylaxis is uncertain. However, prophylactic antimicrobials may be considered for:

(1) Debilitated patients who are to have surgery, e.g. those with severe anaemia, blood dyscrasias, or diabetes—some diabetic patients show a lessened resistance to infection, and this is especially true of uncontrolled diabetes mellitus;

(2) Patients who have had radiation to the jaws and for whom, unfortunately, oral surgical procedures are required—any irradiated area must be considered as having lowered vitality and poor resistance to infection;

(3) Patients on prolonged steroid therapy for whom surgery is to be undertaken—prolonged steroid therapy weakens natural defence mechanisms against infection (see Chapter 18) but antimicrobial cover is certainly not

required for all such patients, and much will depend on circumstances at the time (e.g. the extent of the operation);

(4) transplant patients who require oral surgical procedures, as they will be receiving an immunosuppressant drug, e.g. cyclosporin, steroids, or azathioprine, and could therefore be liable to infection.

It must be emphasized that the prophylactic use of antimicrobials to prevent postoperative infection is an uncertain measure, even in the conditions listed above. If used, the agent of choice should be given just prior to surgery in order to allow peak plasma concentrations to be reached at the time of operation. The cover should be continued for three to seven days; exactly how long must depend on the clinical judgement of the operator.

DRUG RESISTANCE

Antimicrobial drugs are not active against all micro-organisms; each has its own spectrum of activity that depends to a large degree on its mechanism of action. The phenomenon whereby certain micro-organisms are resistant to a particular antimicrobial agent, referred to as drug resistance, is an important and complex one. Various mechanisms may be concerned with the development of drug resistance in the therapeutic use of antimicrobial agents. These will be considered under three main headings—selection, mutation, and transmission.

Therapeutic selection

In certain instances a bacterial population will consist of some strains that are naturally resistant to a particular drug and others that are sensitive. In the course of therapy the sensitive strains are eliminated leaving the resistant strains to flourish. The strains may be resistant because they are drug-tolerant or drug-destroying. Drug-tolerant bacteria are able to grow in the presence of an antibiotic; sometimes these may actually become physically dependent upon the antimicrobial. Drug-destroying bacteria are able to grow in the presence of the drug because they possess mechanisms that inactivate it. The main example of this type is the penicillinase-producing staphylococcus.

Mutation

It seems beyond dispute that the exposure of certain organisms to certain antimicrobials leads to a degree of drug resistance. In the early days of antimicrobial therapy it was generally believed that the development of drug resistance was due to mutation, and the best-known evidence to support this notion comes from the method of replica plating. This method involves successive plating of a particular culture, followed by sensitivity testing, and it shows that organisms never before exposed to a particular antibiotic nevertheless contained some insensitive cells. Other evidence indicates that drug-resistant bacteria can arise by adaptive mechanisms. Whatever the final mechanism, one fact seems clear, namely, that with some antibiotics, for example polymyxin, drug resistance does not seem to develop. On the other hand, when it is liable to occur, for example with streptomycin, then special steps must be taken to reduce the risk to a minimum, e.g. (see above) by combination therapy. Some organisms may develop drug resistance within a matter of hours (to streptomycin) or days (to erythromycin) but fortunately, in the majority of organisms, resistance develops more slowly.

Transmission of genetic material from one organism to another

The genetic control of cell activity may be altered if the genetic composition of a bacterial cell is changed. This composition may be modified by the arrival of genetic material from external sources, mainly in one of two ways—transduction or conjugation.

Transduction

In transduction, plasmids, which are extra-chromosomal particles of genetic material, are transferred to the micro-organism by means of bacteriophage (a virus that infects bacteria). If the material so transferred contains a gene for drug resistance, the bacterial cell newly infected by the virus may become resistant to the antimicrobial agent. This mechanism was first demonstrated in a staphylococcus that originally had been sensitive to penicillin and was transduced to produce penicillinase and thereby became resistant. It has since been shown that simultaneous transduction of resistance to more than one chemotherapeutic agent may occur. However, the mechanism depends on the existence of a suitable host for the bacteriophage, which, because of its fastidiousness, in general confines the transduction to organisms of the same species.

Conjugation

In episomal transference by conjugation (infectious resistance) it has been found that transfer of drug resistance can occur between organisms of all genera of the Enterobacteriaceae. What conjugation really consists of is the passage of genes from cell to cell by direct contact. As with transduction, the genetic material so transferred consists of plasmids or episomes, which themselves comprise extra-chromosomal genetic particles. In contrast to the more selective transfer of drug resistance, such particles can be passed from one species to another. However, it appears that this type of transference is mainly confined to Gram-negative species. Bacteria capable of transmitting drug resistance by this mechanism can only do so when a second factor is present, known as the 'resistance transfer factor'.

The mechanism whereby an organism, previously drug-sensitive, becomes drug-resistant as a result of episomal transference by conjugation is the formation of an enzyme that inactivates the drug (antibiotic).

It is, of course, of fundamental importance to know whether infectious drug resistance is a permanent feature or whether it is reversible. Fortunately, it appears that provided the affected organism is removed from further exposure to the antimicrobial agent, infectious resistance disappears within a matter of weeks or months. Indeed, if this were not so it would be difficult to understand how the organisms concerned could have retained any sensitivity to the drugs commonly used to treat the infections they cause. It is alarming to find that a high percentage of cultures tested have been shown to exhibit resistance. This finding obviously demands that the greatest care be taken in deciding to use any antimcrobial drug, and also in the prevention of cross-infection between patients.

PENICILLINS

Many types of penicillins are now available. Of those originally isolated, benzylpenicillin was found to be the most suitable for use and its basic properties will now be described, together with the general pharmacodynamics of the group.

Benzylpenicillin

This has a relatively narrow spectrum of antibacterial activity. It is effective against many species of Gram-negative cocci, and also against *Treponema pallidum* and other treponemata. Most Gram-negative bacilli are resistant (e.g. *Escherichia coli; Salmonella typhi; Bacteroides fragilis*); *Bacteroides melaninogenicus* is sensitive.

Amongst susceptible organisms, naturally occurring resistant strains are found. Such strains of viridans streptococci may occur in the mouth together with a majority of sensitive strains, and this poses a hazard for patients with valvular defects of the heart (see p. 213).

There are resistant strains of *Staphylococcus aureus*, resistance being due to their action in forming beta-lactamase (penicillinase), which destroys penicillin. These strains existed before the era of antimicrobials but, in the early days of penicillin, were probably few compared to those staphylococci sensitive to the antibiotic. Today the position is different: the sensitivity of *Staph. aureus* to benzylpenicillin is very variable, with most strains being resistant. In some hospitals there is a high proportion of mutliple resistant *Staph. aureus* strains (MRSA), and this has caused a serious problem.

Pharmacodynamics

Penicillins are bactericidal and interfere with biosynthesis of the bacterial cell wall in susceptible organisms. It is important to realize that there is a striking difference between the cell walls of bacteria and those of mammalian cells. Unlike the mammalian cell wall, the bacterial cell wall is a tough, thick structure, situated external to the cytoplasmic membrane and so acting as a rigid external casing to the organism; this accounts for its remarkable resistance to osmotic damage. If there existed an antimicrobial agent that acted exclusively on the bacterial cell wall, it would have no effect on the mammalian host since there is no counterpart to the bacterial cell wall in the mammal; the nearest to this ideal is penicillin.

A further important factor is the difference between the composition of the cell wall of Gram-positive and Gram-negative organisms, a fact that accounts, in some instances, for the different sensitivities of these main groups of organisms to particular antibiotics. Gram-positive organisms have a thick cell wall that contains a rigid envelope of peptidoglycan, which represents at least 60 per cent of the structure. The cell wall may also contain teichoic and teichuronic acids. Gram-negative organisms have a thin layer of peptidoglycan, which represents not more than 10 per cent of the cell wall, the main components of the wall being lipopolysaccharides and lipoproteins.

Peptidoglycan is synthesized in stages that involve amino acids and the sugar, acetylmuramic acid, which is characteristically found in the bacterial cell wall. The complex is coupled to a molecule of acetylglucosamine and together these form a glycan unit, which is the building brick of the wall. The glycan units are then carried across the cytoplasmic membrane of the bacterial cell by means of a lipid carrier and then incorporated into the cell wall.

The final stage involves the joining of peptides of one layer to the peptides of the next via a peptide link. Penicillins and also cephalosporins prevent the cross-linking of peptide strands, which is the last and vital step in the story of the cell wall. This was once thought to be achieved by blocking the transpeptidase enzyme responsible for this final stage. However, the actual mechanism of penicillin activity is more complex. It is now recognized that there are several penicillin-binding proteins associated with the bacterial cell membrane, which serve different functions, including the final cell wall cross-linking reactions. Each of these penicillin-binding proteins may be involved in the mode of action of this antimicrobial.

Pharmacokinetics

Benzylpenicillin is unstable in acidic conditions, and therefore cannot be relied upon to produce satisfactory clinical results if given by mouth because a high proportion of the original drug is rendered inactive by the acid contents of the stomach. When given by intramuscular injection it is quickly absorbed, the maximum concentration being reached within half an hour and then rapidly falls. In order to maintain a satisfactory plasma concentration, at least 300 mg of benzylpenicillin should be administered intramuscularly every four to six hours. It should also be remembered that tissue concentrations take time to equilibrate with those of plasma.

It is partially bound to plasma protein (46 to 58 per cent) and, although it passes into serious cavities, the concentration is low, especially in the cerebrospinal fluid and joint cavities. When the meninges are inflamed there is increased penetration of the penicillin into the cerebrospinal fluid providing adequate concentrations. The half-life of benzylpenicillin is less than an hour.

The major part (80 per cent) of any dose is excreted rapidly by the kidney due to extensive tubular secretion, and the remaining 20 per cent being via glomerular filtration. This excretion can be delayed by the administration of substances that compete with penicillin for active tubular secretion. Such a drug is probenecid and, by delaying excretion, it prolongs therapeutic plasma concentrations. Benzylpenicillin readily diffuses from the maternal to the fetal circulation.

Less soluble compounds of penicillin delay absorption from the site of injection; an example is procaine penicillin, prepared by the interaction of procaine hydrochloride and benzylpenicillin. The peak concentration of procaine penicillin is reached in 4 hours and thereafter falls over the next 24 hours. Even less soluble compounds are available, such as benethamine penicillin and benzathine penicillin, the effects of which are prolonged up to days or weeks. Unfortunately, the less soluble compounds produce lower plasma concentrations than benzylpenicillin.

Phenoxymethylpenicillin (penicillin V)

This is an oral penicillin that resists destruction in gastric juice and is absorbed from the upper part of the small intestine, although incompletely. Maximum blood concentration is reached in one hour and excretion is as rapid as benzylpenicillin. Administration every four to six hours is necessary to maintain therapeutic concentrations. The range of antibacterial activity is similar to that of benzylpenicillin, but it is somewhat less active against streptococci.

Other acid-resistant penicillins have been introduced, such as phenethicillin. Although more completely absorbed than phenoxymethylpenicillin, they do not seem to offer any real advantages. Phenoxymethylpenicillin is less protein-bound than these later penicillins and consequently there is more antibiotic freely available to diffuse to the site of infection. Phenoxymethylpenicillin remains the acid-resistant penicillin of choice.

Unwanted effects of the penicillins

Penicillin therapy is remarkably free from unwanted effects except for the production of hypersensitivity reactions. Sensitization is often produced by previous treatment but sometimes a history of such contact cannot be established. However, previous exposure to penicillin may not be obvious; an example of occult exposure is the drinking of milk from cows treated with the drug. Penicillin is though to be the most common cause of drug allergy, but this must be considered against the background of its extensive usage. The allergic reactions range from a mild urticaria to a serious anaphylactic shock, which, although rare, may be fatal. The estimated incidence of allergic reactions to penicillin in various areas of the world ranges from 0.7 to 10 per cent.

All preparations of penicillin can bring about hypersensitivity reactions. Although oral preparations are thought to produce reactions much less frequently than parenterally administered penicillin, it must be emphasized that serious reactions have occurred following oral administration. Procaine penicillin is probably the most common offender. All patients who are to receive penicillin, by whatever route, should be questioned as to any previous untoward experience with this drug and offered an alternative antibiotic when necessary.

The penicillins have minimal toxicity. However, intrathecal injection of penicillin G may produce a severe encephalopathy.

Uses

Extremely serious infections of dental origin should be treated by means of benzylpenicillin intramuscularly, 300 to 600 mg every four to six hours, and continued until the infection is overcome. Such a regime would require in-patient care, and usually a dose of 300 mg six-hourly will be found to be adequate.

Most susceptible infections of dental origin can be controlled by the intramuscular injection of 1 ml of fortified procaine penicillin, once or twice daily, followed by the daily injection of a similar amount for four to five days. (Fortified procaine penicillin injection contains both procaine penicillin and benzylpenicillin.) Benzylpenicillin provides a maximal concentration of the antibiotic in the blood within 30 minutes, and the procaine penicillin sustains a therapeutic level over a period of 12 to 24 hours.

For the less severe infections, an oral penicillin, i.e. phenoxymethylpenicillin, 250 mg, four to six-hourly will often suffice. It has been suggested that absorption after a meal is better. Because of the incomplete absorption of the oral penicillins, parenterally administered penicillin is more certain in its effects and should be used for severe infections. As a rule, if the patient treated with penicillin is showing no response within 48 to 72 hours, continued use of the drug is unlikely to be effective in most dental infections.

Penicillinase-resistant penicillins
(e.g. methicillin, cloxacillin, and flucloxacillin)

These are reserved for the treatment of staphylococcal infections, and treatment of such infections should be started with one of these drugs unless the antibiotic sensitivity of the strain is known. However, a staphylococcal infection in dental practice is likely to be rare but serious, calling for supervision in a hospital environment. Methicillin was the first of the penicillinase-resistant penicillins, and it must be administered by injection as it is not acid-resistant. It is probably less active against staphylococci than are cloxacillin or flucloxicillin, and has been implicated in a number of unwanted effects, e.g. granulocytopenia. It finds little use in clinical practice today, having been superseded by the other penicillinase-resistant penicillins. Flucloxacillin is better absorbed from the gut and is to be preferred to cloxacillin for oral therapy.

Broad-spectrum penicillins

(e.g. ampicillin, amoxycillin, becampicillin, ciclacillin, mezlocillin, piperacillin, pivampicillin, talampicillin)

Ampicillin is effective against Gram-positive organisms, although slightly less so than benzylpenicillin. However, it has much greater activity against Gram-negative bacteria. It is destroyed by penicillinases and should not, therefore, be used to treat resistant staphylococcal infections. Ampicillin is acid-resistant and can be administered orally, but for maximal effect it should be given parenterally. Its main use seems to be in the treatment of bronchitis and urinary infections, although many urinary isolates, e.g. *E. coli*, are now resistant to ampicillin.

Skin rashes appear to be more common with ampicillin than with other penicillins, with an incidence of about seven per cent. Most of these rashes are of the maculopapular type and seem unrelated to those of true penicillin allergy. The rashes may develop during the course of treatment or sometimes days after treatment has stopped. Ampicillin rashes tend to occur more frequently in patients suffering from infectious mononucleosis, and the drug should not be administered to such patients. Cross-hypersensitivity probably exists between all penicillins in the susceptible patient. However, the maculopapular rash of ampicillin does not necessarily contra-indicate later treatment with other penicillins.

Amoxycillin has the same spectrum of antibacterial activity as ampicillin. It is related to ampicillin but is more rapidly and completely absorbed from the gastro-intestinal tract. Peak concentrations in plasma are about twice as high as attained by ampicillin after oral administration of the same dose. Another advantage is that absorption does not appear to be affected by food. The half-life of the drug is in the region of six hours. In dentistry, it finds particular use as a prophylactic agent in the prevention of infective endocarditis (see later). Its unwanted effects are similar to those of ampicillin.

Clavulanate

Clavulanate is a beta-lactamase inhibitor, and is combined with amoxycillin in the preparation Augmentin. Clavulanate is not, in itself, antimicrobial but, by preventing the destructiveness of penicillinases, allows amoxycillin to act against resistant staphylococci, which it would otherwise not do.

Other penicillins

Ticarcillin, carbenicillin, azlocillin, and carfecillin are used in infections due to *Pseudomonas aeruginosa*. Others, such as mecillinam and pivmecillinam, are broad-spectrum penicillins, active against a wide variety of Gram-negative bacilli, such as *E. coli, Proteus mirabilis*, and salmonellae. These have no activity against *P. aeruginosa*, penicillinase-producing staphylococci, or enterococci and much less activity against Gram-positive organisms. Mecillinam must be given by injection. Pivmecillinam is an ester of mecillinam and is well-absorbed when given orally. After absorption it is hydrolysed to the active agent, mecillinam. Pivmecillinam has a local irritant effect on the oesophageal mucosa and occasionally causes oesophagitis. These drugs may be indicated in severe infections due to enterobacteria, e.g. *E. coli*, which account for a high proportion of urinary tract infections.

None of these drugs has a place in dentistry.

Cephalosporins

These are closely related chemically to penicillin. They are broad-spectrum antimicrobials with activity against a wide range of Gram-positive and Gram-negative bacteria. The first of the series to be used in Britain was cephaloridine, and it was thought to be resistant to beta-lactamase producing staphylococci, but this is now known not to be the case. It was also nephrotoxic.

The cephalosporins have been divided into three generations, as follows:

(1) first generation—cephalothin, cephalexin, cephazolin, cephradine;

(2) second generation—cefuroxime, cephamandole, cefoxitin, cefaclor;

(2) third generation—cefotaxime, ceftazidine, ceftizomine, and latamoxef.

The first generation has good activity against Gram-positive and Gram-negative bacteria including streptococci, *Neisseria gonorrhoea, Strep. pneumoniae*, and *Corynebacterium diphtheriae*. Their activity against some Gram-negative organisms is variable. They have no activity against *Ps. aeruginosa, Strep. faecalis, Bact. fragilis*, and most of the Enterobacteria.

The second generation of cephalosporins is largely resistant to beta-lactames, and they are much more active against almost all Gram-negative bacilli. Cephamandole is very active against the Enterobacteria and staphylococci.

The third generation of cephalosporins is more active than either of the other two generations against certain Gram-negative bacteria.

Pharmacodynamics

The cephalosporins act in the same way as the penicillins by interfering with the biosynthesis of the bacterial cell wall in susceptible organisms, thereby exerting a bactericidal effect.

Pharmacokinetics

The first cephalosporins, cephaloridine and cephalothin, both had to be administered parenterally. Newer preparations include cephradine (oral and parenteral administration); cephazolin (parenteral); cefuroxime (parenteral); cephamandole (parenteral). Cefadroxil is a new oral cephalosporin. Once absorbed into the circulation the cephalosporins exhibit variable binding to plasma proteins from 20 to 90 per cent (e.g. cephaloridine, 20 per cent; cephalothin, 70 per cent). The cephalosporins are mainly excreted by the kidney, some unchanged and others as metabolites.

Unwanted effects

It seems that the incidence of allergic reactions to cephalosporins is lower than that of the penicillins, the reactions which occur being similar to those caused by the penicillins.

In penicillin-sensitive subjects the use of cephalosporins should be viewed with caution as there is clinical evidence of partial cross-allergenicity between the penicillins and the cephalosporins. It seems that patients with a history of penicillin allergy are predisposed to accelerated reactions to cephalosporins; such reactions suggest that the underlying mechanism is likely to be due to cross-allergenicity, rather than to a generalized and unspecific tendency to drug hypersensitivity. Patients with a history of mild urticaria to penicillins do not seem to be at a great risk of an allergic reaction when given cephalosporins, but a patient with a severe, immediate reaction to penicillin should not be given a cephalosporin. About 10 per cent of patients who are allergic to penicillins react in some way to the cephalosporins.

Cephalosporins have been implicated in renal damage, but this was most commonly due to the original cephaloridine.

Uses

In general terms there appear to be few absolute indications for the use of the cephalosporins, especially in dentistry. Perhaps they can be regarded as 'second line of defence' antimicrobials.

TETRACYCLINES

(e.g. tetracycline, chlortetracycline, clomocycline, demeclocycline, doxycycline, lyme-cycline, methacycline, minocycline, and oxytetracycline)

The tetracyclines comprise a group of closely related, bacteriostatic antimicrobials that provide a 'broad spectrum' of activity against organisms. Susceptible species include Gram-positive organisms, which are also sensitive to penicillin, and many Gram-negative organisms insensitive to penicillin. Tetracyclines are also active against rickettsia (e.g. typhus), brucella, and diseases due to *Chlamydia trachomatis*, causing lymphogranuloma venereum. They are also effective against treponemata and *H. influenzae*. Initially the tetracyclines were effective against aerobic Gram-negative bacilli, but now many species are resistant.

Pharmacodynamics

The majority of the broad-spectrum antimicrobials act by interfering with the synthesis of protein by bacteria. They achieve this by interrupting one or more of the critical synthetic steps in a process which depends upon the sequential coupling of amino acids, brought about through the beautifully co-ordinated activities of messenger RNA (mRNA), ribosomal RNA (rRNA), and transfer RNA (tRNA). In order to describe the various ways in which different antimicrobials interfere with protein synthesis, it is necessary to review briefly the normal mechanisms of bacterial protein synthesis.

The primary information for protein synthesis is stored by DNA, and is transmitted to mRNA during transcription. The actual process of protein synthesis takes place on ribosomes, which consist of rRNA and protein, and which either lie free in the cytoplasm or attached to the cytoplasmic membrane. The cytoplasmic membrane of bacteria corresponds to the membrane of mammalian cells. Each bacterial ribosome, which consists of a 30 S and a 50 S component (the 'S' refers to Svedberg unit, a measure of the relative density as determined by speed of centrifugation), threads itself on to the end of a strand of mRNA where it contains two attachment sites for amino acids. At the same time, the available amino acids become temporarily attached to tRNA, each amino acid having its own specific tRNA, thus ensuring the correct assembling of the amino acids to form the peptide chain. Thus mRNA consists of a long chain of four nucleotides joined in such a way as to provide a codon triplet, each one of which represents a code for a specific amino acid. Similarly, each amino acid is 'recognized' by its specific anticodon triplet, which couples to it and transports it to the appropriate codon triplet site on mRNA when the appropriate acceptor site becomes available. Transpeptidation then takes place, whereby the peptide chain already attached (by means of tRNA) is transferred to the next amino acid thus freeing the carrier tRNA. Translocation of the ribosome now takes place and it moves along mRNA and opens up a new acceptor site, which contains another codon for the next amino acid in the chain. The whole process is then repeated.

The tetracyclines interfere with the transfer of amino acids because they bind to the 30 S component of the ribosome and thus prevent polypeptide synthesis.

Pharmacokinetics

The tetracyclines are generally administered orally, but occasionally by intravenous or intramuscular injection.

Absorption from the gastro-intestinal tract is fairly rapid, but significant amounts are retained in the bowel. Absorption is reduced if the drug is taken with milk or with substances containing calcium, magnesium, iron, or aluminium, all of which chelate with tetracyclines.

The original tetracyclines, i.e. tetracycline, chlortetracycline, and oxytetracycline, produce adequate and maintained plasma concentrations by the administration of 250 mg at six-hourly intervals. They have a half-life of about 6 to 10 hours; the maximal concentration in the plasma is reached in 2 to 4 hours after oral administration, and gradually falls to about half this amount in 9 to 12 hours, and to a very low concentration at 24 hours.

Demeclocycline and methacycline, on the other hand, have half-lives of about 16 hours, and satisfactory plasma concentrations may persist for 24 hours or more.

Doxycycline and minocycline have longer half-lives, being in the region of 16 to 18 hours. Doxycycline, for instance, is given in an initial dose of 200 mg—maximum plasma concentration being reached in two hours—and this is followed by a daily dose of 100 mg.

Tetracyclines are widely distributed in the tissues and they also enter the cerebrospinal fluid. As they chelate with calcium ions, they are localized in bone and teeth. Excretion of the tetracyclines is in the urine and the faeces, but mainly via the kidneys. Clearly, in general terms, the exceretion of these drugs will be affected by the state of renal function. The exceptions are doxycycline and minocycline, where excretion is in the faeces.

Unwanted effects

Hypersensitivity reactions are rarely encountered with the tetracyclines but, where they are, cross-hypersensitivity between the various members of the group will be present. Large doses of tetracyclines given parenterally can damage the liver; pregnant women appear to be particularly susceptible.

Immediately after absorption tetracyclines are built into calcifying tissues and this becomes a permanent, discolouring feature in the teeth. The use of tetracyclines should be avoided during the formative period of the crowns of the teeth. There is a clear linear relationship between the number of courses of treatment with tetracyclines and the discolouration of developing teeth (0 to 12 years). Of the original tetracyclines it appeared that chlortetracycline produced a grey-brown discolouration; yellow staining of varying intensity occurred in patients who had taken tetracycline, oxytetracycline, or demethylchlortetracycline. The third type, a brownish-yellow discolouration, was of mixed origin. Of the earlier tetracyclines the least objectionable staining was produced by oxytetracycline.

In infants, increased intracranial pressure with bulging fontanelles has been observed with tetracycline therapy. This is not a common occurrence and all signs clear up on cessation of treatment.

Gastro-intestinal disturbances may complicate therapy with tetracyclines: some patients complain of abdominal discomfort or a feeling of nausea, and there may even be vomiting or diarrhoea. these effects may result from the direct irritant action of the drug on the intestinal mucosa, or may occur because of an alteration of the gut flora. All antimicrobials have the ability to alter the normal microbial flora of the upper respiratory tract, intestinal tract, and genito-urinary tract, and probably do so to some extent in every individual. Pseudomembranous colitis is a rare, but serious, complication of tetracycline therapy. The colitis is characterized by severe diarrhoea and mucus-containing stools. The cause of this condition is the colonization and multiplication of the organism *Clostridium difficile* in the colon, a process encouraged by the alteration of the normal gut flora by the antimicrobial. *Cl. difficile* produces a toxin that is damaging to the gastro-intestinal mucosa. Tetracyclines are not the only antimicrobials which can produce this serious condition; it may occur with others, e.g. ampicillin, amoxycillin, lincomycin, and clindamycin (see below). The treatment of the colitis is to stop the drug immediately and to administer oral vancomycin or metronidazole, to which *Cl. difficile* is sensitive.

Candida albicans is a normal commensal of mucous membranes. The fungus may cause disease in certain predisposed patients, e.g. diabetics; those with leukaemias or lymphomas; those who have received lengthy treatment with cytotoxic drugs, immunosuppressive drugs, or broad spectrum antimicrobials. Patients who have received a long course of treatment with broad-spectrum antimicrobials, e.g. tetracyclines, may develop an oral candidal infection that has been named 'antibiotic stomatitis'. This condition may follow the use of topical antimicrobials in the mouth. The surface proliferation of *C. albicans*, which is known to occur with the administration of broad-spectrum antimicrobials, increases the chances of it invading the tissues and thereby causing infection. A tetracycline mouthwash is listed in the *Dental Practitioners' Formulary 1986–88*, and its use is recommended for no longer than three days, to be followed by a break of three days before the treatment is recommenced. This recommendation is made to avoid the occurrence of an antibiotic induced oral thrush.

Tetracyclines may cause end-stage renal failure when administered to patients with chronic renal disease. These antimicrobials cause a rise in blood urea, which is often accompanied by deterioration in renal function. While the normal half-life of the original tetracyclines is in the region of 6 to 12 hours, this may be increased to 57 to 108 hours in patients with renal failure. Tetracyclines should not, therefore, be given to patients with impaired renal function. Doxycycline and minocycline are possible exceptions to this general statement. The serum half-life of these preparations is in the region of 18 hours and is not significantly changed in patients with chronic renal failure.

Severe liver damage can occur after very large doses, and this may follow the accumulation of tetracyclines in renal failure. It is also likely to occur following parenteral administration in the third trimester of pregnancy.

Uses

At one time tetracylines were regarded as second-choice antimicrobials to the penicillins in dental practice. This is no longer the case. Indeed, there are few indications for the use of tetracyclines in dentistry. A tetracycline mouthwash is sometimes useful in relieving the painful ulcerations of severe recurrent aphthae, the erosions of lichen planus, and especially for oral hepetic ulceration. For this purpose 10 ml of Tetracycline Mouthwash is held in the mouth for two to three minutes, three times daily for no longer than three days. The rationale of this treatment is obscure; possibly it is effective in reducing any secondary infection. If the treatment is continued for more than three days consecutively, then there is the danger of superinfection with *C. albicans* in susceptible patients.

More recently, tetracyclines have found use in periodontal treatments (see Chapter 11).

ERYTHROMYCIN

This has a narrow spectrum of activity, similar to that of benzylpenicillin, but is more active against *Staph. aureus.* It is a bacteriostatic drug but bactericidal in high concentrations.

Pharmacodynamics

Erythromycin blocks translocation (see mode of action of tetracyclines for information on protein synthesis in bacteria). It binds to the bacterial ribosomal units and prevents translocation, with subsequent blocking of polypeptide synthesis. It is, then, a drug that interferes with protein synthesis within the bacterial cell. Drugs that affect translocation are, for some reason, liable to give rise to resistant mutants. In general, Gram-positive organisms are more sensitive than Gram-negative organisms because their cell walls are more readily permeable to such drugs. The Gram-negative enterobacteria, e.g. *E. coli*, salmonella, are resistant to erythromycin. On the other hand some of the Parvobacteria, such as *H. influenzae* and *Bordetella pertussis* are sensitive to erythromycin. The Gram-negative *Legionella pneumophilia* is also sensitive.

Pharmacokinetics

Erythromycin base is destroyed by acid gastric juices and so is administered in enteric coated tablets. It is absorbed from the upper part of the small intestine. Peak plasma concentrations are reached in about four hours and, to achieve this, the tablets should be taken in the absence of food. However, erythromycin estolate is more acid-stable and is usually given in the form of capsules. It is absorbed to a greater extent than any other oral preparation of erythromycin, and gives peak plasma concentrations within about two hours. Higher concentrations of erythromycin can be achieved by intravenous administration. The half-life of erythromycin is in the order of 1.5 to 2 hours.

Erythromycin is widely distributed throughout the body tissues and two to five per cent of the orally administered drug is excreted in its active form in the urine. Although a proportion of the drug is also excreted in the bile, of which some is reabsorbed, the greater part of it seems to be broken down in the body.

Unwanted effects

In general terms, erythromycin may be counted as one of the safest antimicrobials. All preparations of erythromycin can cause gastro-intestinal upsets such as nausea, vomiting, and diarrhoea; epigastric discomfort is not infrequent. This latter symptom is likely to be very marked if large doses are given.

Hypersensitivity reactions are rare with the base, but the estolate produces a high incidence of cholestatic hepatitis, which is thought to be due to hypersensitivity. This condition starts about 10 to 12 days after the commencement of treatment, and is manifested by abdominal pain, jaundice, and fever. On stopping the drug the symptoms and signs disappear, but re-exposure to the preparation may cause an immediate recurrence of the hepatitis.

Uses

Erythromycin is a useful alternative to penicillin when the patient is known to be hypersensitive to the latter and can, perhaps, be regarded as a second-choice antimicrobial to penicillin. It is generally administered orally and, for most dental infections, a five days course will suffice, the dose being 250 mg six-hourly. Erythromycin stearate should be used for treating infections especially if the course of treatment is to last more than a week. The use of the estolate in dentistry is unlikely to cause hepatitis as a course of treatment is usually not prolonged. Erythromycin also finds a use as a prophylactic agent against infective endocarditis, a subject discussed later in this chapter.

Although erythromycin is a useful drug, it is the drug of choice in relatively few diseases, but is recommended for the treatment of infections caused by L. pneumophilia (Legionnaire's disease).

Cross-resistance to other commonly used antimicrobials does not occur readily, but erythromycin has the disadvantage that some sensitive organisms (e.g. staphylococci and even haemolytic streptococci) may become resistant to it during prolonged therapy.

METRONIDAZOLE

This, given orally, is effective in the treatment of trichomonal infections of the genital tract, and coincidentally, it has been found to be successful in the treatment of acute ulcerative gingivitis and other dental infections (see below). Metronidazole exhibits activity against anaerobic cocci and against anaerobic Gram-negative bacilli, including Bacteroides species.

Pharmacodynamics

The drug inhibits DNA synthesis in organisms. When metronidazole is used in infections, it is reduced to form an extremely unstable and reactive intermediate that is thought to bind to DNA and interfere with further cell replication. This results in very rapid killing of obligate anaerobes.

Pharmacokinetics

Metronidazole is available as tablets and for intravenous infusion. The drug is well-absorbed after oral administration and a mean peak plasma concentration is produced in about 1 to 2 hours; the plasma half-life is about 8 hours. The drug penetrates into body tissues and fluids, and is metabolized in the liver; unchanged drug and metabolites are excreted in the urine.

Unwanted effects

Numerous unwanted effects have been recorded, and these are commonly related to the gastro-intestinal tract, e.g. nausea, vomiting, indigestion, diarrhoea, or constipation. Dizziness and headaches have also been reported. It is not unusual for the patient to complain of a bitter, metallic taste in the mouth. Occasionally skin rashes have occurred. Fortunately, the drug is well tolerated and the untoward effects are not often serious. When metronidazole is prescribed, patients should be instructed not to take alcohol as the drug may produce similar reactions to that of disulfiram (Antabuse) when combined with alcohol, e.g. it will inhibit the alcohol metabolism. Metronidazole also potentiates the effects of warfarin and the other coumarin anticoagulants.

Metronidazole has been shown to be carcinogenic in rodents fed on high doses for a prolonged period, but there does not seem to be evidence that there is such a risk in man. Although there appears to be no risk in administering metronidazole in pregnancy, as with all other drugs it should be avoided if possible, especially in the first trimester.

Uses

In medical practice, metronidazole is used in the treatment of genital infections with *Trichomonas vaginalis*. It is also effective in the treatment of *Giardia lamblia* infections (giardiasis). Addditionally it is used in the treatment of amoebic infections, and in the treatment of anaerobic infections due to Bacteroides species, including *fragilis*. In dentistry, the efficacy of metronidazole in the treatment of acute ulcerative gingivitis is well-established. Metronidazole is the first choice of drugs in the treatment of this condition and is dispensed as 200 mg and 400 mg tablets. One 200 mg tablet is swallowed thrice daily for three days. Discomfort usually decreases after 24 hours and ulcerations are beginning to heal after 48 hours.

As yet, sensitive organisms have not been found to develop resistance to metronidazole, and its use in the treatment of oral conditions does not, therefore, prejudice its efficacy against infections occurring in medical practice.

Metronidazole is probably as effective as penicillin in the treatment of acute pericoronitis, and it may also have wider usages in dentistry. A variety of bacterial species are found in dental abscesses, including a high proportion of obligate anaerobes of which *Bact. melaninogenicus* may well be important. This organism is known to produce tissue-active toxins such as collagenase, hyaluronidase, proteinase, and heparinase. It is possible that these may be concerned in the considerable and extensive inflammatory response which characterizes some acute dental infections. Obligate anaerobes are sensitive to both penicillin and metronidazole and, if they are the cause of a lot of dental infections, a rapid response to either of these antimicrobial agents would be expected. There is evidence that both are equally effective. Perhaps the true nature of many dental infections has not been appreciated because of the problems associated in the past with the isolation of anaerobes. Metronidazole may well be a satisfactory alternative to penicillin in patients with acute dental infections. In acute apical infections, 400 mg tablets should be considered rather than the 200 mg tablets, 400 mg being given twice daily. If as effective as penicillin, metronidazole may be preferred as it produces fewer hypersensitivity reactions. *Bact. fragilis* is not found in dental infections for, although it would respond to treatment with metranidazole, it is penicillin-resistant.

LINCOMYCIN AND CLINDAMYCIN

Clindamycin is a derivative of lincomycin, which it has replaced. Both are active against Gram-positive bacteria, including penicillinase-producing strains of staphylococci. Aerobic Gram-negative bacilli are resistant, but the Gram-negative aerobic *Bact. fragilis*, and *melaninogenicus*, are sensitive. Neisseria and enterococci are resistant to these drugs.

Pharmacodynamics

Lincomycin and clindamycin bind to ribosomal units and prevent translocation with subsequent blocking of polypeptide synthesis in organisms (see Pharmacodynamics of the tetracyclines).

Pharmacokinetics

Clindamycin is available for intramuscular injection or slow intravenous infusion; it is also presented as capsules and as a paediatric mixture. Clindamycin is rapidly and almost completely absorbed after oral administration, and its absorption does not seem to be significantly affected by the presence of food in the gut. It produces peak blood concentrations in about 45 minutes. The half-life of the drug is approximately three hours. After intramuscular injection of the phosphate form, peak plasma concentrations are not achieved until three hours in the adult, and somewhat more swiftly in children. Clindamycin is widely distributed throughout the body and penetrates well into bone.

Most of the drug is metabolized and is excreted as metabolites in the urine and bile. A small amount (10 per cent) is excreted unchanged in the urine and an even smaller amount is found in the faeces.

Unwanted effects

Diarrhoea is the most likely unwanted effect, and incidence of this has been suggested as being anything from as low as 2 per cent to well over 20 per cent. It is likly to be much higher with lincomycin. Unfortunately some patients have developed pseudomembranous colitis, a condition described earlier under Unwanted Effects of Tetracycline, with which it is also rarely associated. This can be a very serious problem and, before the mechanism producing this syndrome was understood, the treatment could even extend to colostomy. Although this condition, often referred to as antibiotic-associated colitis, can occur with other antimicrobials, it seems particularly associated with clindamycin, whether used orally or parenterally. Its occurrence seems to be unrelated to dosage, and it can arise any time during treatment or even after discontinuation of treatment. If it does occur, then the drug should be stopped and the condition treated with oral vancomycin or metronidazole to which *Cl. difficile*, the causative organism, is sensitive.

Allergic reactions may occur, and skin rashes are observed in a number of patients. There are more and rare serious reactions, such as Stevens–Johnson syndrome (severe, febrile erythema multiforme; see Sulphonamides below). Interestingly, clindamycin is an antimicrobial that inhibits, or interferes with, neuromuscular transmission and could, therefore, potentiate the effect of certain neuromuscular block agents, e.g. tubocurarine.

Uses

Clindamycin is a very effective drug in many infections, but the high incidence of diarrhoea and the possible occurrence of antibiotic-associated colitis must limit its use. It is especially useful in the treatment of infections caused by Bacteroides species, and in particular those due to *Bact. fragilis.* It should be reserved for infections caused by such organisms and, occasionally, for staphylococcal bone infections after bacteriological identification. The drug of first choice for such bone infections is likely to be flucloxacillin, and there appears to be very little indication for the use of clindamycin in dentistry.

ANTIFUNGAL ANTIMICROBIALS
(e.g. nystatin, amphotericin, imidazole agents)

Fungi are not sensitive to the antimicrobials used against bacterial infections, e.g. penicillin, tetracyclines, erythromycin, and others. Fortunately, up to now, systemic fungal infections have been rare in Britain, for they are serious diseases and difficult to treat. On the other hand, superficial infections by *C. albicans* are not uncommon and are usually trivial, but they tend to persist and may be troublesome in susceptible patients. As we have seen, oral candidiasis may occur as a response to treatment with certain drugs; for example corticosteroids, antibiotics (especially tetracyclines), and immunosuppressive agents.

A number of antifungal drugs are now available for local or systemic use, and one or two have found favour in dentistry; these are now described.

Nystatin

This is effective against *C. albicans* and some other fungi.

Pharmacodynamics

Nystatin is active against yeasts and fungi but inactive against bacteria. This selective toxicity is due to the presence of ergosterol in the cytoplasmic membrane of fungi and yeasts, which is not present in bacterial membranes. A hydrophobic interaction between nystatin and the membrane ergosterol molecule disrupts the osmotic function of the membrane, with consequent death of the fungi.

Pharmacokinetics

Nystatin is not absorbed from the skin or mucous membranes. It is, therefore, used for its local effect in the treatment of candidiasis on the skin or any part of the alimentary tract.

Unwanted effects

These are exceedingly rare. The occasional patient feels nauseated after oral administration. There have been no reports of hypersensitivity reactions. The drug has a very unpleasant taste.

Uses

Nystatin is used primarily to treat fungal infections caused by *C. albicans*, which produces thrush, denture stomatitis, antibiotic stomatitis, and some forms of mucocutaneous candidiasis(-osis).

In treating most oral candidal infections, one pastille of nystatin (100 000 units) is allowed to dissolve in the mouth, and four pastilles are prescribed each day for periods varying from one week to four weeks (e.g. denture stomatitis and angular cheilitis, two to four weeks; thrush and conditions following drug therapy, one to two weeks). In treating candidal leukoplakia, a chronic lesion, the daily regime advocated may have to be continued for many months.

Patients who have denture stomatitis should be advised to leave out their dentures as much as possible and to keep them in a cleansing agent such as sodium hypochlorite solution (Milton). It is understandable that many patients are reluctant to leave out their dentures for any length of time, so a compromise is to smear the fitting surface of the denture with an antifungal ointment (such as nystatin ointment, or amphotericin ointment) before insertion of the denture.

Persistent candidiasis, in spite of treatment, may point to some underlying predisposition. For instance, oral candidiasis is a common complication of leukaemias, especially where immunosuppressive drugs have been used.

Candidal vaginitis is a commonly transmitted sexual disease and generally responds to treatment with local applications of nystatin.

Amphotericin B

This is effective against a number of fungi, including Candida species. Its mode of action is thought to be like that of nystatin, and it has no effect on bacteria.

Pharmacokinetics

Amphotericin is little absorbed from the gastro-intestinal tract and probably not at all from the unbroken skin. It is used locally for the treatment of conditions for which nystatin could be used. Amphotericin B is available for intravenous injection, when it can be used for the treatment of systemic fungal infections, e.g. candidal septicaemia, histoplasmosis. The metabolism of the intravenously administered drug seems to be unknown, but the drug is excreted in an inactive form in the urine, and there is also biliary excretion.

Unwanted effects

The parenteral use of the drug is associated with a host of unwanted effects; these include fever, nausea, and vomiting. Some undesirable effects on the kidney are almost inevitable; a rise in blood urea may occur.

Uses

Amphotericin B is one of the relatively few antimicrobials effective against systemic fungal infections and is, therefore, a valuable weapon in the medical armamentarium, particularly as nystatin is too toxic to be used systemically. In dentistry, it is used for the same purposes as nystatin, so amphotericin B (10 mg) lozenges may be used locally in the mouth as an alternative to nystatin. In severe infections the dose may be doubled. Amphotericin B ointment can be substituted for nystatin ointment.

Imidazole agents
(e.g. miconazole, ketoconazole, clotrimazole)

The particular drug used in dentistry is miconazole. Miconazole and clotrimazole may be used topically; miconazole and ketoconazole may be used systemically. Their mode of action is similar to nystatin, and these drugs alter the permeability of the cytoplasmic membrane.

Pharmacokinetics

Miconazole is available for oral and parenteral administration. It has a lot of unwanted effects when given intravenously and is not the drug of choice as an antifungal for systemic use.

Ketoconazole is available for oral administration, and peak plasma concentrations appear about two hours after an oral dose of 400 mg. Metabolism of the drug occurs in the liver, and most is excreted as metabolites in the urine.

Unwanted effects

Although the most commonly encountered unwanted effects with parenteral ketoconazole are nausea and vomiting, other untoward effects have occurred, e.g. headache, photophobia, rash, and thrombocytopenia. Hepatic toxicity occasionally produces hepatic dysfunction. Unwanted effects when miconazole is used intravenously are frequent, e.g. anaemia, anaphylactoid reactions, central nervous-system involvement (hallucinations, blurred vision).

Uses

Ketoconazole finds a use in the treatment of systemic fungal infections and candidiasis. It is also useful as a prophylaxis in patients who are on immunosuppressive therapy and also in the treatment of such patients who have chronic candidal leukoplakia. A once-daily dose of ketoconazole (200 mg tablet) is taken with food, and the treatment is continued for one to two weeks after symptoms have disappeared and cultures are negative.

Miconazole has found a place in dentistry, and its primary use is topical. Miconazole tablets (250 mg) are available, and the dose regimen is 250 mg six-hourly. The drug is also presented as a sugar-free oral gel (25 mg/ml). The application of the gel is thought to be useful in the treatment of candidal leukoplakia or chronic mucocutaneous candidiasis.

OTHER ANTIMICROBIAL AGENTS

There are many of these, some carefully reserved for the treatment of particular infections. For example, *streptomycin* finds its principal use in the management of tuberculosis (see below), whilst *chloramphenicol* is one of the drugs of choice in typhoid fever, where the seriousness of the complaint overrides the dangers of its use. Chloramphenicol is a dangerous drug because it can produce irreversible bone marrow aplasia; it has no place in general dental practice.

Neomycin sulphate

This is a member of a group of drugs collectively referred to as aminoglycosides. This group also includes gentamicin, kanamycin, netilmicin, streptomycin, and tobramycin. They are particularly effective against many Gram-negative bacillary organisms but, in addition, streptomycin is effective against *Mycobacterium tuberculosis*. Neomycin is not a drug that is used parenterally because it may cause renal damage and is liable to produce deafness; auditory changes may even occur after topical administration. Nevertheless, neomycin alone, or in combination with other drugs, did once achieve some popularity in dermatological preparations. This era seems to have passed and few preparations are listed in the *British National Formulary*. Neomycin combined with a steroid as a cream or ointment was sometimes suggested as being helpful in treating the symptoms of herpes labialis. Various combinations of neomycin with other drugs have been used in dentistry; for example, Cicatrin powder (essentially neomycin and zinc bacitracin) on wounds to prevent postoperative infection. The topical use of neomycin is not without its dangers and it is a fairly frequent cause of allergic sensitization, usually in the form of skin reactions of the delayed type. Such preparations are no longer used in dentistry.

Fusidic acid

This is a drug that is effective against staphylococci, although resistant strains do emerge *in vivo*, if rather slowly. Fusidic acid ointment is listed in the *Dental Practitioners' Formulary*, and it is suggested that this be used in the fissures of angular cheilitis where *Staph. aureus* has been isolated.

Vancomycin

This antimicrobial is mainly active against Gram-positive bacteria. Clostridia species are inhibited by it. It is available for intravenous use and also as a powder for oral use. It is not absorbed from the gut, and so when given orally its use is really as a topical application. By oral administration it may treat antibiotic-associated colitis (500 mg as a loading dose followed by 125 mg six-hourly). It is painful on intravenous injection and should, therefore, be given by slow intravenous infusion. Vancomycin is only used to treat serious infections, such as certain staphylococcal infections (e.g. septicaemia, endocarditis), where the patient is allergic to penicillinase-resistant penicillins. It is also recommended as a prophylaxis against infective endocarditis in special circumstances (see later).

Quinolones

These comprise a group of drugs that act by inhibiting the bacterial enzyme DNA gyrase. The group includes nalidixic acid and cinoxacin. Both of these drugs are active against most Gram-negative bacteria but excluding *P. aeruginosa*. Gram-positive bacteria are predominantly resistant. The main use of quinolones has been in the treatment of urinary infections. More recently a new quinolone, ciprofloxacin, has been introduced, which is a broad-spectrum antimicrobial with activity against both Gram-positive and Gram-negative aerobes. It would appear to have a low incidence of unwanted effects. Like other quinolones, its most common unwanted effects are gastro-intestinal disturbances, e.g. abdominal discomfort and nausea. Concomitant administration of ciprofloxacin with theophylline may lead to elevated plasma concentrations of the latter, with an increased risk of adverse reactions related to theophylline, i.e. CNS stimulant effects. The earlier quinolones had no place in dentistry, but ciprofloxacin could well find a use because of its wider range of activity. Experience with this drug will surely establish its significance, if any, for dental practice.

Anti-tuberculous drugs

These include streptomycin, isoniazid, rifampicin, ethambutol, and pyrazinamide. An important point about rifampicin is that it is an enzyme inducer, and so hastens the metabolism of many other drugs, including prednisone, digoxin, propranolol, the oral contraceptives, and the oral anticoagulants. Clearly the effectiveness of these drugs may be reduced. Oral contraceptives may also be affected by other antimicrobials, e.g. ampicillin and tetracyclines, but perhaps not by enzyme induction; this subject is discussed in Chapter 22.

PROPHYLAXIS: THE PREVENTION OF INFECTIVE ENDOCARDITIS

The dental treatment of patients with valvular defects of the heart poses a special problem. Patients with congenital heart defects, with a history of rheumatic fever or chorea, or those who have undergone valvular cardiac surgery, may all be predisposed to infective endocarditis. Those with a past history of infective endocarditis should be regarded as a special high-risk group. The disease is caused by direct infection from the blood stream with bacteria colonizing the heart valves. Before the era of antimicrobials, infective endocarditis was almost invariably fatal; even today mortality is about 30 per cent, and patients are left with severely damaged hearts in spite of prolonged treatment with antimicrobials. There is a changing pattern in the disease, as now the older patient is affected rather than the young. Rheumatic fever causing residual heart lesions is no longer the main scourge in the young patient, but rather congenital heart defects. In the pre-antimicrobial era a high percentage of cases of infective endocarditis were caused by viridans Streptococci, organisms found in the mouth, and today such streptococci are still heavily implicated.

Transient bacteraemias follow many dental procedures. In the normal patient these are of little moment, for the bacteria are quickly removed from the bloodstream by the body's defences. However, in the predisposed patient, organisms may be implanted on an abnormal heart valve with perpetuation of the bacteraemia from an endocardial focus. The dental treatment of such patients should be undertaken as follows.

History

All patients attending for dental treatment should be questioned for any history of heart disease, previous rheumatic fever, or chorea. There is not complete agreement as to which patients should be considered at risk; not all would accept that one with a history of rheumatic fever, but with no apparent residual heart defects, should be so regarded. If such a patient attends for elective treatment it would be desirable to have the opinion of a cardiologist as to whether antimicrobial cover was required or not. If the same patient attends for emergency treatment, then they should be regarded as 'at risk' until vouchsafed otherwise by a cardiologist. It is important, anyway, to establish a positive history of rheumatic fever, for an indefinite history could have the patient being recorded as a potential risk without justification.

A patient who has had a myocardial infarction or coronary by-pass surgery is not regarded as 'at risk'.

Treatment plan

Those at risk should be encouraged to maintain a high standard of oral care. The teeth must be restored where necessary and periodontal disease prevented. If this state cannot be achieved, either because of indifference on the part of the patient, or because of the inherent quality of the dental tissues, extractions should be contemplated. It must be remembered that dental tissues may be the source of bacteraemias even in the absence of dental procedures. It must also be emphasized that the edentulous patient is not free from risk of infective endocarditis. Ulcers due to ill-fitting dentures may be the cause of a bacteraemia, and such ulcers should receive early attention.

Although it is agreed that any dental procedures may cause a bacteraemia, the emphasis must be on what should be regarded as a 'significant bacteraemia'. After all, chewing and toothbrushing could cause bacteraemias!

The use of antimicrobial agents

In order to prevent the occurrence of infective endocarditis in those patients considered to be at risk, antimicrobial cover should be provided when certain dental procedures are undertaken. A Working Party of the British Society for Antimicrobial Chemotherapy produced a report, published in the *Lancet* of 11 December 1982, on the subject of 'The Antibiotic Prophylaxis of Infective Endocarditis'. This report was not merely concerned with dental problems but a summary of the report, appertaining to the practice of dentistry, was published in the *British Dental Journal* (Cawson 1983). The Working Party report indicated that 'a risk of infective endocarditis appears to be associated only with extractions or scaling or surgery involving the gingival tissues'. This is a positive statement, but there are bound to be 'grey' areas in which clinical judgement will have to be exercised. For instance, in endodontic treatment it seems that a bacteraemia will not be produced so long as instrumentation is contained within the root canal. Instrumentation beyond the apex is likely to produce a bacteraemia and, in spite of the apparent margin of safety, many—perhaps most—endodontists would consider that root canal therapy should be undertaken under antimicrobial cover, and preferably completed at one visit.

The fact is that relatively few patients with infective endocarditis will give a recent history of dental treatment. Furthermore, it is impossible to know how effective are prophylactic antimicrobial regimens in preventing the occurrence of infective endocarditis. Nevertheless, in spite of all the ignorance surrounding the subject, the occurrence of the disease is so serious that it is generally agreed that prophylaxis must be provided for some patients.

The antimicrobial regimens for patients predisposed to infective endocarditis are as follows:

1. Dental treatment under local anaesthesia:
   (a) patients not allergic to penicillin.

Adults—3 g amoxycillin orally one hour before the operation. The drug should be given with either the dentist or the dental nurse present. This is done simply to ensure that the antimicrobial is taken by the patient. For *children* under ten years, half the adult dose; and for children under five years, quarter of the adult dose. For children over ten years, the dosage is as for the adult.

This regimen applies to patients with prosthetic heart valves as well as those with natural valvular disease. The patient who has a properly functioning prosthetic valve is no more likely to get infective endocarditis following on dental procedures than one with damaged natural valves. However, if the patient with prosthetic valves does have an attack of infective endocarditis then it is likely to be severe with a poorer prognosis.

(b) Patients allergic to penicillin.

Adults—1.5 g erythromycin stearate given orally under supervision, 1 to 1.5 hours before the dental procedure, followed by a second dose of 500 mg orally 6 hours later. For *children* under ten years, half the adult dose; for children under five, quarter of the adult dose; and for children over ten years, the dosage is as for the adult.

These regimens will cover most problems faced in general dental practice. The 3 g of amoxycillin is a high dosage and seems to provide adequate plasma concentrations for the critical period of 10 hours following the dental procedure. The reason why two doses of erythromycin are recommended is because absorption of erythromycin is less predictable and the initial dose, although quite large in itself, is not equivalent to the 3 g dose of amoxycillin. However, a 1.5 g dose of erythromycin is about the maximum that can be tolerated by patients without causing nausea.

At one time an alternative to amoxycillin was suggested if the patient had been taking a penicillin recently. It is now thought that high-dose (3 g) regimens of amoxycillin are appropriate, even for patients who have recently taken a penicillin.

2. Dental treatment under general anaesthesia;
   (a) patients not allergic to penicillin.

Adults—1 g of amoxycillin intramuscularly before induction and 500 mg of oral amoxycillin, six hours later. *Children* under 10 years, half the adult dose. Amoxycillin given intramuscularly is painful, and 1 g is about the maximum that can be tolerated. An alternative is to give 3 g of oral amoxycillin, four hours prior to induction, followed by another 3 g of oral amoxycillin as soon as possible after the dental treatment.

These regimens are not suitable for patients with prosthetic heart valves.

(b) patients who are allergic to penicillin.

Intravenous vancomycin and intravenous gentamicin are recommended for these patients, but these drugs are not available to dental practitioners under the *Dental Practitioners' Formulary*. Such patients should be referred to hospital.

A special problem exists for patients with prosthetic heart valves who require a general anaesthetic, and for patients who have had endocarditis. For those with prosthetic valves, a regimen using intramuscular amoxycillin (1 g) and intramuscular gentamicin (1.5 mg/kg) is recommended immediately before induction, followed by oral amoxycillin (500 mg), six hours later. For the patient who has had a previous attack of endocarditis, whether attending for local or general anaesthesia, a similar regimen of intramuscular amoxycillin and intramuscular gentamicin is recommended. All such patients should be referred to hospital for dental treatment, for these are at special risk. Whenever particular problems present themselves, the patient's physician should be consulted.

As the onset of endocarditis may be insidious, patients should be advised to report any untoward symptoms of signs to their medical practitioner. Endocarditis may develop in spite of prophylaxis and the position has been summed up in the *British Medical Journal* (Leading Article) of 20 October 1973:

Infective endocarditis presents a complex problem both in temperate and tropical countries. The role of immunological and other factors in the patient is uncertain. When we consider the large number of people at risk who have dental extractions or other procedures without any antibiotic cover, the incidence of the disease must be remarkably small. In two-thirds of patients no precipitating cause is detectable. The host's immunological response is probably more important than the infection, but in our present state of ignorance it remains obligatory to give prophylactic antibiotics for those at risk.

SULPHONAMIDES

These were discovered in Germany in 1935, where it was shown that a red dye, prontosil, would cure streptococcal infections in mice. Within a short period, researchers in France and England found that this substance was broken down in the body to two components, one of which, sulphanilimide, was therapeutically active. This was the real beginning of antibacterial chemotherapy and since that time many improvements have been made. Sulphonamides have a wide range of activity against both Gram-positive and Gram-negative organisms, for example streptococci. pneumococci, *H. influenzae, Vibrio cholerae, N. meningitidis, E. coli, N. gonorrhoeae.* Unfortunately, many organisms have become resistant to the sulphonamides and this, at one time, included the gonococci. However, in recent years there has been a gradual re-emergence of sensitive strains of gonococci due to the fact that the drug has not been used for some time in the treatment of gonorrhoea. On the other hand, there has been a gradual emergence of resistant strains of meningococci, and sulphonamides cannot be relied upon to treat meningococcal meningitis.

Pharmacodynamics

The sulphonamides are bacteriostatic drugs, inhibiting the growth and multiplication of sensitive organisms, thus allowing the natural defence mechanisms of the body to deal with the existing infection without being overwhelmed.

Para-aminobenzoid acid (PABA) is an essential metabolite of bacterial cells and sulphonamides are competitive antagonists of PABA. Para-aminobenzoic acid is required for the synthesis of folic acid; the sulphonamides inhibit competitively the enzyme responsible for the incorporation of PABA into the precursor of folic acid. The organisms affected by sulphonamides are those which synthesize their own PABA; those which utilize pre-formed PABA are not affected. Fortunately the mammalian cell, which also requires PABA, utilizes preformed PABA.

Local anaesthetics that are derivatives of PABA, e.g. procaine, amethocaine, could, in theory, interfere with the antibacterial action of the sulphonamides. As discussed in Chapter 7, the presence of such local anaesthetics could make available the PABA and so redress the balance in favour of the bacteria. However, local anaesthetics with formulae that do not have a PABA moiety, e.g. lignocaine, prilocaine, do not antagonize the sulphonamides even theoretically.

Pharmacokinetics

Most sulphonamides are readily absorbed from the gastro-intestinal tract after oral administration, the small intestine being the main site of absorption. There are exceptions to this general statement, for there are some sulphonamides that are not absorbed and are used topically in the bowel.

The sulphonamides are widely distributed throughout the body and they cross the blood-brain barrier to enter the cerebrospinal fluid, more so when the meninges are inflamed. They also readily cross the placenta and enter the fetal circulation. The sulphonamides are mainly metabolized in the liver to acetylated forms. The drug is excreted in the urine unchanged or as metabolites.

Unwanted effects

The sulphonamides produce a high incidence of these, and this was especially marked with the earlier products. Nausea, with or without vomiting, headache, and malaise were all quite common with the earlier sulphonamides but are rarely seen today.

The most serious effects of the sulphonamides are on the bone marrow. A degree of polymorphonuclear leucopenia is not uncommon but is of little importance in itself. However, agranulocytosis does occasionally arise and sometimes, although very rarely, an haemolytic anaemia. The mechanism of these is not fully understood; they may be manifestations of hypersensitivity. Probably there is very little danger if the treatment is not continued for more than 10 days, although this is not an absolute. After withdrawal of the drug, it may take weeks or months for the granulocytes to return to normal levels; nevertheless, recovery does normally occur. Aplastic anaemia, where all functions of the bone marrow are depressed, is a very rare occurrence indeed.

There are hypersensitivity reactions with the sulphonamides, and their incidence tends to vary with the preparation used; the long-acting sulphonamides are particularly implicated. Skin rashes of various sorts may appear— urticarial, pemphigoid, purpuric, and petechial rashes are all possibilities. Serum sickness-type syndrome may occur after some days of treatment, with fever, joint pains, and rashes. Stevens–Johnson syndrome, a severe form of erythema multiforme, may occur and may present with blisters in the mouth and on the skin. The long-acting sulphonamides e.g. sulfametopyrazine, sulphadimethoxine, and sulphamethoxypyridazine, are most likely to be those concerned. Toxic effects due to accumulation are likely to occur with these preparations. Cawson and Spector (1985) describe the essentials of the syndrome in this way: 'the most striking and characteristic feature is the swollen, cracked, bleeding and crusted lips'. There may be ocular involvement. Although an extremely unpleasant condition, it is rarely fatal.

Renal damage from sulphonamides is likely to be rare these days but was not so in the past, when preparations, particularly the acetylated forms, tended to be less soluble than those used today. These insoluble forms appeared as crystals in the urine (crystalluria), and deposition of crystals in the kidney, ureters, or bladder could lead to obstruction and renal failure. Sulphadiazine, though still used, is poorly soluble, and may cause crystalluria.

Uses

A number of groups of sulphonamides can be described; namely, those that are:

(1) readily absorbed, widely distributed, and quickly excreted, e.g. sulphaurea, sulphafurazole, sulphadiazine, sulphadimadine;

(2) readily absorbed, widely distributed, and slowly excreted (long-acting), which include sulfametopyrazine and sulphadimethoxine;

(3) poorly absorbed, e.g. phthalylsulphathiazole, calcium sulphaloxate, sulphagaunidine;

(4) for topical application, e.g. sulphacetamide.

Urinary infections may be treated with sulphadimidine, sulphaurea, or sulphafurazole, being rapidly absorbed and excreted. However, these are less commonly used today because superior antimicrobials are available. Sulfametopyrazine and sulphadimethoxine are used for the treatment of chronic bronchitis. Indeed, the main usage for the sulphonamides is in the treatment of urinary infections and bronchitis.

The poorly absorbed sulphonamides have been used for preoperative bowel sterilization and for the treatment of some intestinal infections, but they are no longer recommended for these purposes.

Sulphadiazine is not available in Britain in tablet form except in combination with other drugs. However, it is available for intramuscular or intravenous injection and has been used prophylactically to prevent the occurrence of meningitis in patients at risk who have had maxillofacial injuries with leakage of cerebrospinal fluid. As pointed out previously, many strains of meningococci are now resistant to the sulphonamides. Benzylpenicillin is probably the first-choice antimicrobial for treating meningococcal meningitis. In patients allergic to penicillin, chloramphenicol may be the drug of choice.

Sulphacetamide, as eye drops, is used locally for the treatment of infections.

Trimethoprim-sulphamethoxazole (co-trimoxazole)

Trimethoprim is an antibacterial agent and has a range of activity similar to that of the sulphonamides. Like the sulphonamides, it inhibits bacteria by metabolic deprivation but at a later stage in their metabolism. When trimethoprim is combined with a sulphonamide (sulphamethoxazole) as in the preparation co-trimoxazole, it exerts a bactericidal effect.

A high proportion of the unwanted effects that occur with this combination are due to the sulphonamide element and the majority of unwanted effects refer to skin. Nevertheless there may be various haematological reactions, e.g. aplastic, haemolytic anaemias, as may also occur with sulphonamides. Theoretically, co-trimoxazole could cause a folic-acid deficiency with consequent anaemia, but this is most unlikely to occur in the normal healthy patient given therapeutic doses.

Trimethoprim-sulphamethoxazole is used to treat lower urinary tract infections and is very effective. The combination appears to be particularly useful in the management of chronic and recurrent infections; it is also used for the treatment of exacerbations of chronic bronchitis. It is one of the drugs of choice for the treatment of dysentry (shigellosis) as many of the causative organisms are now resistant to the broad-spectrum penicillins. The combination is useful in the treatment of typhoid and paratyphoid fevers because it seems to be as active as chloramphenicol but with less risk of producing such serious unwanted effects. It may also be useful in the management of the *S. typhi* carrier state.

Co-trimoxazole may be useful in the treatment of severe dental infections, and in sinusitis and sialadenitis. Co-trimoxazole comes in tablet form (480 mg in each tablet), and the dose is 960 mg every 12 hours, although this may be increased to 1.44 g in severe infections. Although the risk of crystalluria is slight, it is desirable when taking this preparation to increase the fluid intake (water).

Sulphasalazine

This preparation is worthy of mention as it is used in the treatment of mild ulcerative colitis, and is a useful prophylactic agent in that condition, maintaining clinical remissions for many patients. Sulphasalazine is broken down in the gut to sulphapyridine and 5-aminosalicylate. It is the salicylate that seems to act as an anti-inflammatory agent in both ulcerative colitis and Crohn's disease.

ANTIVIRAL AGENTS

Introduction

Viral infections differ from other types of infection because viruses are obligate intracellular parasites that require for their survival the active participation of the metabolic processes of the invaded cell. Thus, agents used to destroy viruses may also damage the invaded cell. Few therapeutic measures have been developed that are clinically acceptable; those applicable to dentistry are described in this section.

Acyclovir

This is an analogue of the nucleotide, purine, and its antiviral activity is essentially confined to the herpes virus. The drug can be given orally (200 mg), intravenously, and topically (5 per cent cream).

Acyclovir has a greater affinity (over 200 fold) for viral enzymes than for cellular enzymes. Viral enzymes phosphorylate acyclovir to form the compound acyclo-GMP, which is then further catalysed by cellular enzymes to acyclo-GTP. The latter is a potent inhibitor of viral DNA synthesis, thus inhibiting replication of the virus. (Fig. 10.1).

When given orally, acyclovir has a half-life of 2.5 hours and is poorly bound to plasma protein (15 per cent). The drug crosses the blood–brain barrier and is eliminated by the kidneys.

Unwanted effects arising from oral administration are few, and include nausea and headache. Topical application of acyclovir to mucous membrane can cause a transient burning sensation but this may be due to the polyethylene base.

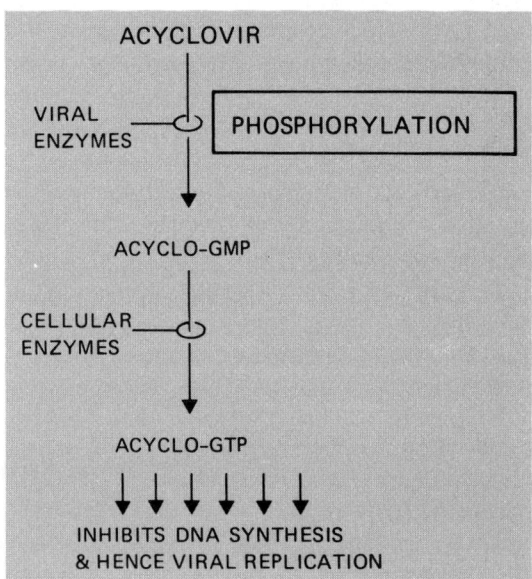

Fig. 10.1. Mode of action of acyclovir.

Uses

Acyclovir is used to treat the following viral infections.

1. *Herpes simplex type I virus:* acyclovir is effective at reducing the symptoms of the mucocutaneous lesions of the face and oropharynx associated with this viral infection.

2. *Herpes simplex type II virus:* this virus causes genital herpes and may also be responsible for meningitis. Primary genital herpes responds to acyclovir, but does not prevent recurrence. The drug is currently being tested for viral meningitis.

3. *Varicella-zoster virus:* Shingles is the principal disease caused by this virus and, in some patients, this is followed by post-herpetic neuralgia. Acyclovir has been shown to reduce the symptoms of the initial attack of shingles, but is of little value in the treatment of the neuralgia.

Idoxuridine

This is an antiviral agent structurally related to thymidine. It is phosphorylated within cells and the triphosphate so formed is incorporated into viral DNA synthesis. The synthesized viral DNA is more susceptible to breakage, and altered viral proteins may result from faulty transcription. Hence idoxuridine is mainly used against DNA viruses (herpes simplex type I, vaccinia, varicella, and cytomegalovirus). Idoxuridine is too toxic for systemic administration and is therefore only used topically.

For management of acute herpetic gingivostomatitis, a 0.1 per cent solution should be used. In young children, the solution should be painted on lesions four to five times a day. Older children and adults can apply a few ml of the solution as a mouthwash, allowing the solution to have maximum contact with the lesions for at least two to three minutes, three times a day.

Idoxuridine is effective in the treatment of herpes labialis, provided it is applied as early as possible. Established cases may respond to idoxuridine 5 per cent in dimethyl sulphoxide solution. The solvent aids the penetration of the antiviral agent into the skin. The solution is applied to the lesions every two hours until they resolve.

Herpes zoster infections may also respond to idoxuridine 5 per cent in dimethyl sulphoxide, provided the solution is applied early in the illness or as soon as the first skin lesions appear. Idoxuridine will reduce the pain associated with herpes zoster and accelerate healing.

Unwanted effects from topically applied idoxuridine are few. The solution has an unpleasant taste and patients may experience stinging when the solution is first applied. Excessive use of idoxuridine in dimethyl sulphoxide may cause maceration of the skin.

Table 10.1. Antimicrobials

Group	Official or approved name	Other names	Spectrum	Drug resistance	Adult dosage	Unwanted effects	Comments
Benzylpenicillin	Benzylpenicillin	Penicillin G Crystapen			300–600 mg, IM, 2–4 times daily	An innocuous drug even in high dosages, apart from hypersensitivity reactions. Hypersensitivity reactions are the most serious hazard—including anaphylactic shock.	Used for treating severe infections and/or relatively insensitive organisms, when high blood levels are required. Rapidly excreted.
	Procaine penicillin	Procaine penicillin G, Depocillin			300 mg, IM, 1–2 daily	Procaine penicillin appears to produce a higher incidence of allergic reactions; phenoxymethylpenicillin a low incidence of reactions.	Effective in all but relatively severe/resistant infections. Lower blood levels maintained for 24 h.
			C+, B+, C−, S. *Proteus mirabilis* and other *Proteus* often sensitive.	Many strains of *Staphylococcus aureus*.			
Acid resistant	Phenoxymethyl penicillin	Penicillin V, Apsin VK, Crystapen V, Distaquaine V-K, Stabillin V-K V-Cil-K			250 mg, orally, 4–6 hourly		Acid resistant. For oral administration. Unsuitable for serious infections because irregular absorption may produce inadequate blood levels.
						N.B. Cross allergenicity is likely to exist between the penicillins.	N.B. Penicillin is usually regarded as first choice antimicrobial in dentistry. Metronidazole may be an alternative (see text).
Penicillins resistant to penicillinase	Methicillin	Celbenin	Penicillinase resistant penicillins reserved for the treatment of staphylococcal infections	A few strains of *Staphylococcus aureus*.	1 g, IM, 4–6 hourly.	Have the same low order of unwanted effects as benzylpenicillin. It has been suggested that methicillin may cause permanent renal damage.	Although active against penicillin sensitive and pencillinase producing strains of *Staphylococcus aureus*, much less active than benzylpenicillin against other penicillin sensitive species. None of these penicillins is effective against infections due to Gram − bacilli. Reserved for the treatment of serious infections due to resistant staphylococci.
	Cloxacillin	Orbenin			500 mg orally, 6 hourly. 250 mg, IM, 4–6 hourly		
	Flucloxacillin	Floxapen			250 mg orally, or IM, 6 hourly		
Broad spectrum penicillins	Ampicillin*	Amfipen Ampilar Penbritin Vidopen	C+, B+, C−, B−, S. Slightly inferior to benzylpenicillin against most Gram+ bacteria.	Many strains of *Staphylococcus aureus*.	250 mg–1 g orally, 6 hourly.	Ampicillin produces a higher incidence of skin rashes than other penicillins. The rash is usually of the maculopapular type and may be unrelated to the usual type of penicillin hypersensitivity. The rash may appear during treatment or days	These penicillins are active against Gram+ bacteria, but are especially effective against Gram − bacteria. In dentistry these drugs should be reserved for infections caused by identified Gram − organisms. In medicine ampicillin, for example,
	Amoxycillin	Amoxidin Amoxil			250–500 mg orally, 8 hourly.		

Class	Drug	Trade names	Indications	Resistance / Spectrum	Dose	Adverse effects	Comments
						(about 5) after the discontinuation of treatment.	has been used for a wide variety of infections, especially urinary tract infections. Amoxicillin used as prophylactic agent.
Carboxypenicillins	Carbenicillin	Pyopen	Pseudomonas infections and infections with Proteus species.	Many strains of Staphylococcus aureus. Strains of Proteus mirabilis which form penicillinase.	5 g, 4–6 hourly. Slow IV injection.	As for benzylpenicillin.	These penicillins are of importance because of their activity against Pseudomonas aeruginosa and certain Proteus species. Ticarcillin is more active against Ps. aeruginosa than is carbenicillin.
	Ticarcillin	Ticar			15–20 g daily in divided doses. IM or slow IV injection.		
Cephalosporins	Cephalothin	Keflin		A degree of susceptibility to staphylococcal penicillinase	1 g. IV, every 4–6 hours.	The incidence of allergic reactions may be lower than that for the penicillins. There is a degree of cross allergenicity between the cephalosporins and the penicillins. Cephalothin, and possibly other cephalosporins, may be nephrotoxic in patients with renal impairment.	A useful alternative to penicillin when the latter cannot be used, other than because of hypersensitivity. Not, as at first hoped, the answer to staphylococcal infections, being susceptible to penicillinase. The second generation cephalosporins (cefuroxime and cephamandole) are less susceptible to inactivation by penicillinases. A third generation (e.g. cefotaxime, ceftazidime, etc.) are more active against certain Gram– bacilli. Cephalosporins find little place in dentistry.
	Cephradine	Velosef		Similar to ampicillin	250–500 mg, orally, 6 hourly. 0.5–1 g. IM, 6 hourly.		
	Cephalexin	Ceporex, Keflex			250 mg, orally, 6 hourly.		
	Cefuroxime, Cephamandole	Zinacef, Kefadol		Less susceptible to penicillinase.			
Tetracyclines	Chlortetracycline	Aureomycin		C+, B+, C– B–, S, R, V. Often inactive against Proteus species and Pseudomonas aeruginosa.		Hypersensitivity reactions are rare. Nausea, vomiting and diarrhoea may occur. Super-infection with resistant strains of Staphylococcus aureus can cause a fatal enterocolitis. Overgrowth of Candida albicans may lead to thrush, glossitis, pruritis ani, etc. Staining of the teeth if administered during the period of calcification of the dental tissues, if given over a long period. May cause terminal renal failure in a stabilized renal failure. Tetracyclines should not be given to patients with renal disease with the exception of doxycycline and minocycline. N.B. Cross hypersensitivity is likely to exist between the tetracyclines.	The development of bacterial resistance has reduced the general usefulness of the tetracyclines. However, they are valuable agents in rickettsia, in some infections produced by mycoplasma and in infections caused by chlamydia (e.g. psittacosis, urethritis). Tetracyclines are also useful in treating exacerbations of chronic bronchitis. They find little place in dentistry other than for recurrent aphthae when they are used topically. May also be used for treatment of juvenile periodontitis. Whenever possible tetracyclines should be avoided during the period of calcification of the teeth because of the staining produced in developing teeth. Tetracyclines should be avoided in patients with ulcerative colitis.
	Oxytetracycline	Chemocycline Galenomycin Imperacin Oxymycin Terramycin Unimycin		Slow development of resistance but many Streptococci are resistant and there is an emerging resistance of Pneumococci. Cross resistance between the tetracyclines.			
	Tetracycline	Achromycin Economycin Sustamycin Tetrabid Tetrachel Tetrex			250–500 mg orally, 6 hourly is the dose range for most preparations. Exceptions: Sustamycin, Tetrabid. Doses for individual preparations should be checked prior to administration. Preparations are available for injection.		
	Doxycycline	Doxatet Doxylar Nordox Vibramycin			200 mg orally on first day. Then 100 mg daily.		
	Minocycline	Minocin			Initially 200 mg orally. Then 100 mg 12 hourly.		

Table 10.1. Antimicrobials

Group	Official or approved name	Other names	Spectrum	Drug resistance	Adult dosage	Unwanted effects	Comments
Erythromycin group (Macrolides)	Erythromycin	Erycen Erymax Erythrocin Erythrolar Erythromid Ilotycin Retcin	Legionnaire's disease C+, B+, C−, S	Develops rapidly; may occur during treatment	250–500 mg orally, 6 hourly	Gastrointestinal upsets (nausea, vomiting, epigastric discomfort, diarrhoea) not uncommon. Hypersensitivity reactions are rare except that erythromycin estolate produces a high incidence of cholestatic hepatitis if given for more than 10 days. In this instance the hepatitis is thought to be due to hypersensitivity.	Similar range of activity to benzylpenicillin. In low concentration it is mainly bacteriostatic, but in higher concentration it exerts a bactericidal effect. It is another alternative in the treatment of infections when the patient is allergic to penicillin, or when prophylaxis is required. It may be useful in the treatment of infections due to penicillin resistant strains of *Staphylococcus aureus*, if sensitivity is established.
	Erythromycin estolate	Ilosone			250–500 mg, orally, 6 hourly		
Lincomycin	Lincomycin	Lincocin			500 mg orally, 3–4 times daily. 600 mg, IM (every 24 h in mild to moderate infections; every 12 h in severe infections).	Hypersensitivity reactions appear to be rare. Diarrhoea is common with both drugs, possibly less so with clindamycin. Cases of pseudomembranous colitis have been reported following the use of both drugs. N.B. Cross allergenicity is likely to exist between lincomycin and clindamycin.	Probably best reserved for the treatment of osteomyelitis as they are thought to penetrate well into bone. It is recommended that these drugs be used with extreme caution, and only where no suitable alternative is available, because of the possibility of pseudomembranous colitis. The colitis is due to a toxin produced by *Clostridium difficile* which is resistant to lincomycin and clindamycin. If diarrhoea colitis occurs the drug should be stopped at once. Treatment of the colitis is by vancomycin or metronidazole, the anaerobic *Cl. difficile* being sensitive to these drugs.
	Clindamycin	Dalacin C	Similar to that of erythromycin	Some strains of *Staphylococcus aureus*.	150–300 mg, orally, 6 hourly, 0.6–2.7 g, IM, daily in 2–4 divided doses.		

Anti-fungals							
	Nystatin	Nystan	Candida albicans. (No antibacterial activity).	Strains of Candida albicans serially subcultured become resistant. Resistant Candida albicans not yet found clinically.	Nystatin pastilles (100 000 i.u. per pastille) 1 pastille sucked 4 times daily. Nystatin tablets (500 000 units per tablet) 1–2 tablets 4 times daily Nystatin ointment. Applied to lesions 4 times daily.	Occasionally produces nausea and vomiting.	It is used locally in the management of candidiasis of the alimentary tract. In treating oral candidiasis (e.g. denture stomatitis, thrush) 1 nystan pastille is allowed to dissolve in the mouth, 4 times daily, for a period of from 1–4 weeks. Dentures should preferably be removed and disinfected. (Tablets are swallowed to treat intestinal infection and the local treatment should be combined with this to help combat the generalized gastrointestinal infection.) If angular cheilitis is present, nystan ointment may be applied to the lesions. Sometimes nystatin is combined with tetracyclines to prevent overgrowth of Candida albicans.
	Amphotericin B	Fungizone (for infusion) Fungilin lozengers, Fungilin tablets, Fungilin ointment.	Candida species. Coccidioides immitis. Blastomyces dermatidis. Cryptococcus neoformans.	Strains of Candida albicans serially subcultured become resistant. Resistant Candida albicans not yet found clinically.	1 lozenge (10 mg) to be dissolved in the mouth 4 times/day for 1–4 weeks. 1–2 tablets (each containing 100 mg). 4 times daily. Amphotericin ointment 3%, applied 4 times/day	Parenterally administered amphotericin B is associated with a large number of unwanted effects, e.g. hypersensitivity reactions, chills, fever, local thrombophlebitis, decreased renal function, and, rarely, irreversible renal failure.	Amphotericin B (Fungizone) is available when it is administered intravenously for the treatment of severe, systemic mycotic disease. Amphotericin B (Fungilin) lozenges and ointment are used for the same purpose as nystatin tablets and ointment, in the treatment of oral candidiasis. Amphotericin tablets are used to combat gut candidiasis. Amphotericin B does not have the unpleasant taste of nystatin.

Table 10.1. Antimicrobials

Group	Official or approved name	Other names	Spectrum	Drug resistance	Adult dosage	Unwanted effects	Comments
Anti-fungals	Miconazole nitrate	Daktarin tablets Daktarin injection Daktarin oral gel	Active against a broad spectrum of fungi.		250 mg, orally, 6 hourly. 600 mg, 3 times daily, by slow IV infusion. Miconazole: Oral Gel 25 mg/ml. 5–10 ml placed in mouth near lesions. Retain and then swallow. 4 times daily.	Unwanted effects are frequent after systemic administration. These include nausea, vomiting, anaemia, hypersensitivity reactions, CNS toxicity. The vehicle carrying the active agent is cremophorel which also produces unwanted effects.	Miconazole is essentially a drug for topical use, it is too toxic for parenteral administration, except in special circumstances. The oral gel seems to be effective in the treatment of denture stomatitis and angular cheilitis. The gel is lightly smeared over the fitting surface of the upper denture and this is done 4 times daily. The fitting surface should be clean and dry prior to the application of the gel. Similarly, the gel may be applied to lesions at the angle of the mouth. Treatment may have to be carried out for a number of weeks.
Nitroimidazoles	Metronidazole	Flagyl	Anaerobic bacteria e.g. *Bacteroides* species (including *Bacteroides fragilis*). Protozoa, e.g. *Giardia lamblia*, *Trichomonas vaginalis*.	Primary resistance is very unusual in sensitive species of anaerobes.	Anaerobic infections: 400 mg orally, 3 times daily. A.U.G.: 200 mg. orally, 3 times daily. Giardiasis: by mouth, 2 g. daily for 3 days. Trichomoniasis: by mouth, 200 mg, every 8 h for 7 days.	Nausea, vomiting, diarrhoea in about 3% of patients. Occasional metallic taste. Dizziness and ataxia may occur, and transient epileptiform seizures with high doses. Peripheral neuropathy may occur after prolonged treatment. A reversible neutropenia sometimes occurs. Disulfiram-like effect with alcohol.	Metronidazole is a very safe drug overall. No teratogenic effects have been noted after the administration of the drug at various stages of pregnancy. Nevertheless the manufacturer recommends avoidance of high-dose regimens during pregnancy and breast feeding. Such regimens are unlikely in dentistry. Alcohol must be avoided when taking metronidazole as the concurrent use will cause some patients to have vomiting and/or headache. Other nitroimidazoles are available, e.g. tinidazole, nimorazole. Metronidazole is useful in the treatment of antibiotic associated colitis (due to *Clostridia difficile*.)

*The ampicillin esters, bacampicillin (Ambaxin), pivampicillin (Pondocillin), and talampicillin (Talpen), produce higher plasma concentrations than ampicillin, and absorption is little affected by the presence of food.
Code: C + = Gram + cocci. C − = Gram − cocci. B + = Gram + bacilli. B − = Gram − bacilli. S = Treponema pallidum. R = Rickettsiae. V = Chlamydiae, e.g. Chlamydia trachomatis.
N.B.: Doses of older penicillins were originally expressed in units, but it is now customary to express doses in mg (or g). e.g. Benzylpenicillin, 250 000 units = 150 mg; Procaine penicillin, 100 000 units = 100 mg.

Interferon

Interferons are glycoproteins produced by the body in response to a viral infection. Their properties include the induction of resistance to viral infections and the regulation of other cell functions. *In vitro* studies have shown that interferon has a broad-spectrum antiviral activity. However, preliminary results from clinical trials suggest that interferon is not as efficacious in viral infections as initially hoped.

REFERENCES AND FURTHER READING

Admadsyah, I. and Salim, A. (1985). Treatment of tetanus: an open study to compare the efficacy of procaine penicillin and metronidazole. *British Medical Journal,* **291,** 648–50.

Bain, R. J. I. *et al.* (1985). Failure of single dose amoxycillin as prophylaxis against endocarditis. *British Medical Journal,* **290,** 316–17.

Ball, A. P. (1982). Clinical uses of penicillins. *Lancet,* **ii,** 197.

Cafferkey, M. T. *et al.* (1985). Occasional Survey: methicillin-resistant *Staphylococcus aureus* in Dublin 1971–1984. *Lancet,* **ii:** 705–8.

Cawson, R. A. (1981). Infective endocarditis as a complication of dental treatment. *British Dental Journal,* **151,** 409.

Cawson, R. A. (1983). A summary of the BSAC Working Party Report: the antibiotic prophylaxis of infective endocarditis. *British Dental Journal,* **154:** 183–4.

Cawson, R. A. (1986). Update on antiviral chemotherapy: the advent of acyclovir. *British Dental Journal,* **161,** 245–52.

Cawson, R. A. and Spector, R. G. (1985). *Clinical pharmacology in dentistry,* (4th edn), p. 344. Churchill Livingstone, Edinburgh.

Clinical Pharmacy, In *The Pharmaceutical Journal* (1987), **238,** No. 6418, p. 198.

Cohen, J. (1982). Antifungal chemotherapy. *Lancet,* **ii:** 532–7.

Davies, A. J. and Lewis, D. A. (1984). Rifampicin in non-tuberculous infections. *British Medical Journal,* **289,** 3–4.

Eggleston, D. J. (1980). Procaine penicillin psychosis. *British Dental Journal,* **148,** 73–4.

Gallagher, D. M. and Sinn, D. P. (1983). Penicillin-induced anaphylaxis in a patient under hypotensive anaesthesia. *Oral Surgery,* **56,** 361–4.

Goldberg, A. (1985). Co-trimoxazole toxicity. *British Medical Journal,* **291,** 673.

Gould, I. M. and Wise, R. (1985). Third generation cephalosporins. *British Medical Journal,* **290,** 878–9.

Hay, R. J. (1985). Ketoconazole: a reappraisal. *British Medical Journal,* **290,** 260–1.

Holbrook, W. P., Willey, R. F., and Shaw, T. R. D. (1983). Prophylaxis of infective endocarditis. *British Dental Journal,* **154,** 36–9.

Hood, F. J. C. (1978). The place of metronidazole in the treatment of acute oro-facial infection. *Journal of Antimicrobial Chemotherapy,* **4,** (suppl. C), 71–3.

Kucers, A. (1982). Good antimicrobial prescribing. *Lancet,* **ii,** 425–9.

Lacey, R. W. Hawkey, P. M., Devaraj, S. K., Millar, M. R., Inglis, I. J. J., and Goodwin, P. G. R. (1985). Co-trimoxazole toxicity. *British Medical Journal,* **291,** 481.

Leading article (1985). Fifty years of sulphonamides. *Lancet,* **i,** 378.

Leading article (1985). Born-again vancomycin. *Lancet,* **i,** 677–8.

Leading article (1985). What's to be done about resistant staphylococci? *Lancet*, **ii**, 189–90.

Leading article (1985). A nasty shock from antibiotics? *Lancet*, **ii**, 594.

Leading article (1985). Decline in rheumatic fever. *Lancet*, **ii**, 647–8.

Leading article (1985). Antibiotic care for cardiac surgery. *Lancet*, **ii**, 701–2.

Leading article (1985). Antibiotic-induced neutropenia. *Lancet*, **ii**, 814.

Levy, S. B. (1982). Microbial resistance to antibiotics. *Lancet*, **ii**, 83–8.

Martin, M. V., Farrelly, P. J., and Hardy, P. (1986). An investigation of the efficacy of nystatin for the treatment of chronic atrophic candidosis (denture sore mouth). *British Dental Journal*, **160**, 201–4.

McGowan, D. A. and Hendry, M. L. (1985). Is antibiotic prophylaxis required for dental patients with joint replacements? *British Dental Journal*, **158**, 336–8.

McGowan, D. A. Nair, S., MacFarlane, T. W., and MacKenzie, D. (1983). Prophylaxis of experimental endocarditis in rabbits using one or two doses of amoxycyllin. *British Dental Journal*, **155**, 88–90.

Mitchell, D. A. (1986). A controlled clinical trial of prophylactic tinidazole for chemoprophylaxis in third molar surgery. *British Dental Journal*, **160**, 284–6.

Mitchell, L. (1984). Topical metronidazole in the treatment of 'dry socket'. *British Dental Journal*, **156**, 132–4.

Morell, P., Hey, E., Mackee, I. W., Rutter, N., and Lewis, M. (1985). Deafness in preterm baby associated with topical antibiotic spray containing neomycin. *Lancet*, **i**, 1167–8.

Morris, G. K. (1985). Infective endocarditis: a preventable disease? *British Medical Journal*, **290**, 1532–3.

Neu, H. C. (1982). Clinical uses of cephalosporins. *Lancet*, **ii**, 252–5.

O'Grady, F. (1973). *Current antibiotic therapy*, p. 7. Churchill Livingstone, Edinburgh and London.

Orme, M. L'E. and Black, D. J. (1986). Drug interactions between oral contraceptive steroids and antibiotics. *British Dental Journal*, **160**, 169–70.

Phillips, I. (1982). Aminoglycosides. *Lancet*, **ii**, 311–15.

Reeves, D. (1982). Sulphonamides and trimethoprim. *Lancet*, **ii**, 370–3.

Renson, C. E. (1983). Infective endocarditis—prophylaxis and prevention. *Dental Update*, **10**, 254–8.

Roberts, J. Bianco, M. M., and Fine, J. (1985). Report of a case: fatal anaphylactic reaction to oral penicillin. *Journal of the American Dental Association*, **110**, 505–6.

Roe, F. J. (1977). Metronidazole: review of uses and toxicity. *Journal of Antimicrobial Chemotherapy*, **3**, 205–12.

Sanderson, P. J. (1984). Common bacterial pathogens and resistance to antibiotics. *British Medical Journal*, **289**, 638–9.

Schifter, S., Agaard, M. T., and Jensen, L. (1985). Adverse reactions to vancomycin. *Lancet*, **ii**, 499.

Sterry, A. K., Langeroudi, M., and Dolby, A. E. (1985). Metronidazole as an adjunct to periodontal therapy with sub-gingival curettage. *British Dental Journal*, **158**, 176–8.

Therapeutics (1985). Antibiotic treatment of streptococcal and staphylococcal endocarditis. Report of a Working Party of the British Society of Antimicrobial Chemotherapy. *Lancet*, **ii**, 815–17.

Walker, D. M., Stafford, G. D., Huggett, R., and Newcombe, R. G. (1981). The treatment of denture-induced stomatitis. *British Dental Journal*, **151**, 416–19.

Watson, C. J., Walker, D. M., Bates, J. F., and Newcombe, R. G. (1982). The efficacy of topical miconazole in the treatment of denture stomatitis. *British Dental Journal*, **152**, 403–6.

Wheeley, M. St.G. (1986). Effect of antibiotics on oral contraception. *British Medical Journal*, **292**, 903.

Wise, R. (1982). Penicillins and cephalosporins: antimicrobial and pharmacological properties. *Lancet*, **ii**, 140–3.

Wroblewski, B. A., Singer, W. D., and Whyte, J. (1986). Carbamazepine–erythromycin interaction. *Journal of the American Medical Association*, **255**, 1165–7.

11

Pharmacological control of dental caries and periodontal disease

INTRODUCTION

DENTAL caries and periodontal disease are the two principal diseases that affect the morbidity of the dentition. Microbial plaque is the main aetiological factor in both diseases, although diet and the host response play vital roles. The incidence of dental caries can be considerably reduced by fluoride; more recently, attention has focused on the development of a vaccine against dental caries. Mechanical removal of plaque is the basis for controlling periodontal disease but, although desirable, this is often impracticable because of the high degree of motivation and dexterity required to make a mouth plaque-free. Research has been concentrated on the development of chemical methods for inhibiting plaque formation. This chapter discusses the various pharmacological methods for controlling dental caries and periodontal disease.

DENTAL CARIES

This is caused by a biological interaction between bacteria, diet, and the tooth surface. There is now overwhelming evidence that refined carbohydrates are broken down by acid-producing bacteria, which in turn produce further acid causing demineralization of the enamel surface. Streptococci of the *mutans* type are the main bacteria implicated in dental caries, which produce lactic acid from dietary carbohydrates.

The relationship between fluoride and dental caries was first realized in the early part of this century. Since then many epidemiological studies have demonstrated unequivocally the role of fluoride in preventing dental caries (for review see Murray and Rugg-Gunn 1982).

Mode of action of fluoride in reducing dental decay

The precise mode of action is uncertain; fluoride probably acts via several mechanisms including an effect on enamel structure, an alteration in tooth morphology, and an action on bacterial plaque.

Fluoride and enamal structure

Enamel is mainly composed of crystals of hydroxyapatite, which readily loses its hydroxyl group in the presence of fluoride to form fluorapatite. Hydroxyapatite crystals dissolve more easily than fluorapatite in acid due to the presence of voids caused by disordered arrangement of the hydroxyl group. Fluoride thus makes apatite crystals less soluble in acid by two mechanisms. Firstly, crystals of fluorapatite have less voids than crystals of hydroxyapatite, thus reducing solubility (Gron *et al.* 1963). Secondly, fluoride displaces carbon and magnesium ions from apatite crystals; such displacement improves the crystalline structure. There is a greater concentration of fluorapatite on the surface of enamel, which further reduces enamel solubility (Weatherell *et al.* 1972).

Fluoride also has an effect on the remineralization of enamel after acid attack, causing an increase in the formation of the more stable fluorapatite. Thus the enamel surface will be more resistant to future acid attack (Brown *et al.* 1977; Koulourides *et al.* 1980).

Fluoride and tooth morphology

It has been shown that fluoride ingested during dental development slightly alters the shape of teeth resulting in wider fissures and more rounded cusps (Forrest 1956). Enamel and dentine are also thinner due to altered matrix formation caused by impaired protein synthesis (Kruger 1970). However, it is unlikely that these actions of fluoride are of any great clinical significance and may only have a slight effect on the incidence of pit and fissure caries.

Fluoride and plaque

Research has shown that fluoride has a dual effect on plaque, causing an inhibition of formation and a reduction of enzymic action within formed plaque. The early phase of plaque formation depends upon the integrity of the dental pellicle, which is derived from salivary protein. Fluoride reduces the precipitation of protein from saliva on the enamel surface. However, the value of this mode of action of fluoride for causing a reduction in caries is uncertain (Jenkins 1978).

Much interest has been focused on the action of fluoride on plaque metabolism, in particular anaerobic glycolysis. Low concentrations of fluoride (1 to 2 p.p.m.) are capable of inhibiting acid production in plaque. Furthermore, plaque can concentrate fluoride, although it is easily leached out. Repeated exposure of plaque to fluoride (either in toothpastes or rinses) maintains the concentration of fluoride in the plaque (Birkeland *et al.* 1971).

Pharmacokinetics of fluoride

Fluoride is passively absorbed from the stomach, stored in skeletal tissue, and excess is excreted via the kidney, sweat, and faeces. The placenta acts as a partial barrier to fluoride, which depends upon the maternal concentration of fluoride. Thus, the efficacy of therapeutic fluoride given to the pregnant mother to enhance the baby's teeth is uncertain.

Fluoride administration

Fluoride can be administered systemically via the water supply, tablets, drops, milk, and salt, or topically in the form of solutions, gels, varnishes, and toothpastes.

Water fluoridation

Early epidemiological studies in areas with natural fluoride in the water supply clearly demonstrated its anticaries effect. In areas with no natural fluoride in their water supply, the addition of fluoride up to 1 p.p.m. causes a significant reduction in the incidence of dental caries. Fluoride so added has the additional benefit of serving a large population at minimal cost.

Fluoride tablets and drops

These are either the sodium or calcium salt, or the acidulated phosphate salt of fluoride; dosage is between 0.5 to 1 mg per day. The effectiveness of fluoride tablets depends upon the age at which the child commences treatment; the earlier, the greater the percentage reduction in caries. Overall results from several studies indicate that this form of fluoride therapy produces a 40 to 80 per cent reduction in the incidence of dental caries (Murray and Rugg-Gunn 1982). Compliance with home-administered fluoride is poor but school-based programmes might overcome this problem.

Fluoridized milk

Milk is widely dispensed in schools and would thus seem a good vehicle for delivering fluoride. Furthermore, absorption of fluoride is not affected by the Ca^{2+} present in milk (Ericsson 1958). There have been few studies to support the effectiveness of fluoridized milk in controlling dental caries, and other methods of fluoride delivery may be more acceptable. The amount of fluoride added to milk, in the form of sodium fluoride, is the equivalent of receiving 1 mg F/per day.

Fluoridated table salt

Salt, like water and milk, is another excellent vehicle for dispensing fluoride. Concentrations of fluoride in salt vary between 200 to 350 mg F/kg salt. Although widely used on the continent of Europe, there have been few studies of the efficacy of this method of fluoride delivery for controlling dental caries. However, what findings there are suggest that fluoridated salt is an effective method for controlling dental caries, but not as good as fluoride in the water supply (Murray and Rugg-Gunn 1982).

Fluoride solutions

These can be classified into two types: aqueous solutions of sodium or stannous fluoride, or the acidulated phosphate fluoride system.

Sodium and stannous fluoride

Sodium fluoride was the first topically applied fluoride solution. In clinical use, a 2 per cent solution is applied to dried teeth for three minutes, usually three to four times per year. The long-term efficacy (over four years or more) of this method of fluoride application is uncertain, but short-term results indicate a caries reduction of between 30 to 50 per cent.

Stannous fluoride has been shown to be more effective than sodium fluoride at reducing enamel dissolution by acid. In clinical practice, an 8 to 10 per cent stannous fluoride solution is used, but such a solution is unstable and each new application requires a fresh solution. A further disadvantage of stannous fluoride is the staining of teeth, especially at the margins of restorations.

Acidulated phosphate fluoride

This system was developed after studies had shown that the uptake of fluoride by enamel was enhanced by reducing the pH (Bibby 1947). Clinical trials have demonstrated that a 1.23 per cent acidulated phosphofluoride solution causes a 20 to 40 per cent reduction in caries activity. The acidulated solution has to be applied to dried teeth for four minutes, usually twice a year. Application of the solution can present a problem with young children who have a copious salivary flow. Acidulated fluoride solutions cause nausea and sometimes vomiting if swallowed. This problem can be overcome by applying the solution in the form of a gel or by using a tray that fits closely to the teeth.

Fluoride varnishes

Fluoride applied in the form of a varnish allows of longer contact between the enamel surface and fluoride ions. Proprietary fluoride varnishes include Duraphat, Elmex, Protector, and Epoxylite 9070, which are usually applied twice a year. The effectiveness of this mode of applying fluoride is uncertain, and claims of caries reduction show marked variation between studies. Evidence suggests that this method of applying fluoride is the least effective (Hodge *et al.* 1980; Mainwaring and Naylor, 1983).

Fluoride toothpastes

Fluoride in toothpaste is the commonest and easiest method of applying topical fluoride. Nearly all brands of toothpaste sold in the UK contain fluoride, usually sodium monofluorophosphate. Regular use of a fluoride toothpaste causes a 30 per cent reduction in the incidence of dental caries. Recently, the effectiveness of sodium monofluorophosphate has been enhanced by the addition of either sodium fluoride or calcium glycerophosphate to the toothpaste.

Mouth rinses

A sodium fluoride solution at a concentration of 100 to 200 p.p.m. is widely used as a mouth rinse. The efficacy of this method of applying fluoride depends upon the frequency of rinsing, which is usually recommended once a week. Supervision at schools offers an ideal opportunity to carry out such a programme.

Unwanted effects of fluoride therapy

These can be classified as effects on skeletal tissue and effects on the teeth.

Effects of skeletal tissue

A high regular intake of fluoride (greater than 8 p.p.m.) can lead to skeletal fluorosis, which is characterized by an increase in bone density, especially in the lumbar spine and pelvis, and an increase in the thickness of long bones. In severe cases, calcification of the ligaments occurs. Histologically, skeletal fluorosis resembles osteomalacia but, biochemically, the plasma calcium and phosphate levels are normal. The strength of fluorotic bone is poor, and spontaneous fractures are common (Nordin 1973).

Effect on teeth

Excessive fluoride intake will cause dental fluorosis. The clinical appearance can range from white patches in the enamel to severe hypoplasia of the whole tooth. Dental fluorosis can develop if the daily fluoride intake exceeds 2 p.p.m.

Fluoride overdose

The various fluoride preparations are readily available to the public and overdose can arise, especially in young children consuming excess tablets or drops. The lethal dose of sodium fluoride for man is 5 g. Signs and symptoms of overdose include abdominal pain, vomiting, and diarrhoea. Fluoride overdose is treated by gastric lavage to reduce further absorption.

PHARMACOLOGICAL CONTROL OF PERIODONTAL DISEASE

Introduction

Periodontal disease is caused by bacterial plaque, although various systemic factors can modify the inflammatory response of the periodontal tissues to bacterial toxins. The disease can be prevented by either inhibiting the formation of plaque on the tooth surface or by complete plaque removal before inflammatory changes occur in the gingival tissues. Complete plaque removal by mechanical means may be possible in well-motivated individuals, but the majority of people leave plaque on some part of the tooth surface after brushing. Much attention has, therefore, been focused on chemical means to inhibit plaque formation; inhibitory agents can be categorized into the following groups: enzymes, antiseptics, antibiotics, oxygen-releasing agents, and fluoride.

Enzymes

The major part of bacterial plaque (70 per cent) comprises micro-organisms, and the remainder is an intermicrobial matrix of protein and carbohydrate. Enzymes are utilized to break down the plaque matrix and disperse micro-organisms. Enzymes that have been used to 'destroy' plaque include mucinases, extracts from dried pancreas (containing trypsin, chymotrypsin, carboxypeptidase, amylase, lipase, and nuclease), and dextranase. These have to be incorporated into chewing gum and toothpastes. However, their efficacy in plaque control is poor, and although *in vitro* findings showed promise, clinical trials produced indifferent results and a high incidence of unwanted effects. The present consensus of opinion does not favour the use of enzymes as a method for controlling plaque formation and periodontal disease (Hull 1980).

Antiseptics

Many antiseptic mouthwashes can affect the bacterial flora in the mouth and the development of plaque. However, their inhibitory effect is often short, and repeated use is required. Antiseptics used for controlling plaque are the biguanides and the quarternary ammonium compounds.

Biguanides

The main biguanide used for controlling plaque is chlorhexidine (see Chapter 9); alexidine is also used. Biguanides are effective against both Gram-positive and Gram-negative micro-organisms. Chlorhexidine destroys bacteria by being adsorbed onto the cell wall, which leads to damage of the permeability barriers. High concentrations cause precipitation and coagulation of the bacterial cytoplasmic contents. It is used as a mouthwash (0.2 per cent aqueous solution), with 10 ml being applied twice daily, or as a toothpaste gel (0.5 to 1 per cent).

Regular twice-daily rinsing with 10 ml chlorhexidine causes an 85 to 95 per cent reduction in salivary bacteria. Bacterial counts return to normal within 48 hours after cessation of the rinses (Loe and Schiott 1970).

Chlorhexidine, although used for inhibiting plaque formation, has no effect on subgingival plaque except by direct irrigation into periodontal pockets (Flotra *et al.* 1971). An important property of chlorhexidine is its ability to bind to various oral surfaces, including tooth enamel, the pellicle, and salivary protein.

Chlorhexidine is mainly used after periodontal surgery where mechanical plaque-control methods may be difficult to achieve until final healing has occurred (Davies 1976). Chlorhexidine mouthwash has also been shown to be useful in the management of aphthous ulceration and denture stomatitis (Addy 1977; Budtz-Jorgensen and Loe 1972).

Unwanted effects

Chlorhexidine has been used for 20 years; as outlined in Chapter 9, most of its unwanted effects are of a local nature. Many patients find the initial taste of this compound unpleasant and repeated use often produces a disturbance in taste, which may last for several hours. Occasional cases of desquamative lesions of the oral mucosa and parotid swelling have been reported, but the incidence is low. The main unwanted effect of chlorhexidine mouthwash or gel is a brown staining of the teeth. Three possible mechanisms may account for this staining; these are as follows—all three mechanisms may contribute to this problem (Eriksen *et al.* 1985):

1. Non-enzymatic browning reactions (Maillard reactions). Carbohydrates and amino acids can act as substrates for the Maillard reaction. These food substances undergo a series of condensation and polymerization reactions leading to the formation of brown pigmented substances known as melanoids. Melanoid production is catalysed by a high pH and by chlorhexidine (Nordbo 1979). The glycoprotein of the acquired pellicle covering the tooth surface may well serve as a substrate for the Maillard reaction.

2. Formation of pigmented metal sulphides. The glycoprotein molecules of the tooth pellicle contains many disulphide bridges. When the glycoprotein is denatured, these bridges split, yielding free sulphydryl groups. These free groups will react with ferric or stannous ions in the diet to form the corresponding brown or yellow metallic sulphides. Chlorhexidine causes denaturation of the pellicle glycoprotein, which may contribute towards the staining potential (Hjeljord *et al.* 1973).

3. Reaction between chlorhexidine and factors in the diet. Many factors may be involved in this reaction (Addy *et al.* 1979). It has been shown that aldehydes and ketones react with chlorhexidine to form coloured products that would attach to a tooth surface. Staining from chlorhexidine is accentuated if there is a heavy consumption of tea, coffee, and red wine, which all contain tannin. Wine causes denaturation of the pellicle glycoprotein; red wine also contains a high amount of iron.

Regular use of chlorhexidine causes thickening of the pellicle, which provides a larger than usual surface area for stain absorption. The thickened pellicle also predisposes towards supragingival calculus formation, which may counteract the benefit of chlorhexidine (Leach and appleton 1981).

Although staining from chlorhexidine is troublesome, the stain can be removed with a rubber cup and pumice paste.

Quaternary ammonium compounds

Mouthwashes containing either benethonium chloride or cetylpyridinium chloride are the main quaternary ammonium compounds used to control plaque. These compounds have chemical and antibacterial properties, and unwanted effects, similar to those of chlorhexidine. However, they are less effective than chlorhexidine as plaque-inhibiting agents (Hull 1980). This difference in efficacy may be due to the poor adsorption of quaternary ammonium compounds.

Antibiotics

As plaque mainly comprises bacteria, many antibiotics have been evaluated as anti-plaque agents. Two widely used for this purpose are tetracycline and metronidazole. However, it must be stressed that antibiotics should only be used for a short time to support conventional periodontal treatment. Continuous prophylactic use of antibiotics in the treatment of periodontal disease is not recommended.

Tetracycline

The pharmacological properties and unwanted effects of this broad-spectrum antibiotic were discussed in Chapter 10. The drug has been administered either systemically, as a mouthwash, or by direct delivery into periodontal pockets as methods of controlling bacterial plaque. Direct irrigation has the advantage of reducing the amount of tetracycline administered (Lindhe *et al.* 1979). Clinical studies have shown that tetracycline therapy significantly reduces bacterial colonization of teeth and periodontal pockets. The drug is particularly useful in cases of juvenile periodontitis where it reduces the micro-organisms *Actinobacillus actinomycetemcomitans* and Capnocytophaga.

Metronidazole

This is effective against obligate anaerobes (see Chapter 10), and studies have shown that systemic administration retards plaque accumulation and the development of gingivitis. The drug has also been used in the treatment of progressive periodontal disease, where it is effective against *Bact. asacharolyticus*, and in juvenile periodontitis against *A. actinomycetemcomitans* and Capnocyto-phaga (Mitchell 1984).

Oxygen-releasing agents

Hydrogen peroxide and sodium peroxyborate (Bocasan) are the main oxygen-releasing agents used in the treatment of periodontal disease. Both are restricted to the treatment of acute ulcerative gingivitis, which is thought to be caused by anaerobic bacteria. It is doubtful if the amount of oxygen released has a significant action on the metabolism of anaerobic organisms during the short period of exposure.

DENTINE SENSITIVITY

Painful symptoms arising from exposed dentine are a common finding in the adult population, with an incidence of 1:7. Exposure of dentine can arise from either removal of enamel or denudation of the root surface. Loss of enamel occurs in attrition, erosion, toothbrush abrasion, or caries. Several factors can cause denudation of the root surface including gingival recession with increasing age, chronic peridontal disease, periodontal surgery, incorrect toothbrushing, and trauma (Dowell and Addy 1983).

Dentine sensitivity (erroneously termed hypersensitivity) is characterized by pain, elicited by various stimuli and disappearing when the stimulus is removed. Some people are sensitive to cold alone; others to touch, sweet, or sour foods, and some to a combination of any of these stimuli. The pain may be so severe that they find eating difficult.

Theories of dentine sensitivity

Precisely how external stimuli are transmitted through dentine to the pulp is not established and, although evidence suggests that dentine is innervated, the extent or magnitude of this innervation is uncertain. There are three theories of dentine sensitivity: (a) the dentinal receptor mechanism; (b) the hydrodynamic mechanism; (c) the modulation of nerve impulses by polypeptides.

Dentinal receptor mechanism

This theory suggests that the odontoblast has a sensory function, perhaps serving as a transducer between external stimuli and the nearby pulpal nerve plexus. Certainly, when there is disruption of odontoblasts, the dentine becomes very sensitive (Brannstrom and Astrom 1964). However, pain-inducing substances, such as potassium chloride, 5-hydroxytryptamine, and histamine, have failed to evoke pain when applied to exposed dentine (Brannstrom 1962). This finding would question the nociceptive role of the odontoblast.

Hydrodynamic mechanism

This is the most widely accepted theory of the cause of dentine sensitivity. Dentinal tubules contain fluid; a blast of air, or hot and cold stimuli, will cause a rapid movement of this within the tubules. this movement will cause deformation of both the odontoblastic process and adjacent nerve fibres. Nerve deformation causes pain (Brannstrom 1966).

Modulation of nerve impulses by polypeptide

Pulpal tissue contains a number of polypeptides that can act as regulators of neural transmission. These include substance P and bradykinin, which may alter the permeability of the odontoblast cell membrane (hyperpolarization). Such hyperpolarization could make the pulp more sensitive to various external stimuli. Thus, substance P and bradykinin may act as modulators of nerve impulses in the pulp (Koreger 1968).

Desensitizing agents

The ideal properties of a desensitizing agent were postulated by Grossman in 1935, and include:

(1) non-irritant to the pulp;

(2) relatively painless on application;

(3) easily applied;

(4) rapid onset of action;

(5) effective permanently;

(6) should not stain the teeth;

(7) consistently effective.

Many agents have been used against dentine sensitivity, and some are discussed below.

Sodium fluoride

This is conveniently applied as a paste, for example Lukomsky's paste, which contains equal parts by weight of sodium fluoride, kaolin, and glycerin. The paste is burnished into the previously dried sensitive area, and left on for about three minutes before the patient is allowed to rinse. Occasionally, paste application may cause marked but transitory pain. Fluoride from the sodium salt will be taken up by the dentine thus making it more resistant to acid decalcification. The fluoride may also lead to an increase in secondary dentine formation, which will block dentinal tubules. Sodium fluoride either in pastes, gels, or mouthwashes has to be applied frequently for maximum effectiveness.

Stannous fluoride

This also reduces dentine sensitivity. In solution it undergoes spontaneous hydrolysis and oxidation, so it is applied in the form of a gel mixed with carboxymethylcellulose or glycerine. Stannous fluoride acts as an enzyme poison and may inactivate enzymic activity within the odontoblastic process. Like sodium fluoride, stannous fluoride induces mineralization within the dentinal tubules, which creates a calcific barrier on the dentine surface.

Sodium monofluorophosphate

This fluoride salt is widely used in toothpastes, but is of uncertain efficacy as a desensitizing agent. It is suggested that monofluorophosphate is hydrolysed by hydroxyapatite on the surface of enamel and dentine. The hydrolysis releases fluoride ions, which are then incorporated into the lattice work of the apatite crystal.

Calcium hydroxide

Although this compound occludes dentinal tubules, its use as a desensitizing agent is uncertain, probably because of its poor adhesion to exposed dentine.

Tresiolan

This comprises a mixture of two siloxane esters, which are immiscible in water. It is a light yellow liquid, marketed in plastic drip bottles. In the presence of moisture, Tresiolan polymerizes, and when applied to the surface of dentine it forms an organosiloxane resinous skin. This skin is probably superficial, although there may be some penetration of the liquid into the surface of the dentinal tubules before polymerization commences. It would appear that this material seals off or plugs the orifices of the dentinal tubules, forming a mechanical barrier against exogenous stimuli.

Tresiolan is applied to the sensitive area by means of a pledget of cotton-wool. The area must be dried before application, and two minutes allowed for the reaction to be complete. It does not cause pain on application, and is not irritant to the oral mucous membrane. As with other densensitizing agents, the action of Tresiolan is not permanent and several applications are usually necessary to produce complete desensitization. The medicament may prove ineffective for some patients.

Strontium chloride

Strontium ions have a strong affinity for calcified tissues, and they also accelerate the rate of calcification. Thus, strontium salts will obliterate the dentinal tubules. Sensodyne toothpaste contains 10 per cent strontium chloride, but the efficacy of this compound in controlling dentine sensitivity is uncertain (Addy and Dowell 1983).

Formaldehyde

Toothpastes containing 1.3 to 1.4 per cent formalin (e.g. Emoform) are used as desensitizing agents, but their unpleasant taste may limit their use. Formalin is thought to precipitate protein in the dentinal tubules and hence reduce sensitivity.

Resins and adhesives

Various of these can be applied to exposed dentine, sealing off the tubules and hence acting as a mechanical barrier to external stimuli. Tooth preparation, such as acid-etching, is required before some of these materials can be applied, so their use should be restricted to the more persistent cases of dentine sensitivity.

CARIES VACCINATION

Dental caries is now recognized as an infectious disease and there has, in recent years, been a revival of interest concerning the use of the body's own defence mechanisms to reduce both the incidence and severity of caries. These mechanisms can, in general, be mobilized by vaccination. Many of the experimental studies in animals have used a vaccine prepared against *Strep. mutans*. The cell wall of this bacterium has many antigens, especially the enzyme glucosyltransferase (GTF), which is responsible for the synthesis of insoluble extracellular mutan. A caries vaccine prepared from Strep mutans, which contains antibodies to GTF, has provided protection against dental caries in animals.

Human caries vaccine

The findings from animal experiments have given impetus to the development of a caries vaccine that can be used both safely and efficaciously in man. However, there are certain drawbacks. For example, caries in the experimental animal was induced by infection with *Strep. mutans*, thus assuming a direct causal relationship between dental caries and that bacterium. In man, this association is less clear and, if a vaccine were to eliminate *mutans*, other bacteria might take on a cariogenic role. Problems have also been encountered of a possible cross-reaction between antigens from the cell wall of *Strep. mutans* and human heart tissue.

A human caries vaccine could easily be incorporated into the general vaccination programme, but dental caries is not a life-threatening disease, and other preventive methods are available for reducing its incidence. If there is any element of doubt as to the safety of a vaccination, then public opinion would be against such a procedure. The future of a caries vaccine for use in man is still questionable (Sims 1985).

REFERENCES

Addy, M. (1977). Hibitane in the treatment of aphthous ulceration. *Journal of Clinical Periodontology*, **4**, 108–16.

Addy, M. and Dowell, P. (1983). Dentine hypersensitivity—a review. Clinical and *in vitro* evaluation of treatment agents. *Journal of Clinical Periodontology*, **10**, 351–63.

Addy, M., Prayitno, S., Taylor, L., and Codogan, S. (1979). An *in vitro* study of the role of dietary factors in the aetiology of tooth staining associated with the use of chlorhexidine. *Journal of Periodontal Research*, 14, 403–10.

Bibby, B. G. (1947). A consideration of the effectiveness of various fluoride mixtures. *Journal of the American Dental Association*, 34, 26.

Birkeland, J. M., Jorkjend, L., and von der Fehr, F. R. (1971). The influence of fluoride rinses on the fluoride content of dental plaque in children. *Caries Research*, 5, 169–79.

Brannstrom, M. (1962). The elicitation of pain in human dentine and pulp by chemical stimulation. *Archives of Oral Biology*, 7, 59–62.

Brannstrom, M. (1966). Sensitivity of dentine. *Oral Surgery*, 21, 517–26.

Brannstrom, M. and Astrom, A. (1964). A study on the mechanisms of pain elicited from the dentine. *Journal of Dental Research*, 43, 619–25.

Brown, W. E., Gregory, T. M., and Chow, L. C. (1977). Effect of fluoride on enamel solubility and cariostasis. *Caries Research*, 11(suppl. 1), 118–41.

Budtz-Jorgensen, E. and Loe, H. (1972). Chlorhexidine as a denture disinfectant in the treatment of denture stomatitis. *Scandinavian Journal of Dental Research*, 80, 457–64.

Davies, R. M. (1976). Use of hibitane following periodontal surgery. *Journal of Clinical Periodontology*, 4, 129–35.

Dowell, P. and Addy, M. (1983). Dentine hypersensitivity—a review. Aetiology, symptoms and theories of pain production. *Journal of Clinical Periodontology*, 10, 341–50.

Ericsson, Y. (1958). The state of fluoride in milk. *Acta Odontologica Scandinavica*, 16, 51–7.

Eriksen, H. M., Nordbo, H., Kantanen, H., and Ellingsen, J. E. (1985). Chemical plaque control and extrinsic tooth discoloration—a review of possible mechanisms. *Journal of Clinical Periodontology*, 12, 345–50.

Flotra, L., Gjermo, P., Rolla, G. and Waerhaug, J. (1971). Side effects of chlorhexidine mouthwashes. *Scandinavian Journal of Dental Research*, 79, 119–25.

Forrest, J. R. (1956). Caries incidence and enamel defects in areas with different levels of fluoride in the drinking water. *British Dental Journal*, 100, 195–200.

Gron, P., Spinelli, M., Trautz, O., and Brudevold, F. (1963). The effect of carbonate on the solubility of hydroxyapatittite. *Archives of Oral Biology*, 8, 251–63.

Grossmann, L. (1935). A systematic method for the treatment of hypersensitive dentine. *Journal of the American Dental Association*, 22, 592–602.

Hjeljord, L. G., Sonju, T., and Rolla, G. (1973). Chlorhexidine–protein interactions. *Journal of Periodontal Research*, 8(suppl. 12), 11–16.

Hodge, H. C., Holloway, P. J., Davies, T. G. H., and Worthington, H. V. (1980). Caries prevention by dentrifices containing a combination of sodium monofluorophosphate and sodium fluoride. *British Dental Journal*, 149, 193–204.

Hull, P. S. (1980). Chemical inhibition of plaque. *Journal of Clinical Periodontology*, 7, 431–42.

Jenkins, G. N. (1978). *The physiology and biochemistry of the mouth*, (4th edn). Blackwell, Oxford.

Koulourides, T., Keller, S. E., Manson-Hing, L., and Lilley, V. (1980). Enhancement of fluoride effectiveness by experimental cariogenic priming of human enamel. *Caries Research*, 14, 32–9.

Kroeger, D. C. (1968). Possible role of neurohormonal substances in the pulp. In *Biology of the dental Pulp organ* (ed. S. B. Finn), pp. 334–46. Alabama Press, Birmingham University, Ill.

Kruger, B. J. (1970). The effect of different levels of fluoride on the ultrastructure of ameloblasts in the rate. *Archives of Oral Biology*, **15**, 109–14.

Leach, S. A. and Appleton, J. (1981). Ultrastructural investigation by energy dispersive X-ray micro-analysis of some of the elements involved in the formation of dental plaque and pellicle. In *Tooth surface interactions and preventitive dentistry*, pp. 65–79. IRL Press, London.

Lindhe, J., Heijil, L., Goodson, J. M., and Socransky, S. S. (1979). Local tetracycline delivery using hollow fibre devices in periodontal therapy. *Journal of Clinical Periodontology*, **6**, 141–49.

Loe, H. and Schiott, C. R. (1970). The effect of mouthrinses and topical application of chlorhexidine on the development of dental plaque and gingivitis in man. *Journal of Periodontal Research*, **5**, 79–83.

Mainwaring, P. J. and Naylor, M. N. (1983). A four-year clinical study to determine the caries inhibiting effect of calcium glycophosphate and sodium fluoride in calcium carbonate base dentifrices containing sodium monofluorophosphate. *Caries Research*, **17**, 267–76.

Mitchell, D. A. (1984). Metronidazole: its use in clinical dentistry. *Journal of Clinical Periodontology*, **11**, 145–58.

Murray, J. J. and Rugg-Gunn, A. J. (1982). *Fluoride in Caries Preventions* (2nd edn). Wright, Bristol.

Nordbo, H. (1979). Ability of chlorhexidine and benzalconium chloride to catalyze browning reactions *in vitro*. *Journal of Dental Research*, **58**, 1429.

Nordin, B. E. C. (1973). *Metabolic bone and stone disease*. Churchill Livingstone, Edinburgh.

Sims, W. (1985). *Streptococcus mutans* and vaccines for dental caries: a personal commentary and critique. *Community Dental Health*, **2**, 129–47.

Weatherell, J. A., Robinson, C., and Hallsworth, A. S. (1972). Changes in the fluoride concentration of the labial enamel surface with age. *Caries Research*, **6**, 312–24.

12

Haemostasis and haemostatic agents

HAEMOSTASIS

SEVERAL factors play an integrated role in the arrest of haemorrhage after a tooth extraction or dental surgery. These include the ability of vessel walls to contract, the adhesion and aggregation of platelets, the ability of blood to coagulate, and the breakdown of blood clot (fibrinolysis). A variety both of diseases and drugs can affect these factors. However, in the context of this Chapter only the effect of drugs will be discussed.

Vessel wall contraction

In the early stages of injury, contraction of the smooth muscles in vessel walls is an important factor in the control of haemorrhage. This vasoconstriction is only of short duration (usually 5 to 20 minutes) but can be prolonged by topical or local infiltration of adrenaline.

Platelets

These are non-nuclear cells with a cytoplasm rich in granules. They are formed by the fragmentation and detachment of delicate processes from the megakaryocyte. The normal platelet count in man is in the range 150 000–400 000 cells/ml, and their half-life is 7 to 10 days. Platelets have an essential role in haemostasis: when a blood vessel is cut or damaged, they rapidly adhere to the exposed sub-endothelial tissues, especially collagen. This platelet adhesion is followed by the release from the platelet granules of adenosine diphosphate (ADP) and the powerful pro-aggregating substance, thromboxane A_2 (TXA$_2$), (Hamburg et al. 1975). Both ADP and thromboxane induce further platelets to stick to each other (platelet aggregation) to form a platelet plug. The plug will arrest haemorrhage, but it must be further stabilized by fibrin. Fibrin formation is stimulated by the exposed cut collagen, platelet membranes, and chemicals released by the platelets themselves, such as 5-hydroxytryptamine and platelet phospholipid (Walsh 1974).

Blood coagulation

This is a complex process that involves the initiation and interaction of several factors in blood and damaged tissues (Fig. 12.1). The basic framework of blood coagulation is the activity of thromboplastin (Factor III) on prothrombin (Factor II) to form thrombin, which in turn converts fibrinogen (Factor I) to fibrin. Fibrin is further polymerized by Factor XIII.

Thromboplastin activity can be generated in two ways—by an intrinsic system (blood thromboplastin), or an extrinsic system (tissue thromboplastin). Activation of the intrinsic system occurs when blood contacts an abnormal surface. This leads to the sequential activation of Factors XII, XI, IX, VIII, and X. Activated Factor X (Xa) together with Factor V and phospholipids derived from platelets result in the formation of thromboplastin (Fig. 12.1). The extrinsic system is

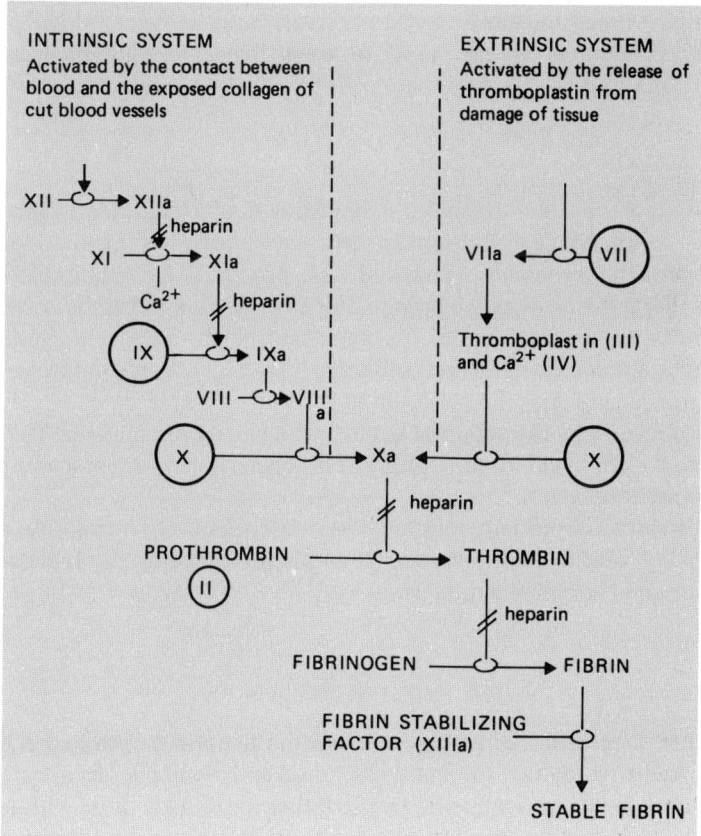

Fig. 12.1. Schematic representation of the blood clotting cascade (factors in circles are dependent on vitamin K for their synthesis, and are affected by warfarin).

activated by tissue damage, which results in the release of a tissue factor rich in phospholipid. The tissue factor, together with Factor VII, activates Factor X. The sequence of events is then the same as in the intrinsic system.

Calcium ions (Factor IV) are essential for many of the stages of blood coagulation and help to accelerate the reaction between thrombin and fibrinogen.

Vitamin K

Vitamin K is a fat-soluble vitamin that is essential for the normal hepatic biosynthesis of several factors required for blood clotting (II, VII, IX, X). The pharmacology of vitamin K is dealt with in more detail in Chapter 19.

The main use of vitamin K is the correction of hypoprothrombinaemia—either congenital, or drug-induced by the coumarin group of anticoagulants (see later). Excessive bleeding from patients on these anticoagulants can be corrected by an intravenous injection of 10 to 20 mg vitamin K. Careful monitoring of the prothrombin time and anticoagulant levels are necessary following this procedure. Vitamin K is also used to treat hypoprothrombinaemia of the newborn.

Fibrinolysis

The final state of haemostasis—the breakdown of blood clot by proteolytic enzymes—is known as fibrinolysis. Extravascularly, as in the case of a haematoma, the proteolytic enzymes are produced by white blood cells. Intravascularly, blood clots are broken down by plasmin, which is derived from the plasma protein, plasminogen. The conversion of plasminogen to plasmin may be caused by either tissue or blood activators (Fig. 12.2). The tissue factor has not been identified, but may be released as a result of tissue damage. The blood activator is formed by the action of kinases on a blood pro-activator. The kinases are liberated from blood, tissues, and certain bacteria (e.g. streptococci produce streptokinase (see later)).

Fibrinolysis can be influenced by a whole range of factors; for example, age, sex, diet, smoking, altitude, and exercise. It can be inhibited by the inactivation of plasmin by the protein, α_2 antiplasmin.

ANTICOAGULANTS

These either directly or indirectly interfere with the normal clotting mechanisms of blood, and thus reduce the incidence of thrombo-embolic disorders. Hence, patients likely to be receiving anticoagulant therapy include those with a history of myocardial infarction, cerebrovascular thrombosis, venous thrombosis, and pulmonary embolism. Those on renal dialysis also receive anticoagulant therapy prior to and during dialysis.

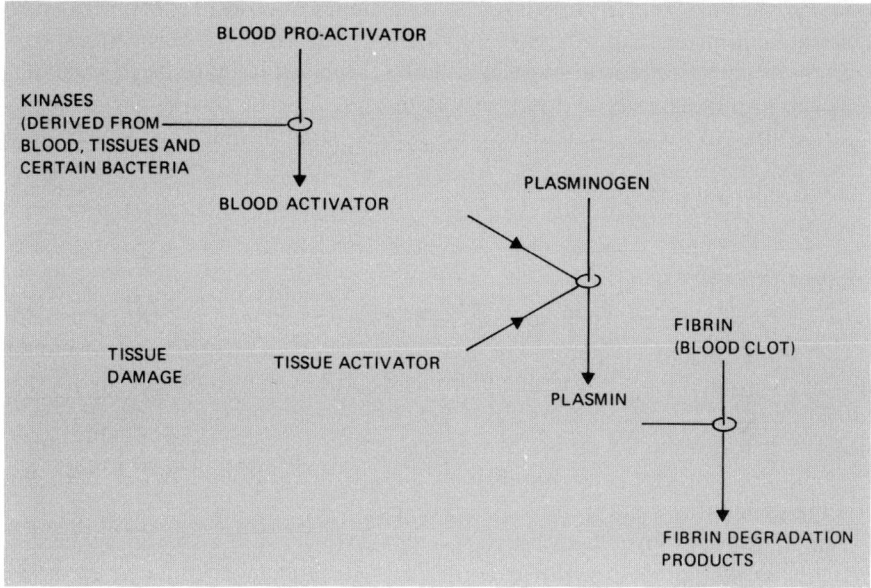

Fig. 12.2. Schematic representation of the various stages involved in fibrinolysis.

Heparin

This glycosaminoglycan occurs in minute amounts in mast cells, but its physiological function is unclear. The drug was 'accidentally' discovered in 1916, although its widespread use as an anticoagulant did not occur until the early 1940s. The synthetic drug is the only effective direct-acting anticoagulant, that is it is immediately effective on fresh blood.

Pharmacodynamics

Heparin interferes with blood coagulation in two ways, both of which are due to the formation of a plasma co-factor (antithrombin III). Firstly, antithrombin III neutralizes several of the activated clotting factors, namely XII, XI, IX, X, II, and XIII. Secondly, antithrombin III inactivates thrombin by forming an irreversible complex with the clotting protein. The activity of antithrombin III is related to the dose of heparin—the lower the dose, the greater the activity particularly against thrombin.

Pharmacological properties

Heparin must be administered parenterally as it is very poorly absorbed from the gut because the drug is highly ionized. It is metabolized in the liver by the enzyme heparinase, and the metabolites excreted via the kidney. After intravenous infusion, the half-life of heparin is one to three hours. Low doses of heparin can be given subcutaneously, but high doses should be given via an intravenous drip. Intramuscular injections of heparin should be avoided because large haematomas can form at the site of injection.

In addition to the anticoagulant properties of heparin, the drug also causes a reduction in plasma concentration of triglycerides. This is of little or no therapeutic value.

Unwanted effects

Haemorrhage is the principle unwanted effect associated with heparin; it usually occurs from the gastro-intestinal or genito-urinary tract. Hence, heparin should not be given to any patient with a bleeding disorder or ulceration of the gastro-intestinal tract. Careful monitoring of the patient's prothrombin time whilst on heparin therapy should minimize the problem of haemorrhage. Prothrombin time is now reported as the British Comparative Ratio (BCR), and the recommended therapeutic range is 2.0 to 4.0.

A mild transient thrombocytopenia is reported to occur in about 25 per cent of patients receiving heparin. However, in a few, thrombocytopenia can be severe and deaths have occurred. Platelet counts should be carried out at regular intervals for all those on heparin therapy.

Commercial preparations of heparin are obtained from animal tissues, and care should be exercised in their use on patients with any history of allergy. Long-term heparin therapy can cause osteoporosis and alopecia.

The anticoagulant effects of heparin can be reversed by the specific antagonist, protamine sulphate, at the dose regime of 1 mg of protamine for every 100 units of heparin. Protamine acts by combining with heparin to form a stable complex that has no anticoagulant properties. This complex is formed through heparin being electronegative and protamine electropositive.

Coumarin anticoagulants

This group, also known as the oral anticoagulants, includes warfarin sodium and phenindione. Coumarin anticoagulants are derived from a substance found in the spoiled sweet clover plant.

Pharmacodynamics

Coumarin anticoagulants are antagonists to vitamin K. Hence they will reduce the synthesis of the vitamin K-dependent clotting factors (II, VII, IX, and X). Because of the varying rate of synthesis of these factors, there is a delay of 8 to 12 hours before a therapeutic response can be obtained after a coumarin anticoagulant. Many factors can affect the activity of these anticoagulants, including diet, small-bowel disease, pyrexia, age, pregnancy, and liver disease.

Pharmacological properties

Warfarin sodium, which is the archetype of the coumarin anticoagulants, is rapidly absorbed and extensively (98 per cent) bound to plasma protein. Its plasma half-life is 35–37 hours. The drug is metabolized in the liver, and the metabolites are excreted in the urine and faeces. Coumarin anticoagulants differ from heparin in that they are effective when given by mouth and have a much longer duration of action.

Unwanted effects

Haemorrhage is the most common unwanted effect, and regular monitoring of the prothrombin (BCR) time (which assesses the efficacy of the anticoagulant) is essential for patients on these drugs. Haemorrhagic problems include haematuria, ecchymosis, epistaxis, and gingival bleeding (O'Reilly 1976). Such problems are treated by withdrawal of the drug, followed by the oral or intravenous administration of vitamin K (10–20 mg) depending on the severity of the haemorrhage. Withdrawal of anticoagulant therapy must be done in consultation with the patient's physician.

Drug interactions

Coumarin anticoagulants are frequently implicated in drug interactions that can either increase or decrease the anticoagulant response. Drugs that increase this response include aspirin, metronidazole, and co-trimoxazole.

Aspirin should not be given to patients on coumarin anticoagulant therapy: as few as one or two aspirin tablets can impair platelet function by blocking the release of ADP and the powerful aggregatory substance, thromboxane A_2 (see earlier). As a consequence of these properties of aspirin, there is a weak and poorly formed platelet plug; the impairment of platelet function, together with the impairment in blood coagulation, can lead to a fatal haemorrhage. Other aspirin-like drugs, such as non-steroidal anti-inflammatory agents (see Chapter 5), may also affect platelet aggregation, and should similarly be avoided in patients on coumarin anticoagulants. Aspirin also displaces warfarin from the plasma-protein binding site, the result being an enhancement of the anticoagulant effect of warfarin.

Metronidazole and co-trimoxazole interfere with the pharmacokinetics of warfarin, resulting in an increase in the drug's half-life. Hence concomitant administration of these antimicrobials with warfarin will enhance the anticoagulant effect.

Barbiturates are the main group of drugs that decrease the anticoagulant response of warfarin. Barbiturates cause an induction of hepatic microsomal enzymes, which increase the metabolism of the anticoagulant. This increase in clearance causes a decrease in hypoprothrombinaemia.

Vitamin C in massive doses can reduce the hypoprothrombinaemic effect of coumarin anticoagulants in some patients. The mechanism of this interaction is unclear, but vitamin C may reduce the absorption of these drugs.

ANTITHROMBOTIC DRUGS

Antithrombotic or antiplatelet drugs decrease thrombin formation. Aspirin has been widely investigated for this purpose; other antithrombotic drugs are dipyridamole and sulphinpyrazone.

Aspirin and platelet aggregation

Aspirin causes an increase in bleeding time by reducing platelet aggregation (O'Brien 1968; Weiss et al. 1968). The haemostatic response to aspirin shows marked inter-individual variation (Seymour et al. 1984). Aspirin inhibits the release of ADP from platelets and prevents aggregation by irreversibly blocking (acetylating) the platelet cyclo-oxygenase enzyme system (Roth et al. 1975). This prevents the formation of the powerful platelet aggregating substance, thromboxane A_2. The anti-aggregatory effect of aspirin lasts for the life-span of the platelet (7 to 10 days), and a single dose of 600 mg may produce detectable effects on platelet aggregation and bleeding time for several days. Normal platelet aggregation is only restored when new platelets are released into the circulation.

In addition to the action on platelet cyclo-oxygenase, aspirin also inhibits the synthesis of vessel-wall prostacyclin (Vane 1978). It is thought that prostacyclin inhibition occurs with higher doses of aspirin (over 1 g per day). Furthermore, vascular endothelial cells are less sensitive to aspirin than are platelets, so cyclo-oxygenase activity in vessel walls can be quickly restored (Preston et al. 1981).

Use of aspirin in the prevention of thrombo-embolic disorders

There has been much interest in the use of aspirin in the prevention of thrombo-embolic disorders such as transient ischaemic attacks (TIAs), myocardial infarction, cerebrovascular disease, and venous thrombo-embolism. However, there remains much controversy as to the most suitable dose of aspirin for such conditions. The confusion has arisen from reports claiming that large doses of aspirin inhibit both thromboxane and prostacyclin biosynthesis, whereas low doses of aspirin selectively inhibit platelet thromboxane synthesis.

Aspirin (600 mg per day) has been shown to be effective in reducing the incidence of TIAs (Fields 1983), but its efficacy in preventing myocardial infarction is equivocal (Elwood 1983; Lewis et al. 1983). Further studies are therefore required, with perhaps different dose regimes, to determine whether aspirin is of any value in preventing such life-threatening conditions.

DENTAL MANAGEMENT OF PATIENTS WITH HAEMOSTATIC PROBLEMS

Haemostatic problems that the dental surgeon is likely to encounter can be broadly classified into three groups:

(1) impaired platelet function;

(2) vascular defects;

(3) impaired coagulation.

In all patients with haemostatic problems, careful treatment planning and consultation with their physician are essential. When surgery is required, such patients are best treated in a Dental Hospital or Oral Surgery Department. Every attempt should be made to obtain adequate haemostasis during the operative procedure (i.e. by suturing and packing sockets).

Impaired platelet function

This may be due to a reduction in platelet count (thrombocytopenia), or impaired aggregation resulting from drug therapy.

Thrombocytopenia occurs when the normal platelet count (range 150 000–400 000 cells/ml blood) falls below 100 000 cells/ml. It can be caused by a variety of factors such as radiotherapy, connective tissue disease, or leukaemia. In patients with a low platelet count (less than 50 000 cells/ml blood), a platelet transfusion may be necessary just prior to a dental surgical procedure (i.e. tooth extraction or periodontal surgery). If the thrombocytopenia is due to immune destruction of platelets, as occurs in idiopathic thrombocytopenic purpura, then corticosteroids need to be administered, either instead of or with the platelet infusion.

Drugs that cause impairment of platelet aggregation and an increase in bleeding time include aspirin and non-steroidal anti-inflammatory drugs (see above), sodium valproate, and phenytoin. When tooth extractions are carried out on patients taking these drugs it is a wise precaution to suture and pack the socket and hence minimize the risk of post-extraction haemorrhage.

Vascular defects

Those that can cause impairment of haemostasis are associated with vitamin C deficiency (ascorbutic) and long-term corticosteroid therapy. Vitamin C is essential for collagen synthesis and a deficiency causes scurvy. Ascorbutic patients have increased capillary fragility, which can cause bleeding problems after surgery. Long-term corticosteroid therapy can cause both a thrombocytopenia and an inadequate constriction of the small vessels after surgery. Both factors can lead to haemorrhagic problems. Patients undergoing dental surgery with such vascular defects can present with these problems of haemorrhage. Usually this can be controlled by pressure, suturing, and packing.

Impaired coagulation

This can be due to either an inherited coagulation defect (for example, haemophilia, von Willebrand's disease, or Christmas disease) or to anticoagulant therapy.

Haemophilia

This is a sex-linked, inherited coagulation disorder that usually affects only males. Patients have a reduced Factor VIII activity, which can be corrected by replacement therapy of freeze-dried Factor VIII (cryoprecipitate). Any dental procedures that involve haemorrhage, such as extractions or scaling, will put the haemophiliac patient at risk. All dental procedures should be carefully planned and carried out with Factor VIII cover. The dose of Factor VIII is dependent upon the severity of the hameophilia. Factor VIII cover may need to be repeated as it is only effective for 12 hours. Other drugs used in conjunction with Factor VIII include the anti-fibrinolytic agent, epsilon aminocaproic acid, which reduces the Factor VIII requirements. This drug should be started pre-operatively and continued until all risk of haemorrhage has ceased.

Christmas disease

This is associated with a deficiency of Factor IX; clinically, the disease is identical to haemophilia. Factor IX is derived from plasma, but is not present in cryoprecipitate. The half-life of Factor IX is greater than that of Factor VIII, so replacement therapy is given at longer intervals. The dental management of patients with Christmas disease is the same as for haemophiliacs.

Von Willebrand's disease

This is an inherited disorder associated with both a prolonged bleeding time and a deficiency of Factor VIII, although the latter shows marked individual variation. When Factor VIII levels are low, replacement therapy is necessary if surgery is to be carried out on these patients.

Anti-coagulant therapy

Heparin

Heparinized patients are usually confined to hospital; this group will include those with recent thrombo-embolic disorders and those undergoing renal dialysis. The anticoagulant effects of heparin will last for four to six hours after a single dose. If an emergency extraction is needed on a heparinized patient it should be carried out when the anticoagulant effect is minimal. Patients on continuous heparin therapy should be given intravenous protamine sulphate at the dosage of 1 mg per 100 units of heparin. Monitoring the patient's prothrombin time (BCR) is essential.

Coumarin anticoagulants

If elective surgery, such as removal of an impacted lower third molar, is required for patients on coumarin anticoagulants, consultation with the patient's physician is essential, so that dose regimes can be altered. Prothrombin activity should be measured prior to surgery. Usually, vitamin K (5 mg) is given the day before surgery, or 2.5 mg vitamin K given orally for two days before surgery. The 5 mg dose of vitamin K will bring the prothrombin activity from the so-called 'therapeutic range' of 25 per cent of normal, up to the normal range (90–100 per cent activity). The 2.5 mg dose regimen of vitamin K will bring the value to 50 to 60 per cent of normal activity. The prothrombin activity will return to its previous level of 25 per cent in about four days.

Emergency single extractions can be carried out on patients taking coumarin anticoagulants, provided their prothrombin time does not exceed 2 to 2.5 times the normal value. Sockets should be packed and sutured. If haemorrhage does occur, the anticoagulant effect can be reversed by intravenous vitamin K (phytomenadione, 10–20 mg).

FIBRINOLYTIC DRUGS

This group of drugs promotes the breakdown of thrombi by activation of plasminogen to form plasmin. Examples include streptokinase and urokinase. Fibrinolytic drugs have a prolonged effect on haemostasis and can cause extensive problems if not used carefully.

Streptokinase

This is a protein derived from β-haemolytic streptococci, which interacts with the pro-activator of plasminogen. The combination of pro-activator and strepto-kinase catalyses the conversion of plasminogen to plasmin. Bleeding from the site of injection is a common problem associated with streptokinase administration. Streptokinase is used to treat acute pulmonary embolism and deep vein thrombosis. The drug is extremely expensive, which imposes restrictions on its routine use.

Urokinase

This is a proteolytic enzyme that activates the conversion of plasminogen to plasmin. The drug is as active as streptokinase and is used in patients who are allergic to the streptokinase.

ANTIFIBRINOLYTIC DRUGS

These encourage the stabilization of fibrin by inhibiting plasminogen activation. Examples include epsilon-aminocaproic acid or the more potent, tranexamic acid.

Antifibrinolytic agents may be useful in controlling persistent haemorrhage after tooth extraction, in conjunction with local measures. However, their main use is in haemophiliacs as an adjunct to Factor VIII therapy. Unwanted effects associated with antifibrinolytic drugs include nausea, diarrhoea, and hypotension.

THE MANAGEMENT OF POST-EXTRACTION HAEMORRHAGE

A careful and detailed history should be taken from all patients presenting with a post-extraction haemorrhage. This is essential to ensure that there is no underlying systemic disease or drug therapy (e.g. aspirin or anticoagulant therapy) contributing to the haemorrhage. If the patient has a predisposing problem, then the appropriate treatment should be carried out as previously outlined.

Most cases of post-extraction haemorrhage are due to tears in the mucoperiosteum around the tooth socket. In the majority of such cases, a suture will effectively control the haemorrhage. Further aids to haemostasis can be obtained by placing an absorbable material in the socket. These materials are made of either cellulose, alginate, gelatin, or fibrin, and provide a network that activates the clotting mechanisms.

Surgicel (oxidized regenerated cellulose) is the most widely and easily applied resorbable material. It is available in strips and can be cut and placed in the tooth socket. Surgicel resorbs within 7 to 10 days, and foreign-body reactions are rare.

REFERENCES

Elwood, P. C. (1983). British studies of aspirin and myocardial infarction. *American Journal of Medicine*, **74**, 50–4.

Fields, W. S. (1983). Aspirin for prevention of stroke. *American Journal of Medicine*, **74**, 61–5.

Hamberg, M., Svenson, J., and Samuelsson, B. (1975). Thromboxanes: a new group of biologically active compounds derived from prostaglandin endoperoxides. *Proceedings of the National Academy of Sciences U.S.A.*, **72**, 2994–8.

Lewis, H. D. *et al.* (1983). Protective effects of aspirin against acute myocardial infarction and death in men with unstable angina. *New England Journal of Medicine*, **309**, 396–403.

O'Brien, J. R. (1968). Aspirin and platelet aggregation. *Lancet*, **i**, 204–5.

O'Reilly, R. A. (1976). Vitamin K and the oral anticoagulant drugs. *Annual Review of Medicine*, **27**, 245–61.

Preston, F. E., Whipps, S., Jackson, C. A., French, A. J., Wyld, P. J., and Stoddard, C. J. (1981). Inhibition of prostacyclin and platelet thromboxane A_2 after low dose aspirin. *New England Journal of Medicine*, **304**, 76–9.

Roth, G. J. and Majerus, P. W. (1975). The mechanism of the effect of aspirin on human platelets I: acetylation of a particular fraction protein. *Journal of Clinical Investigation*, **56**, 624–32.

Seymour, R. A. *et al.* (1984). A comparative study of the effects of aspirin and paracetamol (acetaminophen) on platelet aggregation and bleeding time. *European Journal of Clinical Pharmacology*, **26**, 567–71.

Vane, J. R. (1978). Inhibitors of prostaglandin, prostacyclin and thromboxane synthesis. *Advances in Prostaglandin and Thromboxane Research*, **4**, 27–44.

Walsh, P. N. (1974). Platelet coagulant activities and haemostasis: a hypothesis. *Blood*, **47**, 597–605.

Weiss, H. J., Aledort, L. M., and Kochwa, S. (1968). The effect of salicylates on the haemostatic properties of platelets in man. *Journal of Clinical Investigation*, **47**, 2169–80.

PART II

GENERAL DRUGS

13

Autonomic nervous system

GENERAL ORGANIZATION

THE autonomic nervous system consists of two main parts:

(1) central

(2) peripheral, which in turn consists of;

   (i) sympathetic (thoracolumbar outflow; lateral horn cells T1–L2);

   (ii) parasympathetic (craniosacral outflow: cranial nuclei 3, 7, 9, and 10; lateral horn cells, sacral 2–4.

Classically, the peripheral autonomic nervous system has been considered to be exclusively efferent. However, it is clear that certain *afferent* nerves form an essential functional part of the system; for example, visceral afferent, vagal afferent, and nociceptive fibres, which travel with specific nerves. These afferent nerves form the afferent arm of various important autonomic reflexes. Thus, the afferent fibres from the viscera consist mainly of non-myelinated fibres and form the primary afferent neurones in autonomic reflex arcs that are concerned with respiratory, vasomotor, and other functions. Integration of these reflexes takes place initially in the spinal cord but their overall integration takes place centrally, particularly in the hypothalamus.

Central autonomic nervous system

The organization of the central autonomic nervous system is illustrated diagrammatically in Fig. 13.1. The 'head' of the central autonomic is the hypothalamus. It receives its input from somatic and visceral afferent fibres and, after functional integration of this information, controls those organs and systems that it supplies via the sympathetic and parasympathetic outflows. The hypothalamus contains many nuclei, of which those located posterolaterally are mainly sympathetic in function, whilst those anteromedially are mainly concerned with the parasympathetic system. The hypothalamus also has important connections with the pituitary gland (hypophysis), limbic system, thalamocortical system, and brain stem. Furthermore, it receives and integrates information about the milieu from receptors sensitive to temperature, ionic concentration (osmolarity), and hormone concentration. Through these interac-

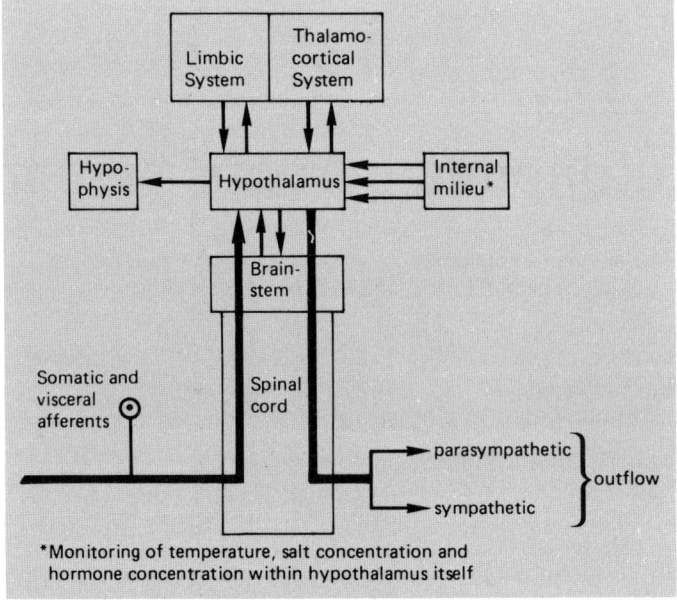

Fig. 13.1 The organization of the central autonomic nervous system

tions it is responsible for the regulation of visceral, metabolic, and endocrine functions, which include the following:

Cardiovascular system	Respiration
Swallowing	Feeding
Vomiting	Metabolism
Temperature	Micturition
Defaecation	Sexual function
Emotions	Sleep
Endocrine mechanisms	

Thus it can be seen that the autonomic nervous system, through its central and peripheral parts, is responsible for controlling those vital body functions that require constant monitoring and adjustment, not only to control the internal milieu but to adapt it to rapidly changing requirements and environmental conditions.

Drugs acting upon the autonomic nervous system may be divided into two broad categories. first, those designed to act upon some part of it; for example, adrenoceptor blocking drugs, antimuscarinic drugs. Second, drugs not designed to act upon the autonomic nervous system but that nevertheless, through lack of specificity, produce various actions upon it that manifest themselves as unwanted effects; for example, antimuscarinic effects of tricyclic antidepressants, hypotensive action of neuroleptics (antipsychotics).

Peripheral efferent parts of the autonomic nervous system

The efferent pathways of the autonomic nervous system, both sympathetic and parasympathetic divisions, transmit impulses to the effector cells from central connections. The peripheral efferent portions of the system comprise preganglionic and postganglionic neurones (Fig. 13.2). The preganglionic neurone arises from cells of central origin and ends at the ganglion. From cell bodies within the ganglion fibres arise that pass to the effector cells, and these fibres comprise the postganglionic neurone.

The sympathetic outflow is limited to the thoracic and upper lumbar segments of the spinal cord. Between the first thoracic and second lumbar segments (inclusive), the grey matter of the spinal cord has lateral horns. The sympathetic neurones have their cell bodies in these horns, and the preganglionic fibres pass out via the anterior nerve roots. These fibres enter the sympathetic chain, which runs on either side of the spinal cord. This chain extends for the whole length of the spinal cord; it has a swelling or ganglion associated with each spinal segment with the exception of the cervical region, where there are only three ganglia (superior, middle, and inferior cervical ganglia). The preganglionic fibres may run up or down the sympathetic chain before synapsing with a postganglionic fibre in one of the ganglia. Each postganglionic fibre leaves the chain and runs to its

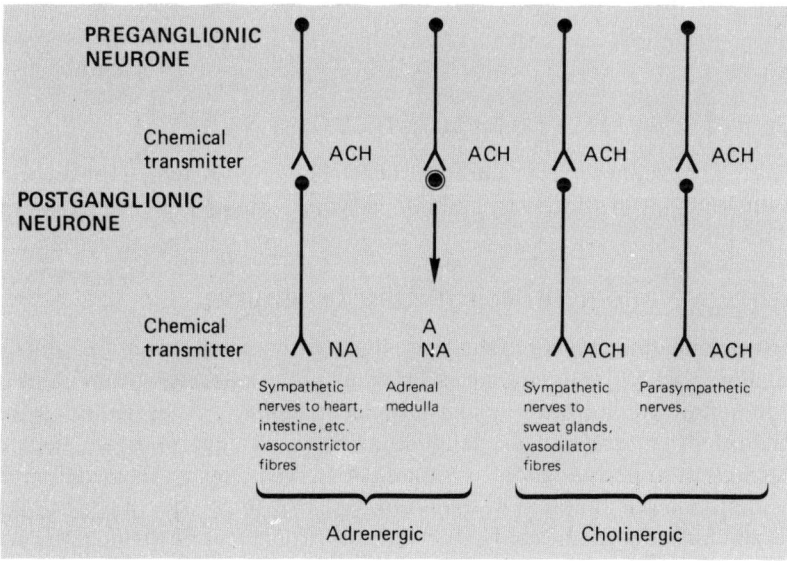

Fig. 13.2. Diagrammatic representation of the neurones of the autonomic nervous with their related chemical transmitters. Left: adrenergic; right: cholinergic. Note that although nerves to the sweat glands are anatomically part of the sympathetic nervous system, pharmacologically they are included with the cholinergic division (ACH = acetylcholine; A = Adrenaline; NA = noradrenaline).

destination in a mixed motor and sensory nerve. The cranial sympathetic fibres run in the outer coat (adventitia) of blood vessels—the internal carotid and external carotid arteries, and their branches.

In the parasympathetic nervous system the nerves leave the central nervous system (CNS) in the spinal region only at the second, third and fourth lumbar segments but, in addition, there is an important outflow in some of the cranial nerves that arise from the brain itself; thus the parasympathetic system has a craniosacral outflow. By far the most widely distributed cranial nerve is the tenth cranial nerve or vagus, which supplies the contents of the thorax and the abdomen.

A gap, called a synapse, exists between the preganglionic and the postganglionic neurones, and a similar junction occurs between the postganglionic neurone and the autonomic effector organ, so that there must be a mechanism for bridging these junctions. It is generally agreed that transmission at synapses is performed by chemical mediators or transmitters. The transmitter liberated at all preganglionic nerve endings, and at parasympathetic post-ganglionic nerve endings, is acetylcholine. Adrenergic transmission, which occurs between postganglionic sympathetic nerve endings and the effectors innervated by them, is mediated by noradrenaline. Noradrenaline is important in the maintenance of normal sympathetic tone, not only by virtue of being a chemical transmitter, but also as a result of being released in appropriate amounts from the adrenal medulla into the general circulation.

SYMPATHETIC NERVOUS SYSTEM

The adrenal medulla secretes a number of catecholamines, which are associated with the functioning of the sympathetic nervous system.

Occurrence and synthesis of catecholamines

Three catecholamines occur in the body: these are dopamine, noradrenaline, and adrenaline; a fourth, isoprenaline, is a product of the laboratory. Adrenaline and noradrenaline are secreted by the adrenal medulla; noradrenaline is found concentrated in granules in postganglionic sympathetic neurones; and dopamine is also present in postganglionic sympathetic nerves. Dopamine, noradrenaline, and adrenaline are all found in the brain.

Noradrenaline is synthesized in the neurones from tyrosine through the action of three enzymes (1) tyrosine hydroxylase, (2) dopa decarboxylase, and (3) dopamine-β-hydroxylase. In the neurone, synthesis stops at the stage of noradrenaline formation but, in the adrenal medulla, a further enzymatic step results in the methylation of noradrenaline to become adrenaline (Fig. 13.3).

Fig. 13.3. The intermediate stages in the formation of adrenaline. Note that the last stage, in which noradrenaline is methylated to adrenaline, only occurs in the adrenal medulla. (From A. Wilson and H. O. Schild (1968). *Applied Pharmacology*, (10th edn), p. 77. Churchill, London.)

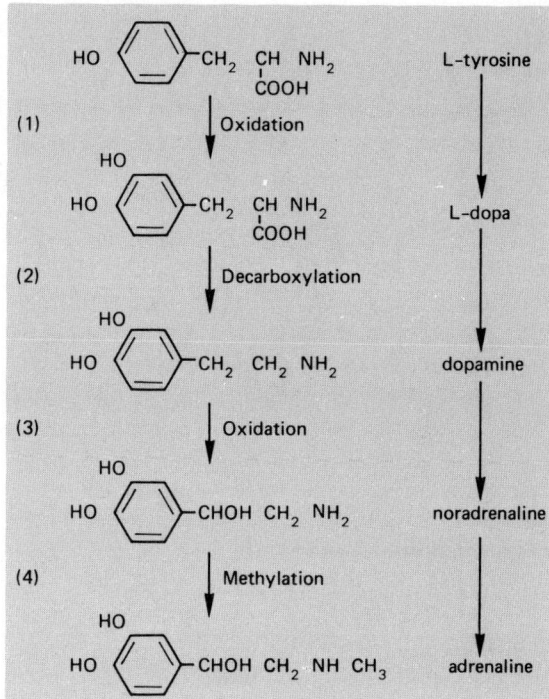

Stages of chemical transmission at synapses

The main stages in synaptic transmission (Fig. 13.4) are as follows:

(1) synthesis of the chemical transmitter from tyrosine;

(2) storage of the chemical transmitter in special granules;

(3) release of the chemical transmitter from storage sites;

(4) activation of post-synaptic receptors leading to stimulation or inhibition of the effector organ;

(5) inactivation of the chemical transmitter, principally through re-uptake into the sympathetic nerve endings.

It is thought that postganglionic sympathetic neurones, adrenal medullary cells, and certain cells in the CNS synthesize catecholamines and store them in granules. The arrival of a nerve impulse at the nerve endings results in the release of the transmitter from the storage granules. The transmitter is released from the postganglionic sympathetic nerve endings and, after diffusing across the synaptic cleft, activates receptors situated on the postsynaptic membrane. This will result

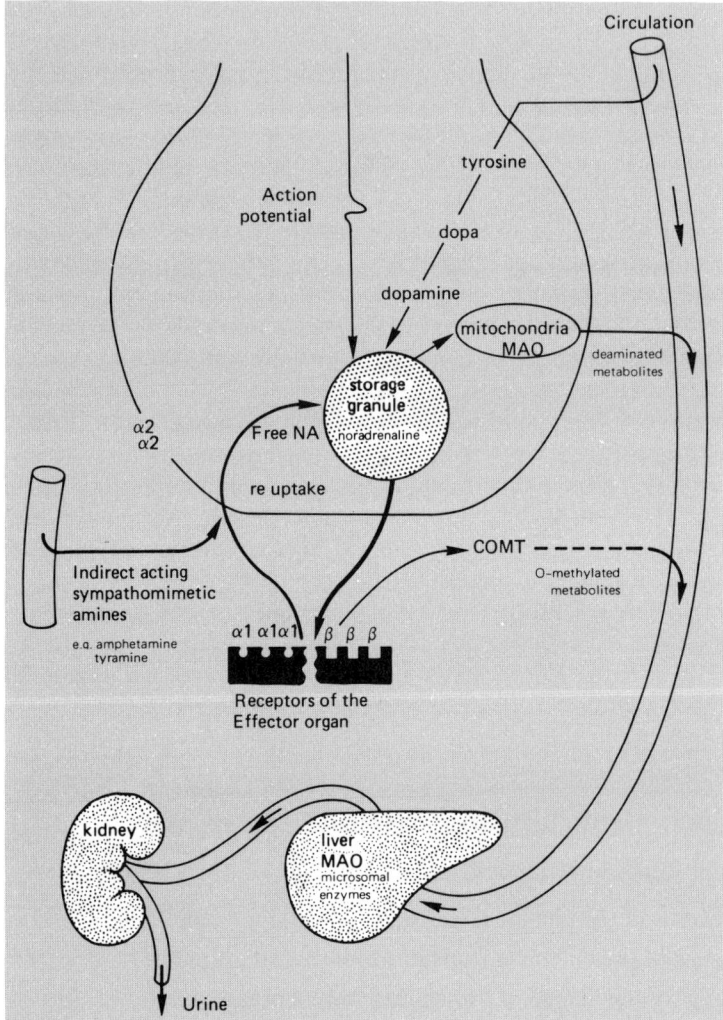

Fig. 13.4. Steps involved in the synthesis, storage, release, and subsequent metabolism of noradrenaline at a postganglionic sympathetic nerve ending (NA = noradrenaline; COMT = catechol-O-methyl transferase; MAO = monoamine oxidase; α = α-receptors; β = β-receptors).

in an action that depends upon the effector organ involved; for example, the contraction of vascular smooth muscle.

There are other amines with actions, like those of the catecholamines, that mimic sympathetic stimulation. At first it was believed that all these drugs acted in the same way as the naturally occurring catecholamines. Later it became clear that, whereas the endogenous adrenaline and noradrenaline act directly upon adrenergic receptors, other drugs (such as amphetamine and tyramine) act indirectly by causing the release of the transmitter substance from the nerve endings. It is now thought that indirectly acting sympathomimetic amines are taken up first by the amine pump (see below), and then by the granule pump, with the result that they displace noradrenaline from its storage sites in the granules (see Fig. 13.4); the noradrenaline so released then acts in the normal way.

Receptors for catecholamines

Postsynaptic receptors for catecholamines are of two types, described as alpha (α) and beta (β) receptors. A number of factors appear to determine the effects produced by a chemical compound that stimulates these receptors. For example, the chemical configuration determines which receptor or receptors will be activated and to what degree. Another factor is the distribution of the α- and β-receptors in the tissues under consideration. For instance, in certain smooth muscles there is a preponderance of β-receptors so that, even if a particular compound is able to stimulate both α- and β-receptors, in these muscles the β effects will predominate. The smooth muscle of blood vessels in skin contains α-receptors, whereas the smooth muscle in vessels supplying the skeletal musculature possesses both α- and β-receptors, although the β-receptors predominate.

Noradrenaline acts mainly on α-receptors whilst isoprenaline acts mainly on β-receptors, whereas adrenaline acts on both. In terms of α- and β-receptor stimulating activity, the relative potencies of noradrenaline, isoprenaline, and adrenaline vary according to the tissue involved, but in general terms are as follows:

	Relative potency on receptors		Selectivity for receptors
	α	β	
Noradrenaline	1	1	α, and β_1, weak β_2
Isoprenaline	1/10–1/50	100	β, slight α
Adrenaline	2–10	10–50	α and β

It should be noted that noradrenaline has a greater selectivity for α-receptors than adrenaline, but weight for weight, adrenaline is the more potent activator of α-receptors.

Distribution of receptors

Alpha receptors (Fig. 13.4) have been subdivided into:

(1) prejunctional receptors, designated as α_2-receptors;

(2) postjunctional receptors, designated as α_1-receptors;

α_1-receptors are mainly located postjunctionally and therefore are responsible for the initiation of postsynaptic events. On the other hand, α_2-receptors are certainly, in part, located on presynaptic nerve terminals; activation of these receptors inhibits the release of noradrenaline. There are also α_2-postjunctional receptors in the CNS, and stimulation of these causes a reduced sympathetic outflow.

Beta receptors have been subdivided into:

(a) β_1-receptors, found chiefly at cardiac sites;

(b) β_2-receptors, found in bronchial smooth muscle, blood vessels of skeletal muscle.

Effects of sympathetic stimulation on various parts

See Table 13.1.

Inactivation of catecholamines

There are at least three ways in which catecholamines are inactivated; by uptake into sympathetic neurones, or by attack from two different enzymes. Sympathetic neurones, as we have seen, have the ability to take up catecholamines, and to bind them within storage granules. This so-called 'amine pump' mechanism is the principal factor in the inactivation of injected catecholamines, and also of noradrenaline released through sympathetic stimulation. The re-uptake mechanism is an example of a very economical use of resources, as noradrenaline released from sympathetic nerve endings is, in the main, re-housed and used again.

At one time the enzyme monoamine oxidase (MAO) was believed to be mainly responsible for the inactivation of catecholamines. Although the main source of the inactivation is re-uptake, it is now clear tht any metabolic degradation is principally through the enzyme catechol-O-methyltransferase. Adrenaline and noradrenaline undergo methylation to become metanephrine and normetanephrine respectively, the reaction being catalysed by catechol-O-methyltransferase. A second step of oxidative deamination is carried out by MAO, to produce 3-methoxy-4-hydroxy-mandelic acid.

A minor route of metabolic degradation of catecholamines involves the same enzymes acting in reverse order—first MAO followed by catechol-O-methyltransferase. These reactions are shown in Fig. 13.5.

Catechol-O-methyltransferase is found outside not within the sympathetic neurone; it also occurs in the liver and kidneys. Monoamine oxidase is widely distributed throughout the body, notably in the mitochondria of sympathetic neurones, the liver, and gastro-intestinal tract. Noradrenaline stored in the granules of sympathetic neurones is not vulnerable to degradation by MAO.

However, noradrenaline that is released, or that leaches out into the neuronal cytoplasm, is metabolized by MOA contained in the mitochondria; thus this enzyme may exert a controlling influence on the total concentration of noradrenaline within the cell.

Table 13.1. The effects of sympathetic stimulation on various parts

	a_1-receptors	a_2-receptors	β_1-receptors	β_2-receptors
Heart				
SA node			Increased heart rate	
AV node and conduction system			Increased conduction	
Atria and Ventricles			Increased strength of contraction. Increased myocardial excitability	
Lungs				
Bronchial musculature (smooth muscle)	Constriction			Relaxation (broncho-dilatation). More evident when muscle is contracted through disease, e.g. bronchial asthma.
Bronchial glands	Secretion decreased			Secretion increased
Arterioles				
Skin and mucosa	Constriction			
Skeletal muscle	Constriction			Dilatation
Coronary	Constriction			Dilatation
Salivary glands	Potassium secretion		Amylase secretion	
Veins	Constriction			Dilatation
Liver	Glycogenolysis—rise in blood sugar			Glycogenolysis
Pancreas				
Islet cells		Decreased secretion		Increased secretion
Stomach				
Sphincters	Contraction			
Motility		Decreased		Decreased
Intestine				
Sphincters	Contraction			
Motility	Decreased		Decreased	Decreased
Eye				
Radial muscle (mydriasis)	Contraction			
Fat cells			Lipolysis	
Uterus (smooth muscle)	Contraction (in pregnancy)			Relaxation
Platelets		Aggregation		

β_1-receptors are predominantly present in the heart and for all practical purposes, the heart has no a-receptors.

As will be seen from Table 13.1 a_1 receptors in blood vessels are concerned with vasoconstriction in the skin and mucosa, coronary vessels, and skeletal musculature. They also mediate the constriction of most sphincters. β_2-receptors are responsible for causing smooth muscle relaxation in many organs, e.g. bronchial, uterine, and intestinal smooth muscle. β_2-receptors are also responsible for vasodilatation in skeletal muscle.

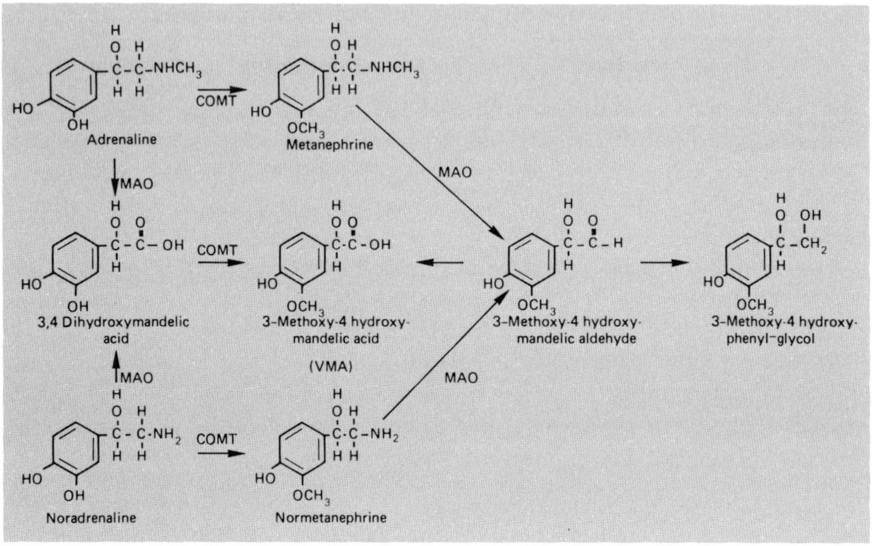

Fig. 13.5. Metabolic pathways for adrenaline and noradrenaline in man (COMT = catechol-O-methyl transferase; MAO = monoamine oxidase). (After Axelrod, 1960.)

SYMPATHOMIMETIC DRUGS

These can be classified as:

(1) directly acting sympathomimetics, e.g. adrenaline, noradrenaline, isoprenaline, phenylephrine, salbutamol, and terbutaline;

(2) indirectly acting, e.g. cocaine, amphetamine, tyramine;

(3) directly acting and indirectly acting (mixed), e.g. ephedrine.

Directly acting sympathomimetics

Adrenaline

Pharmacological actions

Adrenaline is formed by the methylation of noradrenaline in the body; both compounds are directly acting amines.

Adrenaline is destroyed by the acid of the stomach and is, therefore, not effective if taken orally. It is usually given by subcutaneous or intramuscular injection, its effects being produced more rapidly from the intramuscular site. Following injection its various actions become apparent within a minute, and they are:

1. Adrenaline is a powerful cardiac stimulant and acts directly on β-receptors.

There is an increase in the force and rate of contraction of the heart, so that the patient may complain of palpitations.

2. There is a rise in systolic blood pressure due to the increased cardiac output. However, the diastolic pressure shows little change as adrenaline produces vasoconstriction only in the skin, whereas peripheral resistance is decreased by the action of adrenaline on the β_2-receptors of muscle vessels causing dilatation.

3. Adrenaline causes an increased coronary flow through stimulation of β_2-receptors.

4. Adrenaline causes relaxation of bronchial muscles (β_2 stimulation). This bronchodilator action is much more noticeable when the bronchial musculature is contracted, as occurs in asthma or hypersensitivity reactions.

5. Adrenaline has a metabolic effect in that it raises blood sugar by mobilizing glucose from the tissues; it decreases the glycogen content of the liver and skeletal muscles. Adrenaline predominantly affects the α-receptors of the pancreas, resulting in a decrease in the secretion of insulin.

The main function of endogenous adrenaline (Goth 1966) '. . . appears to be the great emergency hormone which stimulates metabolism and promotes blood flow to skeletal muscles, preparing the individual for fight or flight'.

Unwanted effects
The rapid injection of adrenaline, or its use in large amounts, may produce ventricular fibrillation, which can be lethal. The intramuscular injection of 1:1000 adrenaline solution in anaphylactic shock is not without hazard and must be undertaken carefully. Intravenous injection of adrenaline has no place in dentistry.

Uses
(1) It is used to relieve many acute hypersensitivity reactions (see chapter 21).

(2) It is used as a vasoconstrictor in many local anaesthetic solutions (see Chapter 7).

(3) It may be used as a topical haemostatic agent, being applied in a 1:250 concentration.

Noradrenaline
Like adrenaline, noradrenaline is a naturally occurring catecholamine and it can also be produced synthetically. It is, as we have seen, the chemical mediator liberated by postganglionic sympathetic nerve endings and acts directly on effector cells.

The actions of adrenaline and noradrenaline on the cardiovascular system are likely to be quite different when both are administered in small doses. The effects are somewhat similar when large, unphysiological doses are administered. Perhaps the most important action of injected noradrenaline is to produce widespread vasoconstriction of the arterioles by stimulation of α_1-receptors. The

β_2-receptors in the vessels of the skeletal musculature are not affected and these vessels are not dilated. There is then an increase in both systolic and diastolic blood pressure, with an increased mean pressure. Intravenous infusions of noradrenaline have been used in the treatment of shock associated with trauma, or haemorrhage. the rationale of this treatment is doubtful, for such shock will already have initiated intense peripheral vasoconstriction.

Noradrenaline is a powerful vasoconstrictor and can cause a reflex bradycardia (except in the presence of an antimuscarinic drug (e.g. atropine), when it can cause a tachycardia). For these reasons its use as a vasoconstrictor in local anaesthetic solutions is contraindicated because of its pressor effects.

'The main function of noradrenaline appears to be the maintenance of normal sympathetic tone and adjustment of circulatory dynamics' (Goth 1966).

Isoprenaline

This is a synthetic catecholamine that has powerful β actions, but is almost devoid of α actions. It is well-absorbed from the buccal mucosa and respiratory tract. Isoprenaline relaxes smooth muscle, including that of the bronchial tree, and so can be used as a bronchodilator. It may be administered by aerosol inhalation, or as a 20 mg tablet sucked until the asthmatic attack is over, when the remainder of the tablet is ejected. Unfortunately, isoprenaline is a non-selective adrenoceptor stimulant and overdosage by inhalation can be dangerous due to the induction of ventricular arrhythmias.

Phenylephrine

This is a non-catecholamine, but is closely related to adrenaline chemically. It acts directly but mainly on α_1-receptors. The drug is a powerful vasoconstrictor and so produces increased peripheral resistance to blood flow with a consequent rise in systolic and diastolic pressures.

Phenylephrine, in nasal drops, is used locally to produce vasoconstriction of the nasal mucous membranes. Such use as a nasal decongestant is not without its hazards. Phenylephrine is a substrate for MAO and so, in the patient taking monoamine oxidase inhibitors (MAOI), phenylephrine will not be metabolized and so may produce a significant rise in blood pressure because of its vasoconstrictor effects.

Salbutamol

Salbutamol is a selective β_2-adrenergic stimulant and so it produces bronchodila-tation with considerably fewer cardiovascular effects than, for example, isoprenaline. Nevertheless it may produce tachycardia, but this is seldom a problem when delivered by aerosol inhalation. Its use in asthma is well-established; generally it is taken by mouth as a 4 mg tablet, or administered in an aerosol. It can also be given by slow intravenous injection (250 μg) in severe attacks.

Terbutaline

This is an effective bronchodilator and a selective β_2-adrenoceptor stimulant. It is administered orally or by aerosol inhalation, although it can also be given parenterally.

Indirectly acting sympathomimetics

Amphetamine

This drug acts indirectly in that, following uptake into the sympathetic nerve ending, it causes displacement of noradrenaline from storage sites in the synaptic vesicles. As the actions of noradrenaline are profound on α_1-receptors, but minor on β_2-receptors, the effects of amphetamine, like other indirectly acting sympathomimetics, are marked on receptors related to the peripheral vasculature. Consequently, in human beings, the oral administration of amphetamine raises both systolic and diastolic pressures.

The main interest of amphetamine is its effect on the CNS. It is said to abolish fatigue and restore energy and alertness; it certainly does not improve intelligence or skills. By its stimulant effect, amphetamine may seem to give an elevation of mood. For this reason it has been used in the treatment of depressive illness and can be classified as a psychomotor stimulant. Prolonged use of the drug is invariably followed by mental depression and fatigue. Dependence to amphetamine-like drugs often occurs, and they have little place in medical practice. The amphetamines may be useful in the rare disease called narcolepsy, in which the sufferer has uncontrollable attacks of sleepiness, for these drugs do produce wakefulness. Indeed, taken much after 4.0 p.m. they will usually prevent sleep at night.

Dexamphetamine sulphate combined with amylobarbitone was once used for the treatment of depressive illness, the two drugs potentiating each other. This combination produces the substance called 'Drinamyl', better known as 'purple hearts'.

Apart from their past use in psychiatric medicine, amphetamine-like drugs have been used as appetite suppressants in the treatment of obesity. Such use is hardly justified considering the risks associated with these drugs.

Tyramine

This is an indirectly acting amine, that is it causes the release of noradrenaline from its storage sites and does not itself act directly on receptors. It is to be found in many foodstuffs—mature cheese, broad beans, yeast extracts, yoghourt, and wine—and is a substrate for MAO in the gut and in the liver. It is of interest because when MAOI are administered, they allow tyramine to reach the systemic circulation, causing noradrenaline release from its storage sites. This release may lead to a dangerous hypertension (the so-called cheese reaction), with cerebrovascular catastrophe and death of the patient if not corrected.

Directly acting and indirectly acting (mixed) sympathomimetics

Ephedrine

This compound occurs naturally in some plants but is prepared synthetically for medical use. Ephedrine stimulates both α- and β-receptors as well as acting indirectly; its actions are, therefore, mixed. In some ways, these actions are similar to those of adrenaline, in other ways most dissimilar. It differs from adrenaline in that it is absorbed from the intestinal tract after oral administration and, although its effects are weaker, they are more prolonged. It has a more marked stimulating effect on the CNS.

Ephedrine increases the systolic and usually the diastolic blood pressure, the effect being mainly due to cardiac stimulation. It also produces a mild degree of bronchial relaxation as compared with adrenaline, but the effect is more prolonged. Consequently, it is useful as a bronchodilator in mild chronic asthma (taken in the form of tablets, 15 to 60 mg orally three times daily), but not in a severe acute attack. It is also used as a nasal decongestant in the form of nasal drops. There is a well-established clinical impression that repeated use of ephedrine over long periods leads to some falling off in its efficacy.

Its stimulant effect on the CNS is not so marked as with the amphetamines. Nevertheless, if it is used for the mild asthmatic it should be remembered that the drug may keep the patient awake at night and, under such circumstances, may have to be combined with a suitable hypnotic drug. Its use should be avoided in those taking a MAOI.

ANTAGONISTS OF ADRENERGIC ACTIVITY
(Drugs used in the treatment of hypertension)

The drugs that oppose adrenergic activity may act peripherally, centrally, or both.

Peripherally acting agents—adrenergic neurone blockers

This group comprises several chemical agents with the common property of interfering with the normal function of adrenergic neurones. They can be divided into subgoups according to their mechanisms of action.

(i) Inhibition of transmitter release
(e.g. guanethidine)

Guanethidine is representative of those drugs that selectively block sympathetic transmission in postganglionic sympathetic neurones by interfering with the release of noradrenaline from the nerve endings. It is taken up into adrenergic nerve endings by the same mechanism that rehouses noradrenaline released from sympathetic nerve endings. This drug also decreases sympathetic activity by depleting the stores of noradrenaline at peripheral nerve endings.

Pharmacokinetics

Absorption of guanethidine from the gastro-intestinal tract is very variable, as little as 3 per cent or as much as 30 per cent may reach the systemic circulation. To some extent this variability must account for the wide variations in dosage required between individuals. The drug is metabolized in the liver, and the metabolites and the parent compound are excreted by the kidney.

Unwanted effects

Guanethidine causes postural hypotension, and this is perhaps the most significant unwanted effect; others include a feeling of weakness, and diarrhoea, which is common.

The action of this drug is inhibited by the tricyclic antidepressants and the phenothiazines, which block the uptake of guanethidine into the sympathetic nerve ending. Guanethidine will only act as a hypotensive if it can reach its site of action within the sympathetic neurone.

Uses

Guanethidine is used to treat a moderate to a severe hypertension, usually in conjunction with a diuretic. It is not often used today because its effect on blood pressure is affected by postural changes, and because better drugs are now available.

Bethanidine and debrisoquine are similar drugs to guanethidine.

(ii) Depletion of noradrenaline stores
(e.g. reserpine)

Reserpine depletes the stores of noradrenaline and 5-hydroxytryptamine centrally, and also produces a depletion of noradrenaline at the sympathetic nerve endings. It causes the release of noradrenaline from the storage granules in the sympathetic nerve endings into the neuronal cytoplasm, where it is metabolized by MAO. The hypotensive effect of this drug may be due to a combination of these central and peripheral actions, which bring about a reduction in the sympathetic outflow to the blood vessels. Reserpine is virtually obsolete today as it tends to produce too many unwanted effects, especially severe mental depression. However, at one time, it was found to be useful in treatment of hypertension.

Centrally acting agents

Methyldopa

At one time it was thought that methyldopa acted peripherally at postganglionic sympathetic nerve endings, but it is now generally agreed that it acts centrally, producing a reduced sympathetic outflow from the brain. It would seem that methyldopa on entering the central nervous system acts as a substrate for dopa decarboxylase with the formation of α-methyldopamine.

Alpha methyldopamine, by a further enzymatic step, is converted to α-methylnoradrenaline. It seems that this α-methylnoradrenaline is an agonist of α_2-receptors in the CNS, and that stimulation of these receptors inhibits the sympathetic outflow.

Pharmacokinetics

The absorption of methyldopa after oral administration is somewhat variable and incomplete. The maximal blood concentrations are reached in about three hours. It is excreted in the urine unchanged in the main, although some is excreted as metabolites.

Unwanted effects

Methyldopa tends to cause drowsiness and sometimes even a depression. The sedative effect is the most common effect and it will tend to wear off with continued use of the drug. A dry mouth may occur with methyldopa but is rarely of any significance.

In about 3 per cent of patients (Rudd and Blaschke, 1985), transient abnormalities of the liver may occur. Usually, on stopping the drug, the liver function returns to normal but the condition may progress to hepatic necrosis.

Drug-related systemic lupus erythematosus has been reported with the use of methyldopa, as have lichenoid eruptions of the oral mucosa (Hay and Reade 1978).

Uses

The drug is used to treat a moderate to mild hypertension in conjunction with a diuretic. It is perhaps less used today than previously because of its unwanted effects.

Clonidine

This antihypertensive, like methyldopa, seems to stimulate central α_2-adrenergic receptors decreasing the sympathetic outflow from the brain. It may also act peripherally on α_2-(prejunctional) receptors.

Pharmacokinetics

Clonidine is much better absorbed than is methyldopa, absorption being rapid and almost complete. Peak plasma concentrations are reached in one to three hours. The half-life of clonidine is about eight to nine hours when administered orally; it is mainly excreted unchanged in the urine. The metabolites produced in the liver by degradation of that fraction which is not passed out in the urine unchanged, are inactive; they, in their turn, are eventually excreted in the urine.

Unwanted effects

The most frequent of these are dry mouth and sedation, both of which may be severe. They may lessen after the drug has been taken for some time, but a proportion of patients have to discontinue its use for these reasons. A so-called rebound hypertension occurs if clonidine is suddenly withdrawn. This is potentially very dangerous and rather suggests that the drug should not be used in those who are unlikely to comply with prescribing instructions. Parotid pain has been recorded in patients treated with clonidine. (Onesti *et al.* 1971).

Uses

Clonidine is hardly ever used for the treatment of hypertension because of its many unwanted effects. However, in low doses it is used for the prophylaxis of migraine, in the form of 'Dixarit' (See Chapter 14).

Adrenergic receptor (adrenoceptor) blockers

Some of the drugs included in this category have found a special place in the treatment of hypertension, these being those drugs that block β-adrenergic receptors. Other drugs, the α-adrenoceptor blocking drugs have not proved particularly useful in this respect, but they have found a place in the treatment of 'hypertensive crises'.

α-adrenoceptor blocking drugs
(e.g. phenoxybenzamine, phentolamine)

These drugs selectively block α-receptors, leaving β-receptors unaffected. Phenoxybenzamine produces an irreversible type of blockade, whereas the blockade produced by phentolamine is competitive. Phenoxybenzamine essentially blocks α_1-receptors whereas phentolamine blocks both α_1- and α_2-receptors.

It might be thought that such drugs would be useful in the management of hypertension but, generally speaking, this has not proved to be the case, and there appear to be few clinical uses for them. However, phentolamine has been found to be useful in the treatment of hypertension crises due to phaeochromocytoma. Phaeochromocytoma is a rare tumour of the adrenal medulla that secretes adrenaline and noradrenaline in excess with a resultant hypertension. The hypertension is often paroxysmal but it may be continuous.

Phentolamine is also used in the treatment of hypertensive crises associated with the sudden withdrawal of clonidine (see above), or with the interaction that sometimes occurs between a MAOI and certain foodstuffs containing pressor amines, e.g. cheese.

β-adrenoceptor blocking drugs

These provide competitive and reversible blockade of β-adrenoceptors in the heart, peripheral vasculature, bronchi, liver, and pancreas. They have many clinical applications and have found a special place in the treatment of hypertension. Their mode of action as hypotensives is uncertain. Some β-blockers are non-selective, e.g. propranolol, nadolol; whereas others are relatively selective having a greater affinity for β_1-receptors (cardiac β-receptors) than for β_2-receptors (bronchial and vascular β-receptors). Some β-adrenoceptor blocking drugs are lipophilic, e.g. propranolol; whereas others are water-soluble, e.g. nadolol, atenolol. Furthermore, some β-adrenoceptor blockers are partial agonists in that they possess a degree of intrinsic sympathomimetic activity, e.g. oxprenolol, acebutolol.

Non-selective β-adrenoceptor blocking drugs
(e.g. propranolol, nadolol, oxprenolol, pindolol, timolol)

Propranolol

This was the first β-blocker of clinical significance. It produces specific blockade of β-receptors but is unselective, blocking both β_1- and β_2-receptors. By blocking cardiac β-receptors it causes a reduction in the rate and force of the heart beat so that cardiac output is lowered; this may account, in part, for the decreased blood pressure. Propranolol may also produce its hypotensive effect by antagonizing the action of noradrenaline released from sympathetic nerve endings. It does so by blocking peripheral adrenoceptors. Some beta-blockers also depress plasma renin secretion, e.g. propranolol (see Chapter 15 for discussion on renin and hypertension).

Pharmacokinetics.   When taken orally propranolol is almost completely absorbed. It is a lipophilic drug and is subject to extensive first pass metabolism. The degree of this metabolism varies in different individuals, and the dose regimen has to be adjusted according to individual requirements. Propranolol is extensively bound to plasma proteins (maybe as much as 95 per cent), and ultimately it is almost completely metabolized in the liver before excretion in the urine. Peak plasma concentrations occur in about 90 minutes and the half-life after oral administration is in the order of four hours.

Unwanted effects.   The unwanted effects of propranolol are mainly due to actions inherent in the drug itself. They are side-effects resulting from extension of the main action of the drug at sites additional to those required for therapeutic purposes. For instance, the blockade of β-adrenergic receptors in bronchial smooth muscle may lead to increased airway resistance. This is probably of little importance in the normal individual but, in the asthmatic, it may induce a dangerous bronchospasm.

As propranolol is lipophilic, it readily enters the brain and occasionally produces nightmares, hallucinations, and sleeplessness. Such unwanted effects are much less likely to occur with more water-soluble β-blockers, such as nadolol.

Nadolol

This non-selective β-blocker, unlike propranolol, is water-soluble. It is a long-acting drug, and it is taken orally when it has a half-life of perhaps as much as 20 hours. It is not metabolized to any degree and is, therefore, mainly excreted in an unchanged form in the urine. The consequence of the relatively long half-life of nadolol, as compared with propranolol, means that it has only to be administered once a day when used as an antihypertensive.

Selective β-adrenoceptor blocking drugs
(e.g. metoprolol, atenolol, practolol)

These drugs are relatively cardio-selective. The first of them was practolol: this was an extremely effective drug but, when taken by mouth, it produced many serious unwanted effects such as conjunctival scarring and peritoneal fibrosis. Its use is now severely restricted.

Metoprolol and atenolol are relatively selective β_1-receptor blockers. Although they are regarded as cardio-selective, this selectivity does not offer any absolute protection against bronchospasm in patients with obstructive airway disease.

Metoprolol is rapidly absorbed from the gastro-intestinal tract and undergoes extensive first pass metabolism. Little of the drug is excreted unchanged in the urine. On the other hand, atenolol is water-soluble and is excreted by the kidneys mainly in an unchanged form.

Non-selective α- and β-adrenoceptor blocking drugs
(e.g. labetalol)

Labetalol, an antihypertensive drug, is novel in that it blocks α_1-receptors and also β_1- and β_2-receptors. It is sometimes useful for those patients who do not tolerate the unopposed α effects that occur with β-blockers.

Uses of β-adrenoceptor blocking drugs
In the treatment of hypertension

The β-blockers, as we have seen, are effective antihypertensive drugs and they produce relatively few unwanted effects. If they prove inadequate alone in controlling the blood pressure, usually they are combined with a thiazide diuretic. The actions of all the β-blockers are likely to be similar.

In addition to their use as hypotensive agents, β-blockers have other uses.

In the treatment of angina pectoris

Because of their action on β_1-cardiac receptors, these drugs generally diminish sympathetic drive to the heart. They also reduce heart rate and cardiac output, and the force of myocardial contraction is decreased. They reduce the response of the heart to exercise and, because of the effects on the myocardium, myocardial oxygen requirements are reduced. All of these actions are useful in angina as there is already present an impaired blood supply to the myocardium and the patient gets pain in the chest on exercise.

In the treatment of cardiac arrhythmias

Because of the reduction in sympathetic drive brought about by these drugs in general, the excitability of the myocardium is reduced and so there is less likelihood of arrhythmias occurring.

In the treatment of anxiety states

Beta-blockers are useful in treating those people who experience anxiety in particular situations; for example, public performers, examination candidates. They are used in the management of anxiety when the effects of sympathetic overactivity result in troublesome palpitations, tachycardia, and tremor.

As prophylactic agents in the management of migraine (see Chapter 14)

Some β-blockers, e.g. propranolol, possess weak membrane-stabilizing (local anaesthetic) properties but this effect is not seen at the concentrations achieved during therapy. This property has no therapeutic value.

PARASYMPATHETIC NERVOUS SYSTEM

The peripheral parasympathetic system consists of preganglionic and postganglionic neurones. The chemical transmitter at both the ganglion and the effector junction is acetylcholine.

There are two main types of membrane receptors for acetylcholine, and these are named 'muscarinic' and 'nicotinic'. The reason for this terminology is because the substances muscarine and nicotine were found to stimulate these receptors selectively. Muscarine is obtained from a fungus (*Amanita muscaria*); it has the same actions as acetylcholine released from parasympathetic postganglionic fibres. The muscarinic receptor is, therefore, located at the effector junction of postganglionic parasympathetic fibres. Nicotinic receptors are found on the postsynaptic membrane of all autonomic ganglia, both sympathetic and parasympathetic, and also on the neuromuscular junction. Muscarine has no effects at the autonomic ganglia, but here the activity of acetylcholine can be mimicked by low concentrations of nicotine. In high concentrations nicotine blocks transmission.

Synthesis, storage, release and inactivation of acetylcholine

Cholinergic nerves synthesize acetylcholine from choline; this synthesis requires the enzyme, choline acetylase. Choline is found in lecithin, which is widely distributed in all animal and vegetable foodstuffs. Acetylcholine is stored in synaptic vesicles at the nerve endings and is released when there is electrical activity in the nerve fibres. On release from the nerve ending, acetylcholine is quickly hydrolysed by the cholinesterases of the body to form acetic acid. In man there are thought to be two definite cholinesterases, true cholinesterase and pseudocholinesterase, the true form being primarily responsible for the hydrolysis of acetylcholine.

Parasympathomimetic drugs

Acetylcholine is not absorbed from the gastro-intestinal tract and, even if given intravenously, it is so rapidly hydrolysed by the cholinesterases of the body that its effects are transient. Although it is a subject of physiological interest, it is not used in medical treatments. There are a number of other drugs that have similar actions to acetylcholine and find clinical application.

Carbachol

This is a synthetic substance chemically related to acetylcholine. Although its action is predominately on muscarinic receptors, it also has a high level of activity on nicotinic receptors, particularly at autonomic ganglia. It is not hydrolysed by the body cholinesterases and so its actions are more prolonged than those of acetylcholine. In contrast to acetylcholine, carbachol stimulates selectively the urinary and gastro-intestinal tracts, increasing smooth muscle tone. It has been used to overcome urinary retention due to atonic bladder where there was no obstruction to urinary flow.

Carbachol is sometimes used in ophthalmology, often combined with other substances, in an emollient solution as eyedrops to reduce intra-ocular pressure in glaucoma (a condition characterized by increased intra-ocular pressure).

Occasionally the drug produces a slight tachycardia due to stimulation of nicotinic receptors in sympathetic ganglia. Usually, the muscarinic effects predominate and the effects on the ganglia have little or no clinical significance.

Bethanechol chloride

This substance produces only muscarinic effects and, like carbachol, these are relatively selective being related to the smooth muscle of the gut, the ureters, and the bladder. The drug is available as tablets, and is used to stimulate the urinary bladder.

Pilocarpine

This is a naturally occurring alkaloid with mainly muscarinic action. Pilocarpine is used in ophthalmology for the treatment of glaucoma. When applied to the eye it causes pupillary constriction (miosis) and ultimately a fall in intraocular pressure. In fact, reduction of intra-ocular pressure occurs within minutes of application and lasts for up to eight hours.

These substances act directly on the receptors, but there are others that produce their effect by preventing the destruction of acetylcholine by cholinesterases; these are called the *anticholinesterases*.

Physostigmine

This combines reversibly with cholinesterase and prevents the hydrolysis of acetylcholine at nerve terminals throughout the body. The actions of acetylcholine are, therefore, intensified at their three sites of action: (i) parasympathetic nerve endings (muscarinic); (ii) autonomic ganglia (nicotinic); and (iii) the nerve endings in voluntary muscle (nicotinic). The final picture produced by these three groups of actions is likely to be a mixed one, but the action at the parasympathetic nerve endings usually predominates.

Physostigmine is used in the treatment of glaucoma, often being combined with pilocarpine in the form of eyedrops, to produce a constricting (miotic) effect on the pupil. The effects of physostigmine are more prolonged than pilocarpine, lasting 24 hours.

Neostigmine

This is a synthetic anticholinesterase drug, similar to physostigmine, but with much more effect on the neuromuscular junction. Anticholinesterase drugs, such as neostigmine, are used to enhance neuromuscular transmission in conditions such as myasthenia gravis, which is a disease characterized by weakness of voluntary muscles. Repeated stimulation of a motor nerve in a patient suffering from this condition leads to fatigue of the muscles supplied by the particular nerve. By interfering with the breakdown of acetylcholine this weakness can be alleviated. One troublesome problem with the use of neostigmine is that it possesses a marked muscarinic action so that there may be excessive salivation. However, this can be overcome by the simultaneous administration of atropine.

Examples of other drugs used in the treatment of myasthenia gravis are: pyridostigmine, distigmine, edrophonium. Edrophonium has a very brief action and is used simply for diagnostic purposes.

Irreversible anticholinesterases

There are substances that produce an irreversible complex with cholinesterase so that their duration of action is prolonged and depends upon the rate which new cholinesterase is formed. These are the organophosphorus inhibitors; they are used as insecticides and form the basis of 'nerve gases'.

Parasympathetic blocking drugs

Ganglion blocking drugs

Acetylcholine is the chemical transmitter at both sympathetic and parasympathetic ganglia. Ganglion blocking drugs were the first powerful weapons that became available to lower raised blood pressure. These drugs act by competing with the acetylcholine released at preganglionic nerve endings—an example of competitive antagonism. Unfortunately, because of their lack of selectivity, the ganglion blocking drugs readily produced unwanted effects due to their blocking parasympathetic as well as sympathetic ganglia. Because of the parasympathetic blockade there occurs decreased salivation, urinary retention, and constipation.

Atropine

Atropine belongs to the belladona groups of drugs, which are obtained from *Atropa belladonna*, deadly nightshade.

Pharmacokinetics

This drug is well-absorbed from the gastro-intestinal tract, and it can also be given subcutaneously, intramuscularly, or intravenously. It can also be absorbed through broken skin and when applied locally to the mucosal surfaces of the body.

Atropine quickly disappears from the blood and has a half-life of about 2.5 hours. It is distributed throughout the whole body, traces can be found in maternal milk, and it crosses the placental barrier to enter the fetal circulation. The compound is largely broken down by the liver enzymes but a small fraction of it may be excreted in the urine unchanged, mainly within 12 hours.

Pharmacodynamics

Atropine is an antimuscarinic drug, and the major action of all antimuscarinic drugs is competitive antagonism to acetylcholine and drugs like it. To some extent, competitive antagonism is quantitative and can be overcome by increasing the concentration of acetylcholine at the receptor site. Atropine is very selective in its antagonism, acting at receptors of smooth and cardiac muscle and exocrine glands. Atropine does not antagonize the nicotinic action of acetylcholine on skeletal muscle, and only affects autonomic ganglia in very high dosage.

Pharmacological properties

Atropine diminishes cardiac vagal tone and thus leads to an increase in the heart rate. The amount of acceleration produced will depend upon the degree of inhibition present. The influence of atropine on vagal tone is most noticeable in the young, healthy adult; whereas in infancy and old age, it may cause less cardiac acceleration.

Atropine blocks the action of acetylcholine on glands. In therapeutic doses it does not greatly diminish gastric secretion, but it does dry up the copious salivary secretion induced by parasympathetic stimulation.

Sympathetic activity has little control in the regulation of gastro-intestinal tone and motility, parasympathetic nerves being principally involved. Parasympathetic nerves increase both tone and motility and so atropine diminishes these responses, with a decrease in frequency of peristaltic contractions. Atropine has been used to relieve colicky pain.

The administration of atropine leads to a drying up of secretions in the respiratory tract. Although atropine does produce some degree of relaxation of the smooth muscles of the bronchi and bronchioles, it must be remembered that parasympathetic innervation of the bronchi is slight, and cholinergic mechanisms do not seem to play much part in the causation of attacks of bronchial asthma. Other smooth muscle is also relaxed, notably that of the biliary and renal tracts.

When the parasympathetic nerve supply to the eye is blocked there occurs mydriasis (dilation of the pupil) and cycloplegia (paralysis of accommodation) with inability to see near objects. Local administration of atropine to the eye will produce these effects. Mydriasis, for instance, may be necessary for thorough examination of the retina.

Overdosage with atropine leads to an exaggeration of all the actions described, together with a stimulating effect on the CNS with restlessness, hallucinations, and delirium, and finally coma and death.

Uses

1. Atropine (see Chapter 8) is used as part of preanaesthetic medication to dry up salivary and bronchial secretions. Although this is the primary object of such usage, the very fact that secretions are inhibited may reduce the incidence of laryngospasm during general anaesthesia. The administration of atropine also prevents excessive bradycardia and hypotension caused by halothane. The depression of salivary secretion is particularly important in children because the larynx and trachea are so small and any excessive secretion could seriously impair respiration.

2. The drug is used by local application to dilate the pupil so that a proper examination of the retina can take place. Homatropine is often used for the purpose as its effects are not so prolonged as those of atropine.

3. Atropine has been given orally, often as belladonna alkaloids, to treat peptic ulcer; its value here is open to question. The only pharmacological effect that would seem to be beneficial would be if atropine and like drugs suppressed gastric acid secretion. Atropine has a minimal effect on such secretion, but it may be useful in that it relieves spasm of the stomach and duodenal muscles. It also delays gastric emptying so that the action of antacids may be prolonged. Hence, belladonna alkaloids are often combined with other drugs, such as aluminium hydroxide or magnesium trisilicate, both of which are antacids.

Hyoscine

The actions of hyoscine are essentially the same as those of atropine, except for its action on the CNS where, even in small doses, it has a depressant action leading to some degree of sedation, drowsiness, or even sleep. Although a good pre-anaesthetic agent, elderly people tend to be confused by hyoscine and so it is probably best avoided in their premedication. It has a depressant action on the vomiting centre and has been used as a travel sickness remedy.

REFERENCES

Axelrod, J. (1960). The fate of adrenaline and noradrenaline. In *Adrenergic Mechanisms* (ed. J. R. Vane), pp. 28–39. J. and A. Churchill, London.

Goth, A. (1981) Adrenergic drugs. In *Medical Pharmacology*. (12th edn). Mosby, St. Louis.

Hay, K. D. and Reade, P. C. (1978). Methyldopa as a cause of oral mucous membrane reactions. *British Dental Journal*, **145**, 195–203.

Onesti, G., Bock, K. D., Heimsoth, V., Kim, K. E., and Murguet, P. (1971). Clonidine: a new antihypertensive agent. *American Journal of Cardiology*, **28**, 74–83.

Rudd, P. and Blaschke, T. F. (1985). Antihypertensive agents and the drug therapy of hypertension. In *The pharmacological basis of therapeutics* (7th ed) (ed. L. S. Goodman, A. G. Gilman, T. W. Rall, and F. Murad). Macmillan, New York.

FURTHER READING

Beeley, L. (1984). Drug interactions of beta-blockers. (Editorial). *British Medical Journal*, **289**, 1330–1.

Breckenridge, A. (1985). Treating mild hypertension. (Editorial). *British Medical Journal*, **291**, 89–90.

Faldt, R., Liedholm, H., and Aursnes, J. (1984). Beta-blockers and loss of hearing. *British Medical Journal*, **289**, 1490–2.

Kaplan, N. M. (1983). The present and future use of beta-blockers. *Drugs*, **25**, 1.

Leading article (1985). Beta-blockers in situational anxiety. *Lancet*, **ii**, 193.

Leading article (1985). Treatment of hypertension: the 1985 results. *Lancet*, **ii**, 645–7.

Leading article (1985). Treatment of hypertension in the over 60's. *Lancet*, **i**, 1369–70.

Leading article (1985): The functions of adrenaline. *Lancet*, **i**, 561–2.

Michelson, E. L. and Frishman, W. H. (1983). Labetalol: an alpha- and beta-adrenoceptor blocking drug. *Annals of Internal Medicine*, **99**, 553–5.

Ravid, M., Lang, R., and Jutrin, I. (1985). The relative antihypertensive potency of propranolol, oxprenolol, atenolol, and metoprolol given once daily. *Archives of Internal Medicine*, **145**, 1321–3.

Rubin, P. C. and Reid, J. L. (1983). Alpha-blockers and converting enzyme inhibitors. *British Medical Journal*, **286**, 1192–5.

14

The central nervous system

THIS chapter is mainly concerned with disorders of the central nervous system (CNS) and the therapeutic measures used in their treatment. The following disorders will be considered together with their appropriate treatment: psychoses and related disorders, and antipsychotic drugs; depression and antidepressants; hypnotics and anxiolytics; epilepsy, facial neuralgias, and anticonvulsants; migraine, and drugs used in the prophylaxis and treatment of migraine. Many other drugs act on the CNS but are discussed elsewhere; these include opioids (see Chapter 6) and general anaesthetic agents (see Chapter 8).

PSYCHOSES AND RELATED DISORDERS

Psychosis

This major mental illness is characterized by irrational thoughts and loss of contact with reality, and commonly by delusions and/or hallucinations. It can take a number of forms.

Organic

Damage to the brain caused by injury, infection (for example, encephalitis), pharmacological agents (e.g. lysergic acid diethylamide, LSD), toxicological agents (e.g. ethyl alcohol (ethanol); lead), and degenerative changes (Alzheimer's disease; old age) can all lead to temporary or permanent psychotic changes. From what has been said it will be appreciated that organic psychosis is usually accompanied by detectable anatomical, chemical, or pharmacological changes in the brain.

Functional

By contrast to the organic group, this is not accompanied by obvious anatomical changes in the brain. The results of research carried out over the past two decades have shown that some of these conditions appear to be associated with subtle pharmacological changes in various parts of the brain, although whether these are due to cause or effect still remains to be determined. Nevertheless, pharmacological knowledge so obtained has not only made treatment more rational but has also pointed the way to alternative therapeutic approaches.

There are two subdivisions within the functional group.

1. Schizophrenia

This term encompasses a group of related disorders that are characterized by such features as withdrawal from reality, regressive behaviour, and delusions that include feelings of persecution, which when intense is known as paranoia. Auditory hallucinations are also common.

2. Manic–depressive psychosis

This is characterized by phases of excitement (hypomania) or frank mania; or alternatively by severe depression. When manic–depressive psychosis swings in only one direction i.e. mania or depression, it is often referred to as monopolar, whereas when it may swing from mania to depression it is then referred to as bipolar.

ANTIPSYCHOTIC DRUGS

The term 'antipyschotic' is the now preferred one for a group of drugs that have been previously named 'neuroleptics', and 'major tranquillizers', and also 'ataractics'. The term 'anti-psychotic' is preferred because it indicates the type of disease for which it is used whilst at the same time not attempting to suggest a mechanism of action. The term 'neuroleptic' is not helpful and the term 'major tranquillizers' is liable to be confused with 'minor tranquillizers', which are better named 'anxiolytics'. The term 'ataractic' is obsolete.

Until the early 1950s there was no effective drug treatment of schizophrenia. At that time two new drugs, chlorpromazine and reserpine, arrived upon the pharmacological scene. Chlorpromazine was known to be an antihistamine, whilst reserpine was one of the active principles extracted from *Rauwolfia serpentina*, which had long been used in India for the treatment of high blood pressure, mental illness, and numerous other diseases. Both drugs were found to calm patients suffering from psychiatric illness, and the results of clinical trials soon showed that they produced significant improvement in patients suffering from schizophrenia. Chlorpromazine became the preferred drug because reserpine not only produced undesirable effects on the blood pressure but also induced serious depression in some patients. From then on the pharmaceutical industry decided to concentrate its attention on the phenothiazines, of which chlorpromazine is a member. In spite of many clinical trials of other phenothiazines, chlorpromazine has remained an important therapeutic agent and represents the archetype of antipsychotic drugs.

Classification of antipsychotic drugs

The phenothiazines can be divided into three main groups on the basis of their chemical structure, therapeutic effects, and adverse reaction profiles. This classification is in general use and is also included in the *British National Formulary (BNF)*.

Group 1: chlorpromazine, methotrimeprazine
Characterized by pronounced sedative effects, moderate anticholinergic (antimuscarinic) and extrapyramidal side-effects.

Group 2: pericyazine, pipothiazine, and thioridazine
Characterized by moderate sedative effects, marked anticholinergic (antimuscarinic) effects, but fewer extrapyramidal side-effects than groups 1 or 3.

Group 3: fluphenazine, perphenazine, prochlorperazine, and trifluoperazine
Characterized by fewer sedative effects, fewer anticholinergic (antimuscarinic) effects, but more pronounced extrapyramidal side-effects than groups 1 and 2.

Several other chemical groups of drugs have been found to have pharmacological properties similar to those of the phenothiazines of group 3. These include the following:

 (i) butyrophenones, e.g. benperidol, droperidol, haloperidol, and trifluperidol;

 (ii) diphenylbutylpiperidines, e.g. fluspirilene, pimozide;

 (iii) thioxanthenes, e.g. chlorprothixene, flupenthixol, and zuclopenthixol;

 (iv) oxypertine;

 (v) benzamide, e.g. sulpiride.

As chlorpromazine is the archetypal anti-psychotic drug, the remainder of this section will describe its properties. Then, where appropriate, some of the other phenothiazines and related compounds will be compared briefly with it.

Chlorpromazine

Phenothiazine is a tricyclic compound that forms the nucleus of chlorpromazine and numerous other phenothiazine derivatives. Chlorpromazine has an aliphatic side-chain (CH_2—CH_2—CH_2—N—$(CH_3)_2$), which is attached to the nitrogen atom (position 10) of the middle ring of the phenothiazine nucleus.

Pharmacodynamics

Chlorpromazine possesses a multiplicity of actions and this is reflected in the original proprietary name of 'Largactil', which signifies a large number of actions. thus, it produces the following effects:

1. Central
The compound is a competitive antagonist to dopamine, and this action may be the mechanism whereby it produces its powerful antipsychotic and tranquillizing effects. However, chlorpromazine (and other phenothiazines) also have anticholinergic (antimuscarinic), α-adrenoceptor blocking, antihistamine (H_1), and

anti-5HT (5-hydroxytryptamine) actions but the contribution of these effects to the central properties is still not clear. Hallucinations can be controlled by chlorpromazine whether they are part of schizophrenia or part of another psychotic illness, including that induced by pharmacological agents such as 'magic mushrooms'. Chlorpromazine's sedative effect is best seen in agitated patients. Through its action on the hypothalamus it reduces sympathetic outflow, reduces temperature control so that the body does not respond adequately to hypothermia, and also increases the release of prolactin with the result that menstrual irregularities may occur in women and gynaecomastia in man (see Unwanted Effects below). The well-known extrapyramidal syndrome is due to its dopamine agonist action on the basal ganglia.

2. Peripheral

These include anticholinergic (antimuscarinic), α-adrenoceptor blockade, quinidine-like action on the heart (Class I anti-arrhythmic effect), weak antihistamine (H_1) effects, and local anaesthetic actions. The peripheral anticholinergic (antimuscarinic) action is responsible for many of the side-effects that may occur with chlorpromazine, particularly in high dosage; these are dry mouth, difficulty in accommodation, the possibility of acute glaucoma, dry skin, constipation, and difficulty in micturition. The α-adrenoceptor blocking action produces postural hypotension, nasal stuffiness, and failure of ejaculation. The quinidine-like action is unlikely to cause problems except in those already suffering from cardiac conduction defects and particularly, of course, if they are already taking other anti-arrhythmic drugs. The weak antihistamine (H_1) action is probably not of clinical relevance, whilst the local anaesthetic action, although potent, is not clinically exploitable because chlorpromazine is too irritant to tissues to permit of its use in this context.

Pharmacokinetics

The metabolism of chlorpromazine starts as soon as it passes through the gut wall and the liver, and thus it undergoes extensive first pass metabolism. Numerous metabolites are formed and these vary in pharmacological activity and also toxicity. There is enterohepatic recirculation with little renal excretion of unchanged drug. The plasma elimination half-life is 16 to 30 hours but, after repeated dosage, the therapeutic effect is more prolonged than the plasma half-life would suggest. This is due to the large volume of distribution of chlorpromazine, which becomes sequestered in many tissues where it can remain for weeks or months.

Therapeutic uses

These are conveniently considered under four headings.

(i) Psychiatric uses

Chlorpromazine is used in the treatment of acute and chronic psychoses, e.g. schizophrenia, hypomania, and mania, where its antipsychotic and sedative effects are of great therapeutic value. It is also useful in the treatment of acute organic psychotic states including those due to pharmacological and toxicological agents.

(ii) Anti-emetic

Chlorpromazine is valuable in the treatment and prevention of nausea and vomiting due to drugs; for example, during cancer chemotherapy and radiotherapy. It should be noted that it is not effective for the treatment of motion sickness for which H_1 blockers (with sedative action) or antimuscarinic drugs are needed.

(iii) Terminal illness

It is occasionally necessary to use chlorpromazine, usually as a sedative, to relieve anxiety and associated mental suffering during terminal illness. However, there has been a tendency to over-prescribe chlorpromazine for this purpose, such that the patient becomes over-sedated and confused. The aim of terminal care, now renamed palliative medicine, is to keep the patient alert and pain-free so that the quality of life is preserved as much as possible for the benefit of them and their carers.

(iv) Surgical uses

Chlorpromazine is sometimes used as part of premedication and, more particularly, in order to permit the induction of surgical hypothermia; it has also been used as the neuroleptic in combination with an opioid for the production of neuroleptanalgesia.

Unwanted effects

In view of the multiplicity of actions of chlorpromazine it is hardly surprising that it can produce a large profile of unwanted effects. Many of these are predictable from its known pharmacology and have already been referred to earlier in this section. From a clinical point of view it is convenient to classify these unwanted effects under three headings.

(i) Central effects

Sedation occurs initially but tolerance to this effect occurs fairly rapidly. With high doses, such as are used for the treatment of schizophrenia, extrapyramidal syndromes are frequent; these include Parkinsonism, akathisia (a most unpleasant form of enforced restlessness), and different forms of acute dystonic reactions (Blain and Stewart-Wynne 1985). The condition known as tardive dyskinesia may become a serious problem either during or after prolonged therapy, or rarely after even a short period of administration. It consists of irregular repetitive involuntary movements, typically abnormal writhing often accompanied by protrusions of the tongue with lip-smacking, chewing movements, and also facial grimaces. In addition, so-called choreo-athetoid movements of the extremities may occur with the orofacial dyskinesia. Tardive dyskinesia is more likely in patients given high doses of chlorpromazine (or related drugs) over prolonged periods of time, following which the condition may not be reversible, especially in those aged 50 years or more. The mechanism of tardive dyskinesia is not altogether clear although it is believed to be related to supersensitivity of dopamine receptors in the corpus striatum, which is the result of continued dopamine-receptor blockade. Unfortunately, withdrawal of drug therapy is not necessarily followed by improvement and sometimes leads to exacerbation of this difficult problem, a discussion of which is beyond the scope of this text. Nevertheless, it is important for the dental practitioner to be aware of this problem because the sufferer will obviously cause major problems in relation to dentistry.

(ii) Peripheral autonomic effects

As indicated earlier, these result from blockade of muscarinic receptors and α-adrenoceptors. Effects due to muscarinic blockade may produce an unacceptable degree of dry mouth, disturbance of accommodation, constipation, and difficulty with micturition. These can only be lessened by reducing the dose of the drug or, alternatively, by prescribing a different phenothiazine or related compound. Postural hypotension due to α-adrenoceptor blockade can be troublesome at least initially, and when the drug is given parenterally. The Class I anti-arrhythmic action may produce changes in the ECG including prolongation of the QT interval and alteration of the T wave.

(iii) Miscellaneous

A variety of other effects may occur, including those due to associated endocrine disturbances and those due to immunological mechanisms.

Dopamine-receptor blockade is followed by increased prolactin secretion and this in turn may give rise to menstrual disturbances, galactorrhoea, and gynaecomastia. Hypersensitivity reactions occur only occasionally, and include skin rashes, photosensitivity, pigmentation, and also cholestatic jaundice, which is a dose-independent reaction reported in about 2 per cent of cases. Blood dyscrasias, including leucopenia and agranulocytosis, occur rarely. Prolonged high doses of chlorpromazine have also been associated with retinopathy and granular deposits in the cornea and lens.

Drug interactions

Concurrent therapy with drugs possessing any of the actions of chlorpromazine are a possible cause of drug interactions. These are most likely to occur with other centrally depressant drugs including ethyl alcohol (ethanol). The effects of hypotensive drugs may be potentiated.

Other antipsychotic drugs

There are several other groups of drugs that are chemically different from but pharmacologically similar to the phenothiazines. These include the butyrophenones (benperidol, droperidol, haloperidol, and trifluperidol), diphenylbutylpiperidines (fluspiriline and pimozide), thioxanthenes (chlorprothixene, flupenthixol, and zuclopenthixol), oxypertine and benzamide (sulpiride). Some of these drugs are less sedative than chlorpromazine (flupenthixol and pimozide) whilst haloperidol is useful for the rapid control of acute psychotic states. One of the problems of the treatment of schizophrenia is that of drug-compliance. In order to surmount this problem, depot preparations of flupenthixol and zuclopenthixol have been formulated as esters (decanoate) that are dissolved in vegetable oil in which form they are given by injection as a depot preparation every two to six weeks. The selection and use of antipsychotic drugs is obviously an area for the psychiatrist but, with such a large number of preparations available, there is the need for even the specialist to become highly selective and competent in the use of this important group of efficacious but potentially dangerous drugs.

LITHIUM

The medical use of lithium is not new and, during the last century, it acquired a therapeutic reputation amongst those who took the waters because it was beneficial for the treatment of gout. Prompted by this fame, some doctors began to prescribe it for gout and other conditions but it soon had to be abandoned because of its serious toxicity. Later it was given a trial for the treatment of epilepsy and also to replace sodium in the preparation of salt-free diets for the treatment of high blood pressure. Unfortunately, both these uses had to be abandoned because of its serious, including fatal, toxic effects. The possible use of lithium as a psychotropic drug came to light when Cade (1949) observed that lithium urate caused guinea-pigs to become sleepy. Clinical trials of lithium soon followed, and it was found to be the only specific drug for the treatment of mania although, not surprisingly, experience showed that the concentration of lithium in the plasma had to be maintained between narrow limits if toxicity was not to ensue.

Pharmacodynamics

When lithium salts are administered there is a slow displacement of sodium ions by lithium ions. It has been observed that in patients suffering from depressive illness the intracellular sodium ion concentration is elevated, especially so in those suffering from mania. It has therefore been suggested that the mechanism of action of lithium is by displacement of intracellular sodium, thus allowing this ion to return towards the normal concentration. In practice, lithium carbonate or lithium citrate are the salts used.

Pharmacokinetics

Lithium salts, like sodium salts, are well-absorbed but the lithium ion crosses cell membranes more slowly than sodium or potassium ions and this has important implications for its toxicity (see Unwanted Effects). Therapeutic plasma concentrations lie between 0.8 and 1.3 mmol/l. Plasma concentrations above 1.5 mmol/l are likely to be associated with unwanted effects and, at concentrations above 3 mmol/l, severe overdose occurs. The $T_{0.5}$ is 7–20 hours but increases to 36 hours with old age.

Uses

As already indicated, lithium salts are used for the treatment of mania and, more particularly, for the treatment of manic depression, where it can prevent the unpleasant and serious mood swings that are the major feature of this condition. It is also used for the treatment of unipolar depression but usually only after this has been controlled by the use of antidepressant drugs such as the tricyclics.

Unwanted effects

Lithium has a low therapeutic index therefore, as explained earlier, it is essential for the plasma concentration to be kept within narrow limits. As it is eliminated entirely through the kidneys then factors that alter fluid balance and renal function are likely to precipitate lithium toxicity. Thus, a reduced fluid intake (for example, vomiting) or an increased fluid loss (for example, vomiting, diarrhoea, fever, or diuretic therapy) may precipitate toxic effects.

The features of lithium intoxication are gastro-intestinal (anorexia, nausea, vomiting, and diarrhoea) and CNS disturbances (drowsiness, giddiness, lethargy, ataxia, tremor, inco-ordination, and dysarthria). Severe intoxication may be associated with a toxic psychosis, convulsions, coma, oliguria, and circulatory failure leading to death. Lithium therapy has been reported to be associated with an increased incidence of dental caries (Rugg-Gunn, 1979).

Drug interactions with lithium

Both pharmacokinetic and pharmacodynamic interactions may occur.

Pharmacokinetics

After glomerular filtration, lithium appears to be reabsorbed in the proximal renal tubule and probably also in the loop of Henle (but unlike sodium not in the distal tubule). Furthermore, reabsorption appears to be linked to that of sodium (Beeley, 1986). Thus, sodium depletion due to any cause stimulates proximal tubular reabsorption of both sodium and lithium with a consequent increase in plasma lithium concentration. The converse effect is produced when the sodium load is increased. Thiazide diuretics increase sodium excretion by inhibiting distal tubular reabsorption; there will be a compensatory increase in proximal tubular reabsorption that will affect lithium as well as sodium and thereby increase plasma lithium concentrations. Thus, thiazide diuretics should be avoided in patients on lithium; frusemide is less likely to produce this effect. If a patient on lithium requires a diuretic then the dose of lithium must be reduced by 25 to 50 per cent, and the plasma lithium concentration carefully monitored.

Non-steroidal anti-inflammatory drugs (NSAIDs; Chapter 5) reduce lithium excretion and hence increase plasma lithium concentrations. Those known to produce this effect include ibuprofen, naproxen, diclofenac, piroxicam, indomethacin, and phenylbutazone. Now that ibuprofen is available as an over-the-counter prescription it is important to warn patients on lithium that they should not take this analgesic. Fortunately, aspirin and paracetamol have no effect on lithium excretion.

Theophylline and acetazolamide both increase the excretion of lithium. As indicated earlier, sodium salts also increase in this excretion so that medications containing these substances (sodium bicarbonate, magnesium trisilicate, Gaviscon, Fybogel) are best avoided in these circumstances.

Pharmacodynamics

The antipsychotic drug, haloperidol, may precipitate lithium toxicity as also may the anticonvulsant drug, carbamazepine (see later), particularly when the latter is present in high plasma concentrations. Lithium has neuromuscular blocking properties of its own and may potentiate the effects of both competitive (e.g. tubocurarine) and depolarizing neuromuscular blockers (e.g. suxamethonium). In view of the inevitable disturbances of renal function and fluid balance that are likely to occur during *major* dental surgery, lithium therapy should be temporarily stopped several days before this is undertaken in order to avoid the risk of precipitating lithium intoxication.

DEPRESSION AND ANTIDEPRESSANTS

Mental illness of varying degrees forms a significant part of modern life. Most of us experience, from time to time, swings of moods. These are usually related to the circumstances prevailing at the time. However, some people are prone to recurrent episodes of severe depression during which they become incapacitated and even suicidal. These episodes usually pass, but they may last for weeks, months, or even years unless treated. Some patients have marked swings of mood from depression to the manic state, where there is a marked elevation of mood and the patient becomes agitated. This, as we have seen, is referred to as manic–depressive psychosis (bipolar illness), but more commonly the patient is simply depressed (unipolar illness). The antidepressant drugs are usually divided into the following groups:

(1) tricyclic and related antidepressants;

(2) monoamine oxidase inhibitors (MAOIs);

(3) other antidepressant drugs.

Tricyclic and related (tetracyclic) antidepressants

The tricyclic and related antidepressants can be divided into those with distinct sedative properties in addition to their antidepressant properties, and those with less sedative properties:

(1) tricyclics with sedative properties include: amitriptyline, maprotiline, dothiepin, doxepin, trazodone, and trimipramine;

(ii) tetracyclics with sedative properties include: mianserin;

(2) tricyclics with less sedative properties include: butriptyline, clomipramine, desipramine, imipramine, iprindole, lofepramine, nortriptyline, and viloxazine.

Protriptyline is also a tricyclic antidepressant but has a stimulant action.

Pharmacodynamics

It has been postulated that mental depression is the result of a disorder of amine metabolism. The tricyclic antidepressants, and related drugs, appear to block the reuptake of noradrenaline into central sympathetic nerve fibres. Normally, noradrenaline released from storage granules within a sympathetic neurone is mainly inactivated by being taken back into sympathetic neurones, where it is housed within storage granules and is ready for reuse. When this reuptake mechanism is interfered with, as occurs with most tricyclic antidepressants and related drugs, then there occurs a concentration of released noradrenaline at central synapses. If a depression is somehow related to a central deficiency of noradrenaline, then it would seem that the increase in concentration produced by the tricyclics centrally will help to correct the disorder. It is unlikely that noradrenaline is the only amine involved; others could be concerned, for instance 5-HT. Furthermore, as this blockage of reuptake occurs immediately but the drugs do not relieve a depression for some weeks, it is clear that this inhibition of reuptake cannot be the only explanation. An additional factor, which supports this reservation, is that iprindole interferes very little with the reuptake of released amines. Possibly this enhancement of noradrenaline concentration in the synaptic cleft is only the beginning of a sequence of events that finally relieve the depression.

Pharmacokinetics

The tricyclic antidepressants are well-absorbed from the gastro-intestinal tract after oral administration, and peak plasma concentrations are reached within two to eight hours. They are lipophilic drugs that are widely distributed and highly bound to plasma proteins. The tricyclics are metabolized in the liver with the production of a number of active metabolites. These are eventually conjugated with glucuronic acid and are excreted in the urine. The half-life of these drugs is very variable, ranging from about 16 hours for amitriptyline to 80 hours for protriptyline (Baldessarini 1985).

Unwanted effects

The tricyclic antidepressants have a marked anticholinergic effect so that the patient may be troubled by dry mouth, constipation, urinary retention, and blurred vision. The dry mouth may be severe and is often very troublesome. In some patients a persistent fine tremor occurs, although these drugs rarely cause the extrapyramidal effects seen with some of the phenothiazines.

Drug interactions may occur in that tricyclic antidepressants can reduce the effect of some hypotensive drugs, e.g. guanethidine, bethanidine, debrisoquine, and clonidine. Guanethidine, bethanidine, and debrisoquine are adrenergic-neurone blocking agents (all rarely used today) and their antihypertensive properties depend on the fact that they reach high concentrations within sympathetic nerve endings. These drugs gain access to the neuronal ending by the same pathway that reuptakes released noradrenaline. When this reuptake mechanism is blocked, as occurs with the tricyclics and the phenothiazines, then the antihypertensive is unable to get into the nerve endings and is ineffective. It seems that in some way the tricyclic antidepressants also block the central effects of the hypotensive drug, clonidine.

Theoretically, the use of adrenaline in local anaesthetic solutions could produce a hypertensive episode because, in the presence of tricyclic antidepressants, the main pathway of inactivation, e.g. reuptake, of catecholamines is blocked. In clinical practice this does not appear to occur and it would seem that with the concentration of adrenaline in the local anaesthetic solution (usually 1:80 000), and in the amounts used in dentistry, there is no problem. (Cawson and Spector 1985).

A common cardiovascular effect of the tricyclics is postural hypotension, especially in the older patient. This is partly due to the blockade of peripheral α-adrenergic receptors. The anticholinergic activity of these drugs may also cause a mild sinus tachycardia. The tricyclic antidepressants have a cardiotoxic effect in predisposed patients, e.g. those with existing cardiac problems.

The tricyclic drugs are extremely toxic in overdosage and are dangerous, especially when used in attempted suicide.

Therapeutic uses

The tricyclic antidepressants are generally regarded as the drugs of first choice for the treatment of mental depression. Unfortunately, their antidepressant action is not immediate but begins in about two to three weeks and is not fully effective until six weeks. Low doses are usually prescribed at first and gradually built up until plasma concentrations are sufficient. For instance, amitriptyline by mouth is given initially in 50 to 75 mg doses (elderly patients and adolescents, 25 to

50 mg) daily, and is often prescribed as a single dose at bedtime. The dose is gradually increased to a maximum of 150 to 200 mg daily. The *BNF* [No. 12 (1986)] suggests that after suppression of symptoms the drug should be maintained at the optimum level for at least another month before any attempt is made to reduce the dosage. The drug should not be stopped prematurely and the patient may be maintained on a much reduced dosage for some months in order to prevent occurrence of a relapse. Perhaps the most widely used of the tricyclics are imipramine and amitriptyline.

The patient should not be given an unlimited quantity of these drugs as depressed patients are potential suicides and, in overdosage, the tricyclic antidepressants are extremely toxic. Their progress should be monitored regularly; the first sign of improvement is usually an improved sleep pattern.

The oxazine, viloxazine, probably produces its antidepressant effect in the same way as the tricyclic drugs. It prevents the reuptake of released noradrenaline and so increases the functional availability of the neurotransmitter. Viloxazine is unlike the tricyclic antidepressants in that it has little anticholinergic activity.

Monoamine oxidase inhibitors (MAOIs)

The monoamine oxidase inhibitors include:

(1) hydrazine MAOIs—iproniazid, isocarboxazid, and phenelzine;

(2) non-hydrazine MAOIs—tranylcypromine.

The story of the discovery of MAOIs as anti-depressive drugs is of interest. In the early 50s isoniazid was developed as an antituberculous drug. It was noticed that patients being treated for tuberculosis with isoniazid appeared to be more euphoric than perhaps their condition warranted. The fact that isoniazid inhibited monoamine oxidase (MAO) supported the theory that depression could be a disorder of amine metabolism.

Pharmacodynamics

Monoamine oxidase inhibitors block the breakdown of naturally occurring amines such as noradrenaline, 5-HT, and dopamine. Consequent upon this failure of metabolism, the concentration of noradrenaline and other amines is increased in the CNS. It has been suggested that this increased availability of amines centrally is the reason for their effectiveness in depression. As with the tricyclic antidepressants, the effect of these drugs on amine inactivation is almost immediate whereas the relief of the depression is delayed for two weeks or more. The way in which amines are concentrated centrally differs between MAOIs and the tricyclic antidepressants. Once again, as with the tricyclics, it would seem that the theory of disordered amine inactivation is not the whole story.

Pharmacokinetics

When given orally the MAOIs are readily absorbed from the gastro-intestinal tract. Not a great deal is known about the pharmacokinetics of these drugs but the hydrazine MAOIs are partly inactivated by acetylation. Furthermore, these produce an irreversible block of MAO and so their activity tends to be prolonged. After cessation of treatment it takes about three weeks before new enzymes are formed in adequate amounts.

The response to these drugs is somewhat varied; for instance with slow acetylators of the hydrazine type, patients may find toxicity occurring.

Unwanted effects

There is a wide variety of these, some relatively trivial and some very serious. The MAOIs affect the autonomic nervous system and hypotension is produced. Other disturbances of that system include dry mouth, water retention, difficulty in micturition, and constipation. A very serious effect, although of low incidence, is the occurrence of diffuse hepatocellular damage with the hydrazine derivatives. Perhaps the most alarming and serious of unwanted effects are those occurring due to interactions with other drugs and substances.

The interaction between MOAIs and sympathomimetic amines is well-known, and is an example of how the absorption of one drug may be increased by another. The gastro-intestinal tract contains large amounts of the enzyme MAO, which normally metabolizes and thereby restricts the absorption of any amines that are substrates for it, for example tyramine or phenylephrine. Certain foods also contain amines, especially cheese, Marmite and other yeast extracts, Bovril, pickled herrings, broad beans (as an amine precursor), yoghourt, strong beer, and some wines. When these agents are taken by a patient who is receiving an MAOI drug, there is a considerable risk that a so-called MAOI crisis may develop. In this condition there is a severe headache with a dangerous rise in blood pressure that, in some cases, has progressed to a cerebral haemorrhage or acute cardiovascular collapse (Blackwell *et al.* 1967). From the practical point of view it is vital that all patients on MAOIs be informed that they must avoid such foods as well as sympathomimetic amines, some of which are concealed within various patent medicines.

It is the indirectly acting sympathomimetics, such as tyramine, that often produce this interaction. These can cause the release of noradrenaline from its storage sites within the granules or synaptic vesicles of sympathetic nerve endings. The released noradrenaline acts on α_1-receptors in the peripheral blood vessels causing vasoconstriction and a rise in blood pressure, noradrenaline being a pressor substance. Normally the amine, tyramine, contained in foods is not absorbed to any extent, being broken down by the gut MAO. However, when the patient is taking an MAOI, tyramine is absorbed, so causing noradrenaline release, with a potentiation of the pressor effect of noradrenaline. The treatment of such an hypertensive crisis is by the use of a short-acting α-adrenergic blocking agent such as phentolamine, 5 mg IV or IM, repeated if necessary.

Another potentially very dangerous interaction may result from the use of the opioid, pethidine, in those taking MAOIs. Pethidine is a recent addition to drugs listed in the *Dental Practitioners' Formulary*. If given to a patient on MAOIs it may cause hyperpyrexia, which can prove to be extremely serious. This is not a reaction that could have been predicted on the known pharmacology of pethidine; it appears to be limited to that opioid but perhaps other opioids should be avoided in those taking MAOIs, simply as a precaution.

It has been suggested in the past that local anaesthetic solutions containing catecholamines should be avoided in patients taking MAOIs as they were thought to interact, possibly producing a hypertensive episode. This view was based on a pharmacological misunderstanding as it was thought, at the time, that the main inactivation of catecholamines was by MAO. This is now known to be untrue and so there is no real contra-indication in dentistry to the use of catecholamine-containing local anaesthetic solutions in patients taking MAOIs.

If a general anaesthetic is absolutely necessary, then this should be administered by a specialist anaesthetist.

Therapeutic uses

The MAOIs were, perhaps, the first drugs of real significance in the treatment of depression. They are no longer the first choice of such drugs, having been generally superseded by the tricyclic antidepressants, and they now have a more limited use because of the wide variety of their unwanted effects. They are used when vigorous treatment with the tricyclics has failed. The *BNF* (1986–8 No. 12) suggests that the '. . . phobic and depressed patient with atypical, hypochondriacal, or hysterical features are said to respond best to MAOIs.' The delay in improvement of the depression may, as with the tricyclics, be in the order of a few weeks.

In the past, certain of the MAOIs (e.g. the non-hydrazine—pargyline (Eutonyl)) were used as antihypertensive agents as they affected adrenergic activity by neuronal block. Better and safer drugs are now available and pargyline is no longer listed in the *BNF*.

HYPNOTICS AND SEDATIVES

Hypnotics are drugs that induce sleep. Normal sleep has at least two phases, one with regular respiration (called orthodox sleep) alternating with the second phase, which consists of rapid eye movements (REM sleep) associated with irregular breathing. Hypnotics do not produce normal sleep in that, to varying degrees, they tend to reduce the second phase. As the therapeutic effect of the hypnotic begins to wear off before wakening there is an increase in the frequency of REM periods. Nevertheless, in the total sleep period, the proportion occupied by

REM sleep is reduced. When hypnotic drugs are withdrawn, there is an over-compensatory increase in REM sleep and dreaming is excessive. There may even be nightmares associated with the now increased REM activity.

The number of remedies offered to the healing professions and the public suggest that there is a general problem in achieving sleep. Unfortunately the causes of insomnia are as varied as the individuals and the remedies. What is good for one individual is not necessarily good for another. An unduly stuffy room, an overfilled or empty stomach, a distended bladder, pain or discomfort are all frequent causes of insomnia. Such reasons for lack of sleep can usually be tackled without recourse to the use of 'sleeping tablets'. In contrast, insomnia from severe illness or emotional disturbances, such as worry, fear, or bereavement, are different matters altogether. Such cases may require a sleeping tablet, even if only for a short time. As for the elderly, a tot of brandy at night may be as good a remedy as any. Hypnotics should not be prescribed indiscriminately without some good reason and must be under careful supervision. If the cause of lack of sleep is pain then an analgesic should be prescribed, not an hypnotic. Sleep disturbance is very common in psychiatric illnesses, e.g. depression, and it is the illness itself that needs treatment, rather than having recourse to 'sleeping tablets' as an immediate expedient for any sleeplessness.

Hypnotics will be considered under various headings: chloral derivatives, barbiturates, antihistamines, and benzodiazepines. The usual hypnotic drug prescribed today is one of the benzodiazepines. The barbiturates are no longer discussed in the BNF (1986-8) as drugs to be employed for insomnia but, at one time, they were the most commonly used hypnotics (see below).

Chloral hydrate
(0.5 to 1 g, 30 minutes before bedtime)

This was the first of the synthetic hypnotic drugs. It is very irritant to the empty stomach and should be prescribed as a well-diluted solution, preferably with a strong flavouring agent to disguise the unpleasant taste.

Pharmacokinetics
Chloral hydrate is rapidly absorbed from the gastro-intestinal tract and is quickly reduced to trichloroethanol in the liver by alcohol dehydrogenase. Although chloral hydrate itself may possess hypnotic properties, it is believed that the CNS depression that occurs after its ingestion is mainly due to trichloroethanol; in other words, trichloroethanol is the active metabolite. A variable fraction of chloral hydrate is oxidized in the liver to trichloracetic acid (an inactive metabolite). A fraction of trichloroethanol is reduced but the major part is conjugated with glucuronic acid; the conjugate is eventually excreted in the urine, as is trichloroacetic acid.

Unwanted effects

The main one is associated with its irritant effect on the gastric mucosa, causing the patient to feel discomfort. Allergic reactions may occur; these usually take the form of skin rashes. In very large doses, chloral hydrate is a cardiac depressant and is therefore contra-indicated in patients with severe heart disease. It is also to be avoided in those with marked hepatic impairment.

This drug should not be taken together with alcohol as both substances are metabolized by the same enzyme system (alcohol dehydrogenase).

Uses

Chloral is probably still a useful hypnotic drug for, in therapeutic doses, it has little, if any, cardiovascular effect. It appears to be particularly valuable in young children and in the elderly. Hypnotics in general tend to cause post-hypnotic confusion in the elderly, but chloral hydrate seems to cause less.

The BNF (1986–8) refers to chloral hydrate and chloral derivatives as useful hypnotics. It states that dichloralphenazone and triclofos sodium '. . . cause fewer gastro-intestinal upsets than chloral hydrate'. Dichloralphenazone is a popular preparation containing chloral. It is a complex of chloral hydrate with the antipyretic analgesic, phenazone. The phenazone nucleus has been implicated in the production of rashes and agranulocytosis but this white cell effect does not seem to be a problem with dichloralphenazone. It has the advantage that it is available in tablet form and is easier to take than chloral hydrate itself.

The barbiturates

In the past, these were used extensively as sleeping tablets but today they have been displaced by the benzodiazepines. Initially the benzodiazepines were thought less likely to cause dependence problems than did the barbiturates, but sadly this has not proved to be the case (see Benzodiazepines—Unwanted effects, below).

Barbiturates are classified as:

(1) ultra-short acting, e.g. thiopentone, methohexitone (see Chapter 8);
(2) short-acting, e.g. amylobarbitone, pentobarbitone (100 to 200 mg, 30 minutes before bedtime);
(3) long-acting, e.g. phenobarbitone.

Pharmacodynamics

These drugs probably act at many levels in the CNS, but the reticular activating system is particularly sensitive. This system is a complex of neural pathways that extend in the brainstem from the medulla to the thalamus. It is the activity of this system that maintains consciousness and keeps the individual alert. The barbiturates, and other hypnotic drugs, appear to depress transmission of impulses through inhibition of neurotransmitter release.

Pharmacological properties

The effect on the CNS, as indicated above, is inhibition of synaptic transmission.

Therapeutic hypnotic doses of the barbiturates when given orally have few cardiovascular effects in the otherwise healthy patient. They do cause a slight decrease in the blood pressure and heart rate, but these phenomena occur in normal sleep anyway. The barbiturates do, however, inhibit transmission in autonomic ganglia, and intravenous barbiturates may produce a marked fall in blood pressure in the hypertensive patient.

Barbiturates can produce a dose-related depression of respiration. Hypnotic doses usually cause only a minor degree of this, but larger doses cause severe respiratory depression and, in fact, the cause of death in acute barbiturate poisoning is directly attributable to respiratory failure. Another respiratory effect is the production of laryngospasm with the use of the intravenous agents, particularly thiopentone (see Chapter 8).

Barbiturates are enzyme inducers, that is they stimulate the activity of microsomal drug-metabolizing enzymes in the liver. Phenobarbitone is a potent enzyme inducer and the result of such induction is that the half-life of some drugs may be reduced substantially; those so affected include coumarins, phenytoin, and the antifungal drug, griseofulvin. Probably the most dangerous situation that could arise from this effect occurs after the withdrawal of a drug that is an enzyme inducer. Thus, the withdrawal of phenobarbitone during treatment with one of the anticoagulants may lead to a dangerous intensification of the anticoagulant. effect. This is due to the reduced rate of metabolism of the anticoagulant.

Pharmacokinetics

For hypnotic use the barbiturates are administered orally. Absorption takes place mainly from the intestine, and food decreases the rate of absorption. The intravenous route is employed for anaesthetic induction.

The barbiturates are bound variously to plasma proteins; the more lipid-soluble the drug, the more binding there is. There exists no impenetrable barrier in the body to the diffusion of the barbiturates. Small amounts of barbiturates may appear in the mother's milk after ingestion of large doses, and they cross the placenta to reach the fetus.

Following absorption the most lipid-soluble barbiturates, that is those used intravenously (ultra-short acting barbiturates), are quickly concentrated in the brain, and so they have a very rapid onset of action. Their duration of action is also very short (see below).

Three processes are responsible for the termination of the CNS-depressant action of the barbiturates:

(1) physical redistribution;

(2) metabolic degradation;

(3) renal excretion.

All these processes reduce the drug's plasma concentration and result in its withdrawal from its site of action in the CNS. The immediate fate of the drug does seem to depend on the degree of its lipid solubility. The most lipid-soluble ultra-short acting barbiturates undergo rapid redistribution to muscle and then to fat. Indeed, it is this early redistribution that accounts for their relatively brief action. Following redistribution, thiopentone is almost completely metabolized in the liver and only a very small fraction is eventually excreted unchanged in the urine. In point of fact, although metabolized, the rate of metabolism is relatively slow— perhaps in the region of 10 to 15 per cent per hour, which is far too slow to account for the very short duration of action. The rapid emergence from sleep after administration of a single dose of thiopentone depends on a shift of the drug from the brain to other tissues and is not a result of metabolic degradation. About 30 minutes after the injection of thiopentone, the brain may have given up as much as 90 per cent of the drug to muscle and fat depots. The same comments apply to methohexitone, although the metabolic degradation of this drug is probably quicker than for thiopentone.

The less lipophilic barbiturates (the short-acting and the long-acting) reach the brain tissues more slowly. These compounds are metabolized in the liver and this is the way in which the activity of a short-acting barbiturate is mainly terminated. The long-acting barbiturate, phenobarbitone, is metabolized in the liver but about 25 per cent may be excreted unchanged in the urine. The metabolites of all the barbiturates are eventually excreted in the urine.

Unwanted effects

1. Drowsiness is a common after-effect of the barbiturates as hypnotics. Headache and nausea may also occur.

2. Hypersensitivity reactions do occur, particularly in subjects with an allergic diathesis. They often take the form of skin rashes or localized swellings.

3. Barbiturates produce both physical and psychological dependence and, for this reason, have been discontinued, with few exceptions (e.g. phenobarbitone in epilepsy, see later).

4. Instead of depressing the CNS, sometimes barbiturates stimulate the subject, who becomes excitable. This curious effect is most likely to be seen in geriatric patients.

5. Interactions with other drugs may occur because of hepatic microsomal enzyme induction (discussed under pharmacological properties above).

6. Porphyrias are inherited diseases in which there is an abnormality of porphyrin synthesis. They are associated with the excretion of large amounts of

porphyrins, or their precursors, in the urine. Barbiturates enhance porphyrin synthesis and must not be given to a patient with porphyria; to do so may precipitate a serious crisis with lower motor-neurone paralysis.

Uses

The short-acting barbiturates were popular at one time as hypnotics but, as we have seen, they are now virtually obsolete. Furthermore, these short-acting compounds, e.g. amylobarbitone, butobarbitone, cyclobarbitone, pentobarbitone, quinalbarbitone, are now classified as 'controlled drugs' and the prescription must be written in the form ordered for such drugs (see Chapter 3). This requirement has further discouraged their use.

The long-acting barbiturate, phenobarbitone, finds a place in the management of epilepsy but it is also now listed as a 'controlled drug'. However, the actual form of the prescription is not as demanding as for the short-acting barbiturates in that, although the prescription must be signed and dated by the prescriber, other details required need not be in the practitioner's handwriting.

The ultra short-acting agents, thiopentone and methohexitone, have been discussed in Chapter 8. Although thiopentone is a drug that will control status epilepticus, it must be remembered that methohexitone has convulsant properties and should not be used in patients with a history of epilepsy (Goldman 1966).

Benzodiazepines

These comprise a group of drugs with useful hypnotic, anxiolytic, anticonvulsant, and skeletal-muscle relaxant properties. The use of benzodiazepines as hypnotics will be discussed first, although some of the general properties of these drugs (e.g. pharmacodynamics, unwanted effects) will also be considered at this stage. Examples of the benzodiazepine hypnotics include:

nitrazepam (5 to 10 mg, 30 minutes before bedtime—the dose should be halved for elderly patients);

flurazepam (15 to 30 mg, 30 minutes before bedtime—elderly patients, 15 mg);

lormetazepam (1 mg at bedtime—elderly patients, 500 μg);

temazepam (10 to 30 mg immediately before bedtime—elderly patients, half the dose);

triazolam (250 μg, 15 to 30 minutes before bedtime—elderly patients, half the dose).

Pharmacodynamics

The benzodiazepines probably work centrally in a similar way to older hypnotic–sedative drugs, such as the barbiturates. It does appear, however, that the benzodiazepines are different in that they have a specific anti-anxiety action, which is lacking in drugs such as the barbiturates. The benzodiazepines depress the reticular system, but they also depress the limbic system at much lower doses and this system is associated with emotions. This is not the case with the barbiturates which, as we have seen, depress the reticular system preferentially. It seems that the benzodiazepines potentiate the inhibitory action of the neurotransmitter gamma(γ)-aminobutyric acid (GABA) on neurones. Although the benzodiazepines diminish REM sleep, they do not seem to do so to the same extent as barbiturates.

Pharmacological properties

The effects on the CNS are those of sedation to hypnosis. They also have anticonvulsant properties as well as the anti-anxiety effect. The cardiovascular effect of the benzodiazepines is small although, in large doses, they all decrease blood pressure. A similar picture applies to respiration; the usual hypnotic dose does not affect the normal individual. The benzodiazepines are not inducers of hepatic microsomal enzymes to any extent.

Pharmacokinetics

The benzodiazepines are generally well-absorbed when given orally. Some do not reach the circulation intact, but produce their effects through clinically active metabolites; one such is flurazepam. When the benzodiazepines are given orally, the peak plasma concentration is variably reached within a period of 0.5 to 8 hours (Harvey 1985). The half-life of a preparation does not necessarily give an indication of the drug's duration of action as it may produce metabolites that have their own half-lives. This is illustrated in the list below.

Drug	Half-life (h)		Active metabolite
Nitrazepam	15–38		
Flurazepam		[40–250]	N-desalkylflurazepam
Lormetazepam	10–12		
Temazepam	8–22		
Triazolam	2		

(Figures in brackets are the half-life of the major active metabolite.)

Flurazepam and lormetazepam are no longer available on the NHS.

As with the barbiturates, there is a phase of redistribution to muscle and fat especially with the most lipid-soluble benzodiazepines. This may account for the duration of an hypnotic effect just as much as may metabolism. The benzodiazepines are extensively metabolized in the liver by microsomal enzymes and, in general terms, the metabolites are conjugated with glucuronic acid and excreted in the urine.

Unwanted effects

1. Without doubt the most common unwanted effect of the benzodiazepines, when used as sedatives or anxiolytics, is drowsiness. This is also associated with a decrease in reaction time, which is likely to affect driving ability. Judgment and concentration may both be impaired.

2. Occasionally, in doses that relieve anxiety, there is a paradoxical effect in which excitement is seen, rather than depression. This arises more often in the young and the elderly; occasionally a patient may even become aggressive.

3. These drugs are not so innocuous as they were first thought to be. Treatment for anxiety should be limited to short periods as tolerance may develop within about 4 months of continuous use, and there is also the danger of the development of dependence, which is something thought not to occur when they were first introduced. There is evidence that medication with benzodiazepines for some weeks or more can lead to both physical and psychological dependence, and that cessation of treatment can lead to definite withdrawal symptoms (Drug Newsletter 1985). The withdrawal symptoms may sometimes hardly be distinguishable from the original anxiety state. Symptoms of withdrawal include insomnia; restlessness; lack of concentration; delusions; visual and auditory hallucinations; altered sensations in the skin, mouth, jaw, and tongue—and even toothache.

4. The combination of the benzodiazepines with other drugs that act on the CNS may potentiate depressant effects. Thus they must be used cautiously with, for instance, alcohol.

5. Hypersensitivity reactions may occur but their incidence is low.

Uses

The benzodiazepines are useful in the treatment of insomnia. The prescription of hypnotics is justifiable for short periods (1–3 weeks) to cover a time of stress but it is undesirable that patients should become used to hypnotics and so take them regularly year in and year out.

For those who find difficulty in getting off to sleep, but who sleep well once sleep has ensued, a drug like temazepam should be used; this has a relatively short half-life and no active metabolites. On the other hand, for the patient who readily gets off to sleep, but who wakens early in the morning, a longer-acting preparation may be desirable. Flurazepam is quickly converted to active metabolites and these have a half-life up to many days. Nitrazepam has a half-life in the range 15–38 hours and, unlike flurazepam, its metabolites are inactive. Both of these drugs may be useful for the early waker but they can produce residual effects in the following day, e.g. drowsiness. Flurazepam is no longer prescribable on the NHS.

Antihistamines (H$_1$-blockers)
(e.g. promethazine)

These produce CNS depression when used in therapeutic doses and so the patient is not alert and may feel drowsy. The various preparations provide differing degrees of sedation and the patient's reaction to them is individualized. Promethazine is a popular sedative/hypnotic for children but is not recommended for those under 6 months of age. Its dosage regimen is:

By mouth: adults, 25 to 75 mg at bedtime; children of 6 to 12 months—10 mg, of 1 to 5 years—15 to 20 mg, of 6 to 10 years—20 to 25 mg, at bedtime; or, for daytime sedation, once or twice daily using the lower dose.

ANXIETY AND ANXIOLYTICS

Benzodiazepines

As outlined earlier, the benzodiazepine drugs have specific anti-anxiety properties. Anxiety is a state where the individual feels uneasy and apprehensive, where there is also a feeling of tension accompanied by many bodily complaints e.g. palpitations, headache, dizziness, flushing, sweating, tense muscles. Anxiety may also be a feature of other psychological illnesses, e.g. depression. Appropriate anxiolytic dosages are:

chlordiazepoxide (orally, 10 mg three times daily);

diazepam (orally, 2 mg three times daily increased in severe anxiety to 15 to 30 mg daily in divided doses);

oxazepam (15 to 30 mg (elderly patients 10 to 20 mg) three to four times daily; increased in severe anxiety to 60 mg three times daily as a maximum);

lorazepam (orally, 1 to 4 mg daily in divided doses, increased to 10 mg in severe anxiety).

Pharmacokinetics

Chlordiazepoxide and diazepam were amongst the early benzodiazepines to be prescribed for anxiety. Chlordiazepoxide is rather slowly absorbed after oral administration and it takes several hours for peak plasma concentrations to be reached. On the other hand, diazepam, which is highly lipid-soluble, is quickly absorbed producing a peak plasma concentration in about one hour. Some of these anxiolytic benzodiazepines e.g. chlordiazepoxide and diazepam, are metabolized to produce active metabolites, whereas oxazepam and lorazepam are converted to inactive metabolites. The half-life of these drugs and their metabolites is indicated in the following list, which may be compared with that shown in the section on the Pharmacokinetics of benzodiazepine hypnotics above:

Drug	Half-life (h)	Active metabolite(s)
Chlordiazepoxide	5–30 [36–200]	Desmethylchlordiazepoxide→ demoxepam→nordiazepam
Diazepam	20–100 [36–200]	Nordiazepam
Oxazepam	4–15	
Lorazepam	10–20	

(Figures in brackets are the active half-life of metabolites.)

The metabolites eventually undergo glucuronidation and are excreted in the urine.

Uses (general)

These drugs are used in both chronic and acute anxiety states. All of us will have experienced anxiety at some time or another, and most of us will not have required medication. However, when anxiety persists and interferes with the daily functioning of life, it is then that the use of the benzodiazepines may be considered. Again it must be emphasized that treatment should be limited to short periods as tolerance may occur and dependence may develop within four months or less of continuous usage. Dependence is more likely in patients who have a background of alcohol or drug abuse, and in those with an unstable background.

Drugs such as chlordiazepoxide and diazepam are useful in managing chronic anxiety. They have a long half-life and consequently provide a sustained action. It must be emphasized that such patients require psychiatric treatment.

Other benzodiazepines recommended for anxiety, e.g. oxazepam and loraze-pam, have relatively short half-lives and so do not provide such a sustained activity and are more useful for short acute episodic anxiety.

Uses in dentistry

1. Their anxiolytic effect makes the benzodiazepines useful drugs in pre-anaesthetic medication (see Chapter 8).

2. Intravenous diazepam or midazolam are used to provide sedation as an adjunct to local anaesthesia; the sedation achieved often lasts up to an hour. A useful and characteristic feature of such sedation is the anterograde amnesia produced in over 50 per cent of patients given diazepam, and in nearly 85 per cent of those given midazolam (see Chapter 8).

3. A benzodiazepine is a recommended part of an emergency kit in case of the occurrence of status epilepticus (see Chapter 24). In this situation the anticonvul-sant properties of the benzodiazepines are utilized.

4. The muscle relaxant property of the benzodiazepines may be useful in the

management of temporo-mandibular joint pain and dysfunction, which could well be due to tension in the muscles of mastication.

5. The use of oral benzodiazepines to produce sedation before dental procedures, the day before and again just prior to dental treatment, is recommended by some. It is certainly not as sure a method as providing intravenous administration at the time of treatment (see Chapter 8).

General comments on the benzodiazepines

These anxiolytic drugs are sometimes referred to as 'minor tranquillizers' to distinguish them from antipsychotic drugs, which have been called 'major tranquillizers' or neuroleptics. The terms minor and major tranquillizers should not be used as they do not best describe the actions of drugs to which they refer and, in any case, the benzodiazepines can hardly be regarded as 'minor' drugs.

Although certain benzodiazepines are advised for use as hypnotics, and others as anti-anxiety agents, they all serve the same purpose and perhaps the distinction is somewhat artificial.

Propranolol

The use of propranolol for somatic anxiety, as distinct from central anxiety as discussed above, is referred to in Chapter 13.

ANTICONVULSANTS

The treatment of epilepsy and facial neuralgias

Epilepsy is a term used for a group of CNS disorders having in common the occurrence of sudden and transitory episodes (seizures) of abnormal phenomena of motor (convulsions), sensory, autonomic, or psychic origin. The seizures are nearly always associated with abnormal and excessive discharges from neurones within the brain.

Epilepsy can be classified into partial seizures, which are either focal or local, and generalized seizures, which can be of the convulsive or non-convulsive type (International League Against Epilepsy 1981). Epilepsy has an incidence in the range 3–6 per 1,000 population (Hauser 1978).

Generalized epilepsy is by far the most common type of convulsive disorder and two aspects can be recognized, the petit mal attack and the grand mal attack.

The petit mal attack commonly occurs in childhood and is characterized by a very brief loss of consciousness (5 to 10 seconds), sometimes accompanied by facial twitching. Frequent petit mal attacks may well be a warning sign that a grand mal attack is soon to occur. Petit mal responds to therapy.

The grand mal attack is usually of sudden onset, but is often preceded by an aura. The attack is characterized by loss of consciousness, postural tone, and contraction of skeletal muscles. There is often loss of sphincter control causing urination and defaecation. The attacks usually last from a few seconds to a few minutes, but can progress to the life-threatening status epilepticus (see Chapter 24). After the convulsions the patient regains consciousness, but is very drowsy and disorientated; they often complain of a severe headache and usually want to sleep. The management of a grand mal attack in the dental surgery is discussed in Chapter 24.

Drugs used in the treatment of epilepsy include phenytoin, barbiturates, carbamazepine, ethosuximide, valproic acid, and the benzodiazepines.

Phenytoin

This is probably the anticonvulsant of choice to treat most types of epilepsy. Its anticonvulsant properties are thought to be due to a stabilizing effect on neuronal membranes to the action of sodium, potassium, and calcium ions (Woodbury *et al.* 1982).

Pharmacokinetics

Phenytoin is mainly given orally, but can be given intramuscularly or intravenously. The usual oral dose in adults is approximately 300 mg daily. Absorption of phenytoin from the gastro-intestinal tract is often slow and shows marked inter-individual variation. Absorption is affected by age, body weight, sex, and rate of phenytoin metabolism. Once absorbed, the drug is rapidly distributed through all tissues of the body. Phenytoin is highly protein-bound (90 per cent), mainly to albumin. About 5 per cent of phenytoin is excreted unchanged in the urine; the remainder is metabolized in the liver, and the metabolites are excreted initially in the bile and subsequently in the urine.

Unwanted effect

Phenytoin therapy is associated with a high incidence of these, mainly involving the CNS and gastro-intestinal tract. High plasma concentrations of phenytoin can produce ataxia, nystagmus, tremors, and drowsiness. Behavioural effects can occur, including hyperactivity, confusion, and hallucinations. The gastro-intestinal disturbances include nausea, vomiting, epigastric pain, and anorexia; their incidence can be reduced by taking the drug with meals. Hirsutism is a common problem in young female patients taking the drug. Hypersensitivity reactions occur in two to five per cent of patients taking phenytoin and range from skin rashes to the Stevens–Johnson syndrome. Haematological changes have been also reported and include leucopenia, agranulocytosis, thrombocytopenia, and a megaloblastic anaemia due to folic acid deficiency (Waxman *et al.* 1970).

Of particular interest to the dental surgeon is the effect of phenytoin on the gingival tissues. Approximately 50 per cent of those taking phenytoin experience enlargement (hyperplasia) of their gingival tissues (Angelopoulos and Goaz 1972). The pathogenesis of this problem is still uncertain. The hyperplasia occurs more commonly in the anterior part of the mouth and begins as an overgrowth of the interdental papillae, followed by a spread to other gingival regions. The gingiva usually retain their pink colour and their firm consistency. Histopathologically, the hyperplastic tissue comprises dense bundles of collagen fibres (Hassel et al. 1978).

There is some correlation between the degree of gingival hyperplasia and oral hygiene (King et al. 1976; the incidence of gingival hyperplasia can be reduced by maintaining good plaque control. Severe cases can be treated with surgical excision (gingivectomy). Some epileptic patients on phenytoin therapy have recurrent problems with gingival hyperplasia and often undergo repeated gingival surgery. For these, it may be appropriate to consider changing their anticonvulsant therapy through consultation with their physician (Seymour et al. 1985).

Uses

Phenytoin is the most widely used anticonvulsant; it is occasionally used in the treatment of certain facial neuralgias.

Barbiturates

Phenobarbitone is the only barbiturate used in the treatment of epilepsy. The general pharmacological properties of the barbiturates have been discussed earlier. Most have anticonvulsant properties by limiting the spread of seizure activity and elevating seizure threshold. The usual adult dose of phenobarbitone is 60 to 100 mg daily.

Pharmacokinetics

Phenobarbitone is slowly absorbed from the gastro-intestinal tract, with peak plasma concentrations occurring six hours after dosage. The drug is partly bound to plasma protein (50 per cent). About 25 per cent of phenobarbitone is excreted unchanged in the urine; the remainder is metabolized in the liver and the metabolites excreted in the urine. The plasma half-life of phenobarbitone in adults is about 100 hours.

Unwanted effects

Sedation is the main unwanted effect associated with phenobarbitone, especially in the early stages of therapy; however, tolerance soon develops. In children, the drug can produce hyperactivity and irritability, whilst in the elderly it frequently produces agitation and confusion. Occasional skin rashes and haematological problems are associated with it.

Uses

Phenobarbitone is an effective agent for generalized tonic–clonic seizures.

Carbamazepine

This has anticonvulsant properties, although how they are achieved is uncertain. The drug is structurally related to the tricyclic antidepressants and is particularly effective in controlling grand mal seizures, but not petit mal attacks. Carbamazepine is also used to treat trigeminal, glossopharyngeal, and post-herpetic neuralgia (see later). For the treatment of epilepsy, initial therapy is with a dose of 100 to 200 mg twice daily, which can be increased up to 1200 mg daily until seizures are controlled.

Pharmacokinetics

Carbamazepine is absorbed slowly from the gastro-intestinal tract with peak concentrations occurring four to eight hours after dosage. About 75 per cent of the drug is protein-bound. The main metabolite of carbamazepine is the 10,11-epoxide, which also possesses anticonvulsant properties; this is further metabolized to inactive compounds, which are excreted in the urine.

Unwanted effects

The common ones include drowsiness, visual disturbances, nausea, and vomiting. Serious haematological effects may occur with carbamazepine therapy, and include aplastic anaemia and agranulocytosis; routine haematological screening (every three months) is therefore required for all patients on this drug. Chronic usage of carbamazepine is associated with water retention, which may cause problems in elderly patients with cardiac disease.

Ethosuximide

This anticonvulsant is used primarily for the treatment of petit mal seizures. Its action is due to an elevation of the threshold for electro-shock seizures.

Pharmacokinetics

Ethosuximide is well-absorbed following oral administration, and peak plasma concentrations occur three hours after dosage. The plasma half-life is approximately 45 hours. Twenty-five per cent of the drug is excreted unchanged in the urine; the remainder is metabolized in the liver and the metabolites excreted in the urine. The usual dose of ethosuximide is 20 to 40 mg/kg of body weight.

Unwanted effects

Like other anticonvulsants, the main unwanted effects of ethosuximide are related to the CNS and the gastro-intestinal tract; they include drowsiness, lethargy, euphoria, dizziness, headache, nausea, vomiting, and anorexia. Skin rashes and haematological problems have also been reported with this drug.

Valproic acid

This comparatively new anticonvulsant is structurally related to carboxylic acid. Its mechanism of action is uncertain; it may interact with the central neurotransmitter, GABA, by preventing its uptake in nerve fibres.

Pharmacokinetics

Valproic acid is rapidly absorbed from the gastro-intestinal tract and peak plasma concentrations occur one to four hours after dosage. About 90 per cent of the drug is bound to plasma protein, and it has a half-life of 15 hours. Less than three per cent of valproic acid is excreted unchanged in the urine and faeces; the remainder is metabolized in the liver.

Unwanted effects

About 15 per cent of patients experience gastro-intestinal problems such as nausea, vomiting, and anorexia. The drug also has unwanted effects in the CNS including sedation, ataxia, and tremors. Hepatitis is the most serious problem associated with valproic acid therapy, and the incidence of hepatic failure is 1:20 000–40 000 patients taking the drug. Skin rashes and alopecia have been reported, but these are transitory. Of particular concern to the dental surgeon is the effect of valproic acid on haemostasis. The drug may cause thrombocytopenia, impairment of the secondary phase of platelet aggregation, and an increase in prothrombin (BCR) time (Hassell *et al.* 1979). Thus, some patients taking valproic acid may be at risk from a post-extraction or postoperative haemorrhage. Aspirin should be avoided in those taking valproic acid because it also affects platelet aggregation.

Benzodiazepines

Diazepam, lorazepam, and clonazepam have anticonvulsant properties, but they are not the treatment of choice for epilepsy because of the development of tolerance associated with prolonged use. The benzodiazepines are the first line of treatment for the condition of status epilepticus (see Chapter 24), with either intravenous diazepam or midazolam being the drug of choice.

Anticonvulsant osteomalacia

We have noted that many of the anticonvulsants (especially phenytoin, carbamazepime, and phenobarbitone) are hepatic enzyme inducers, i.e., they enhance the activity of certain enzymes, especially the mixed function oxidases. These hepatic oxidases also increase the catabolism of dietary and endogenously produced vitamin D. Therefore, if there is enhancement of the oxidase enzyme system there will be reduced serum concentrations of 25-hydroxycholecalciferol and, in turn, decreased renal production of the active 1,25-dihydroxycholecalciferol (see Chapter 20). Vitamin D deficiency can therefore occur in patients on anticonvulsant therapy and, if severe, may manifest itself as either rickets or osteomalacia. The problem is more common in the institutionalized elderly patient, who may be on a restricted diet and not often exposed to sunlight. Vitamin D deficiency may also increase the tendency for fits. Patients on anticonvulsant therapy should receive dietary advice and be encouraged to enjoy sunlight.

Trigeminal neuralgia (Tic douloureux)

This condition is characterized by unilateral electric shock-like, brief stabbing pains confined to the distribution of the trigeminal nerve. There is little or no associated sensory loss. The pain is triggered by non-nociceptive stimuli; for example, touch or a current of air.

Treatment of trigeminal neuralgia

Trigeminal neuralgia can be treated either surgically or with drugs.

Surgical treatment

This is a highly specialized area of neurosurgery but, in essence, two main types of operative treatment are in vogue. These are (i) gangliolysis and (ii) suboccipital craniectomy with decompression of the trigeminal nerve (Loeser 1977). Gangliolysis is a destructive procedure and the aim is to produce pain relief with minimal loss of sensation in the region affected by pain. The results indicate that 80 per cent patients will obtain pain relief for one year and in over 50 per cent relief will last for five years.

The alternative procedure, suboccipital craniectomy, is based on the observation that in trigeminal neuralgia the trigeminal nerve is often compressed by a blood vessel or very occasionally by some other local anatomical abnormality. The decompression operation is followed by an 85 per cent long-term success rate (Burchiel *et al.* 1981).

Drug treatment

Two anticonvulsant drugs, carbamazepine and phenytoin (see above), have been shown effective for this condition (Crill 1973). Carbamazepine, a close chemical relative of the tricyclic antidepressant group, controls the lancinating pains in about 70 per cent of patients. It commonly produces unwanted effects including nausea, dizziness, ataxia, somnolence, and slurring of speech; rarely, a fall in the white or red cell count of the blood may occur. The starting dose is 100 mg twice daily; this is increased slowly thereafter until, if necessary, a maximum total daily dose of 1200 mg is reached. It is useful to check the plasma concentration, for which the therapeutic range is 5 to 10 μg/ml (20–40 μmol/l; Tomson et al. 1980). As this drug has a long half-life and also produces auto-induction of drug metabolizing enzymes, it is necessary to wait 14 days after any change in dosage before attempting to measure the plasma concentration if meaningful values are to be obtained. In order to detect any bone marrow changes the haematological picture should be examined at monthly intervals during the first three months of treatment and thereafter at regular three-monthly intervals; the plasma concentration can also be measured. Bone marrow suppression is most likely to occur within the first three months of treatment but whenever it occurs it is an absolute indication for immediate withdrawal of the drug.

Phenytoin is the drug of second choice and is usually less effective than carbamazepine. Unwanted effects occur in about 10 per cent of patients, and include somnolence, dizziness, ataxia, slurring of speech, dermatitis, and gingival hyperplasia (see p. 308). The starting dose is 100 mg three times daily and, as with carbamazepine, the plasma concentration should be checked; the therapeutic range is 10 to 20 μg/ml (40–80 μmol/l) and the $T_{0.5}$ is 12 to 24 hours.

When necessary, other anticonvulsant drugs are occasionally used either alone or in combination with carbamazepine or phenytoin.

Post-herpetic neuralgia

This condition follows a herpes zoster infection (shingles). Pain is a feature of the initial infection but usually only lasts for the duration of the rash. However, some patients experience severe pain for many years after the initial infection, the older age groups being especially susceptible. This continuing severe pain is post-herpetic neuralgia; it frequently has a burning quality and may be spontaneous.

Treatment of post-herpetic neuralgia

This can be (1) physical or (2) pharmacological.

(1) Physical

Transcutaneous electrical nerve stimulation (TENS), which involves the application of electrical shocks at either low (5–10 Hz) or high (100–150 Hz) frequencies, may produce very effective analgesia in some patients. A pair of carbon rubber (or other) electrodes are applied either directly on or adjacent to the painful area, and the strength of shocks adjusted to produce a tingling sensation. The patient is instructed how to use this form of treatment and can then treat him- or herself on a regular basis several times daily. For TENS, patients should be referred to a Pain Relief Clinic where the stimulators are likely to be provided on loan by the National Health Service.

(2) Pharmacological

Selected psychotropic drugs, including anticonvulsants, may be used alone or in combination. A well-tried regime is as follows:

First: start carbamazepine 100 mg 12 hourly orally (e.g. 0800 h and 2000 h) increasing at intervals of several days up to a daily maximum of 1600 mg if required. As detailed earlier, the plasma concentration should be measured to confirm that it lies within the therapeutic range of 5 to 10 mg/l. The concentration should then be checked at three-monthly intervals together with the white cell count.

Second: if carbamazepine at a therapeutic plasma concentration fails to control the pain it should be stopped and replaced by amitriptyline, 25 to 75 mg, at night. This may control the pain on its own or may do so only when combined with sodium valproate, 200 mg twice daily. The plasma concentration of these drugs should be checked every three months; amitriptyline (100–200 μg/ml), sodium valproate (50–100 μg/ml). Adverse effects include: amitriptyline—antimuscarinic, CNS (sedation, paraesthesiae) CVS (tachycardia and other disorders of rate and rhythm), and allergic (skin, cholestatic jaundice, agranulocytosis); sodium valproate (see earlier)—nausea, vomiting, diarrhoea, ataxia, tremor, sedation, thrombocytopenia, temporary hearing loss, hepatotoxicity, false positive test for ketones in urine.

Third: if the combination of amitriptyline with sodium valproate fails to relieve post-herpetic neuralgia then the sodium valproate should be withdrawn and replaced by a neuroleptic such as perphenazine, 4 mg three times a day. Adverse effects include sedation, antimuscarinic effects, extrapyramidal signs and symptoms, hypersensitivity reactions, cholestatic jaundice, endocrine disturbances, and blood dyscrasias.

Migraine

This common condition affects about 5 per cent of the adult population. The characteristic features are periodic headaches (typically unilateral) visual disturbances, and vomiting. Attacks are often preceded by visual disturbances (an aura). During a severe migraine attack, sufferers are usually prostrate and photophobic, which necessitates going to bed in a darkened room.

The aetiology of this condition is still obscure. There is clearly some disturbance in cerebral blood flow. In certain patients, individual food substances rich in tyramine or dopamine may precipitate an attack. Recent attention has focused on the role of 5-HT in migrainous headaches. Prophylaxis against migraine can be achieved with drugs that inhibit the reuptake of 5-HT by platelets. Several types of drugs have been tried; these can be classified as those used in acute attacks and those used for prophylactic purposes.

Treatment of migraine

1. Analgesics

Aspirin is frequently used in the treatment of migraine. However, during a migraine attack, there is gastric stasis and absorption of aspirin is poor. This problem can be overcome by the use of metoclopramide, which will increase the rate of gastric emptying. There is no place for the opioids in the treatment of an acute attack of migraine because of the risk of dependence and their action on gastro-intestinal function (see Chapter 6).

2. Anti-emetics

The nausea and vomiting that often accompany an attack of migraine may respond to an anti-emetic. Metoclopramide is the treatment of choice because of the absence of sedative effects.

3. Ergotamine

Ergotamine is an alkaloid derived from ergot, which is produced by a fungus (*Claviceps purpurea*) that grows on rye and other cereals. It is probably the principal drug used to relieve an acute attack of migraine. Ergotamine blocks both α-adrenergic receptors and 5-HT receptors. It can be given orally, parenterally, rectally, sublingually, or by inhalation. The usual dose regime is 2 mg as soon as the headache starts, followed by 2 mg at half-hourly intervals. The total dose per attack should not exceed 10 mg.

Unwanted effects from ergotamine include peripheral vasoconstriction and paraesthesiae. Gangrene of the fingers has occurred in patients taking this drug. Ergotamine should not be used during pregnancy because it causes contraction of the uterus.

4. Cyproheptadine

This is both a potent H_1 and 5-HT antagonist; it also has tranquillizing properties. Although valuable in the treatment of an acute attack of migraine, its mode of action is uncertain. The usual dosage is 4 mg, followed by a further 4 mg 30 minutes later. Cyproheptadine also has mild anticholinergic properties, and causes dry mouth and blurred vision.

Prophylactic treatment of migraine

Methysergide

This drug is a powerful 5-HT antagonist; it also has anti-inflammatory and vasoconstrictor properties. For the prevention of migraine, methysergide 1 to 2 mg should be taken three times a day with meals. The incidence of unwanted effects is high, and includes gastro-intestinal problems, CNS disturbances, weight gain, oedema, and fibrotic changes in the thorax and abdomen. Retroperitoneal fibrosis limits the use of methysergide and it is mainly used if all else fails.

Other drugs used for the prophylaxis of migraine are pizotifen, which is structurally similar to cyproheptadine; clonidine, an antihypertensive, which at low doses reduces the sensitivity of blood vessels to catecholamines; and propranolol, a β-blocker, which prevents vasodilatation of the cerebral arteries.

REFERENCES

Angelopoulos, A. P. and Goaz, P. W. (1972). Incidence of diphenylhydantoin gingival hyperplasia. *Oral Surgery*, **34**, 898–902.

Baldessarini, R. J. (1985). Drugs and the treatment of psychiatric disorders. In *The pharmacological basis of therapeutics*, (7th edn), (eds. A. G. Gilman, L. S. Goodman, T. W. Rall, and F. Murad). Macmillan Publishing Company, New York, London and Toronto.

Beeley, L. (1986). Drug interactions with lithium. *Prescribers Journal*, **26**, 160–3.

Blackwell, B., Marley, E., Price, J., and Taylor, D. (1967). Hypertensive interactions between monoamine oxidase inhibitors and foodstuffs. *British Journal of Psychiatry*, **113**, 349–65.

Blain, P. G. and Stewart-Wynne, E. (1985). Neurological disorders. In *Textbook of adverse drug reactions*, (3rd edn), (ed. D. M. Davies), Oxford University Press.

Burchiel, K. J., Steege, T. D., Howe, J. F., and Loeser, J. D. (1981). Comparison of percutaneous radiofrequency gangliolysis and microvascular decompression for surgical management of tic doloureux. *Neurosurgery*, **9**, 111–19.

Cade, J. F. J. (1949). Lithium salts in the treatment of psychotic excitement. *Medical Journal of Australia*, **36**, 349–52.

Cawson, R. A. and Spector, R. G. (1985). *Clinical pharmacology in dentistry*, (4th edn). Churchill Livingstone, Edinburgh.

Commission on Classification and Terminology of the International League against Epilepsy. (1981). Proposals for revised clinical and electroencephalographic classification of epileptic disorders. *Epilepsia*, **22**, 489–501.

Crill, W. (1973). Carbamazepine. *Annals of Internal Medicine*, **79**, 79–80.

Drug Newsletter. (1985). Benzodiazepine dependence and withdrawal—an update. *Northern Regional Health Authority Drugs Newsletter*, **31**, 125–6.

Goldman, V. (1966). General anaesthesia for children's dentistry. *British Dental Journal*, **121**, 468–9.

Harvey, S. C. (1985). Hypnotics and sedatives. In *Pharmacological basis of therapeutics*, (7th edn), (eds A. G. Gilman, L. S. Goodman, T. W. Rall, and F. Murad). Macmillan Publishing Company, New York, London, Toronto.

Hassell, T. H., Page, R. G., and Lindhe, J. (1978). Histologic evidence for impaired growth control in diphenylhydantoin gingival hyperplasia. *Archives of Oral Biology*, **23**, 381–4.

Hassell, T. H., White, G. C., Jewson, L. G., and Peele, L. C. (1979). Valproic acid: a new antiepileptic drug with potential side effects of dental concern. *Journal of the American Dental Association*, **99**, 983–7.

Hauser, W. A. (1978). Epidemiology of epilepsy. *Advances in Neurology*, **19**, 313–39.

King, D. A., Hawes, R. R., and Bibby, B. G. (1976). The effect of oral physiotherapy on Dilantin gingival hyperplasia. *Journal of Oral Pathology*, **5**, 1–7.

Loeser, J. D. (1977). The management of tic doloureux. *Pain*, **3**, 155–62.

Rugg-Gunn, A. J. (1979). Lithium treatment and dental caries. *British Dental Journal*, **146**, 136–41.

Seymour, R. A., Smith, D. G., and Turnbull, D. N. (1985). The effects of phenytoin and sodium valproate on the periodontal health of adult epileptic patients. *Journal of Clinical Periodontology*, **12**, 413–19.

Tomson, T., Tybring, G., Bertillson, L., Ekblom, K., and Rane, A. (1980). Carbamazepine in trigeminal neuralgia: clinical effects in relation to plasma concentration. *Uppsala Journal of Medical Sciences*, **31**(suppl.), 45–6.

Waxman, S., Corcino, J. J., and Herbert, V. (1970). Drugs, toxins and dietary amino acids affecting vitamin B_{12} or folic acid absorption or utilization. *American Journal of Medicine*, **48**, 599.

Woodbury, D. M., Penry, J. K., and Pippenger, C. E. (1982). *Anti-epileptic drugs* (2nd edn). Raven Press, New York.

FURTHER READING

Ashton, H. (1984). Benzodiazepine withdrawal: an unfinished story. *British Medical Journal*, **288**, 1135–40.

Catalan, J. and Gath, D. H. (1985). Benzodiazepines in general practice: time for a decision. *British Medical Journal*, **290**, 1374–6.

Farmer, R. and Montgomery, S. A. (1984). Antidepressants and heart disease. *British Medical Journal*, **289**, 559.

Godtlibsen, O. B., Jerko, D., Gordeladze, J. O., Bredsen, J. E., and Matheson, I. (1986). Residual effect of single and repeated doses of midazolam and nitrazepam in relation to their plasma concentration. *European Journal of Clinical Pharmacology*, **29**, 595–600.

Higgitt, A. C., Lader, M. M., and Fonagy, P. (1985). Clinical management of benzodiazepine dependence. *British Medical Journal*, **291**, 688–90.

Leading article (1985). Beta-blockers in situational anxiety. *Lancet*, **ii**, 193.

Lindsey, S. J. E. and Yates, J. A. (1985). The effectiveness of oral diazepam in anxious child dental patients. *British Dental Journal*, **155**, 47–50.

McGimpsey, J. G., Kawar, P., Gamble, J. A. S., Browne, E. S., and Dundee, J. W. (1983). Midazolam in dentistry. *British Dental Journal*, **155**, 47–50.

Morgan, H. G. (1984). Do minor affective disorders need medication. (Leading article). *British Medical Journal*, **289**, 783.

Orme, M. L'E. (1984). Antidepressants and heart disease. (Leading article). *British Medical Journal*, **289**, 1–2.

Power, K. G., Jerrom, D. W. A., Simpson, R. J., and Mitchell, M. (1985). Controlled study of withdrawal symptoms and rebound anxiety after six weeks course of diazepam for generalised anxiety. *British Medical Journal*, **290**, 1246–8.

Singh, A. M., Chemij, M., and Jewell, J. (1986). Treatment of triazolam dependence with a tapering withdrawal regimen. *Canadian Medical Association Journal*, **1–34**, 243–5.

Tyrer, P., Murphy, S., Pates, G., and Kingdon, D. (1985). Psychological treatment for benzodiazepine dependence. *Lancet*, **i**, 1042–3.

15

Drugs used in the treatment of cardiovascular disease

DRUGS ACTING ON THE CARDIOVASCULAR SYSTEM:
1. CARDIAC

Cardiac drugs may act on one or more of the following structures and systems:

1. *Myocardium* Drugs may affect the force or the rate of the heart beat, or both. Changes in the force of contraction are known as inotropic effects (Gk: *inos*, fibre), and changes in rate are known as chronotropic effects (Gk: *chronos*, time). Drugs that increase the force or rate of the heart beat are said to produce a positive inotropic or chronotropic effect whereas those that produce the opposite effect are said to produce a negative inotropic or chronotropic effect, respectively.

2. *Conducting tissue* The rate of conduction through the atrioventricular node (AVN) and the bundle of His may be increased or decreased by certain drugs (either directly or indirectly).

3. *Autonomic control* Activity of the heart may be increased when the output of the sympathetic nervous system is increased; conversely, it may be decreased (inhibited) by activation of the parasympathetic nervous system.

Physiology of the normal heart

Anatomical aspects (see Fig. 15.1)

A normal impulse is transmitted from the sino-atrial node (SAN) to the AVN through atrial muscle. The AVN passes these impulses on over the intraventricular conduction system, which divides into right and left bundle branches. The right bundle runs to the right ventricle, branching only when it reaches the papillary muscles, whilst the left bundle branch divides into three fascicles known as the anterior, posterior, and centroseptal. The terminal branches of the bundle of His reach the myocardium (causing it to contract) via complex Purkinje–myocardial junctions.

Cellular behaviour of cardiac muscle

Fundamental studies, which have elucidated the electrophysiological changes in the heart, have made possible major advances in understanding of cardiac

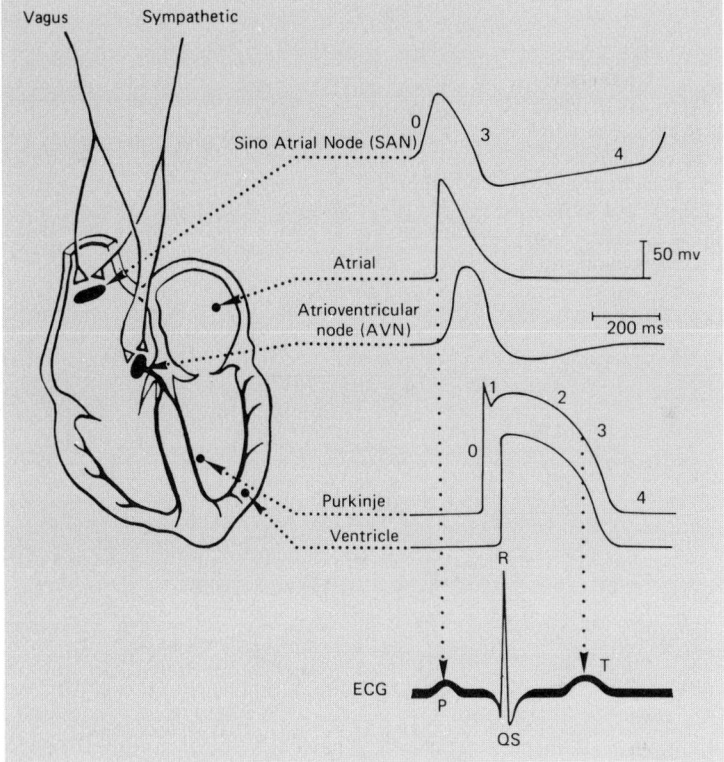

Fig. 15.1. The anatomical layout of the impulse generators and conducting system of the heart, shown in correspondence with an electrocardiogram (ECG).

physiology, both in health and in disease, and also of the effects of cardiac drugs (Noble 1984).

Let us briefly consider the relationship between the action potential (AP), the ionic changes in sodium, potassium and calcium, and the mechanical response of heart muscle (Fig. 15.2).

In cardiac muscle, by contrast with skeletal muscle, the AP lasts as long as the mechanical response, as can be seen by comparing the top and bottom traces in Fig. 15.2. The AP is the result of the movement of sodium, potassium, and calcium ions across the myocardial cell membrane, movements that are dependent upon changes in permeability of cell membrane during the cycle of the AP. Thus, whilst there is an increase in permeability to sodium (second trace), there is a decrease followed by an increase in permeability to potassium ions. There is also an increase in permeability to calcium ions, such that during the plateau of the cardiac AP there is a large influx of calcium ions (slow calcium current). It is for these reasons that the AP in cardiac muscle is so much more prolonged than that in skeletal muscle.

Fig. 15.2. The relationship between electrical and ionic responses of cardiac muscle: from the top downwards the recordings, made from a Purkinje fibre, are of (i) the action potential, (ii) the ionic currents due to sodium (Na$^+$), potassium (K$^+$), and calcium (Ca^{2+}); (after Noble 1979).

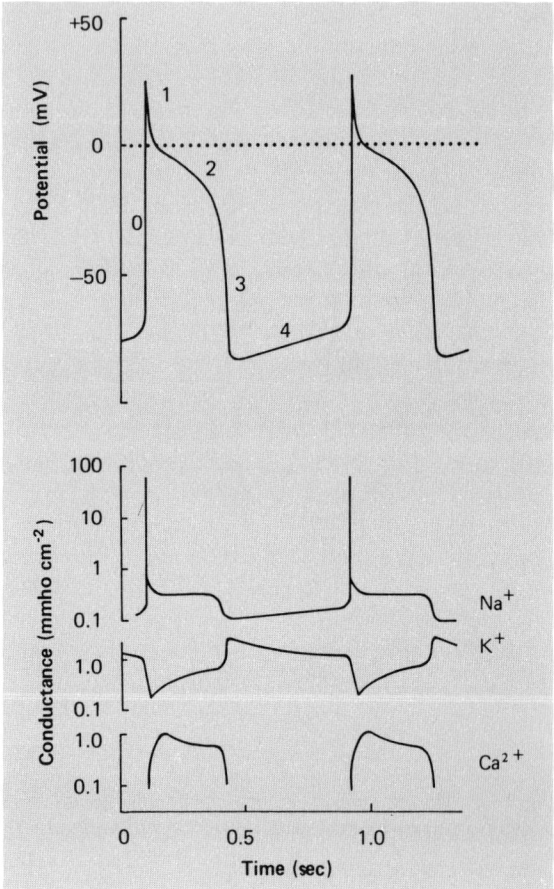

The AP of cardiac muscle, as shown in Fig. 15.2, can be seen to be divided into a number of phases:

Phase 0 is the fast uptake, which represents the rapid depolarization of the membrane potential to a critical threshold of about -60 mV, when the inward current of sodium ions becomes sufficiently large to produce an 'all or nothing' depolarization. It should be noted that the operation of these voltage-dependent sodium channels is transient and, so that they will close again (i.e., become inactivated) within a few milliseconds, the membrane remains depolarized.

Phase 1 consists of partial repolarization, which is a consequence of the inactivation of the sodium current.

Phase 2 consists of a plateau that results from a slow inwards calcium current. The calcium channel, like the sodium channel, is voltage-sensitive but differs from it in that it responds much more slowly. The myocardial contraction is due to the resultant increase in intracellular calcium concentration. It is not quenched by the outward potassium current because the permeability of the muscle cell membrane to potassium is inversely related to the degree of depolarization. Thus, during the plateau of depolarization due to the inward calcium current, the outward potassium current is very small and therefore does not cause any sudden reversal of the membrane depolarization.

Phase 3   is the phase of repolarization and takes place as the calcium current is inactivated. During this phase, potassium permeability rapidly increases with the increase in membrane potential and this accounts for the rapid repolarization (see above under phase 2).

Phase 4   is the so-called pacemaker potential, and differs in various parts of the heart. In nodal and conducting tissues there is a slow depolarization due to an increase in sodium permeability. Furthermore it is most rapid in nodal tissues, and least in the conducting tissues.

In pacemaker cells, such as the SAN and the AVN, the resting potential of the cell is unstable (see Fig. 15.1, phase 4 of recording from SAN), and this accounts for their inherent rhythmicity; as the resting potential rises to the threshold value it fires off another AP, the whole cycle is repeated, and so on indefinitely. In fact, all cardiac cells have some degree of inherent rhythmicity, which is greatest in cells of the SAN and decreases in the order, AVN, His–Purkinje bundle, atrial and ventricular muscle. The result is that if a proximal pacemaker ceases to function or if its impulse is blocked, the next fastest area will take command, usually proximally or distally, in the atrioventricular (AV) junction, or in the bundle of His, or, with more distal disease, in the His-Purkinje system, each with inherently and progressively slower rates.

Autonomic control of the heart

Parasympathetic supply

Parasympathetic cholinergic fibres reach the heart through the vagus to innervate the atrial and nodal tissue. The ventricles are therefore not directly affected by the vagus.

Acetylcholine released at the postganglionic cholinergic nerve endings increases the permeability of the myocardial cell membrane to potassium ions. At the SAN this results in a more negative membrane potential and, therefore, a correspondingly slower rate of rise of the pacemaker potential during diastole, which results in a reduction in heart rate. (NB. The increased potassium permeability allows an increased leak of potassium ions down their concentration gradient out of the cell, which offsets the inward leakage of sodium ions. Excessive vagal activity will stop spontaneous depolarization completely and so stabilize the membrane potential by causing the potassium loss to exceed that of the sodium entry, with the result that the heart stops beating.)

On atrial cells the effect of parasympathetic stimulation is to reduce the duration of the AP by accelerating repolarization. This reduced duration causes a less effective activation of the contractile mechanism of the myocardial cell, which results in a weaker atrial contraction. In addition, there is also a reduction in size of the potentials within the AVN, and the resting membrane potential of the nodal cells may be stabilized. As a consequence, the AV delay is increased and eventually this results in conduction block. It seems likely that all these effects are due to increased potassium permeability of the membrane produced by acetylcholine.

Stimulation of vagal fibres may be produced by such manoeuvres as (i) carotid sinus massage, (ii) eyeball pressure (which can also detach the retina!), (iii) vomiting, and (iv) the Valsalva manoeuvre (forced expiration against a closed glottis and pinched nose). These measures can restore normal sinus rhythm during attacks of paroxysmal supraventricular tachycardia. In the presence of sinus tachycardia these procedures cause a smooth slowing of the pulse but, in atrial flutter (in which the atria contract at approximately 300 per minute and the ventricles follow with a variable degree of AV block), there is a sudden reduction in the ventricular rate as the degree of AV block increases.

Sympathetic nerve supply

Sympathetic nerve fibres running in the cardiac nerves innervate all parts of the heart. Adrenergic stimulation increases the rate of beating of the pacemaker (chronotropic effect) and increases the force of contraction (inotropic effect). There is also an increased conduction rate and ventricular arrhythmia, which may be due to interference with the pattern of repolarization. Adrenaline also increases the force of contraction of the heart and this is associated with an increased concentration of unbound intracellular calcium.

Disorders of cardiac rhythm and anti-arrhythmic drugs

Any such disorder is termed an arrhythmia or a dysrhythmia. An arrhythmia can arise from (i) an abnormality of impulse generation; (ii) an abnormality of conduction; or (iii) a combination of (i) and (ii).

Abnormal impulse generation is caused by an additional pacemaker known as an ectopic focus. Thus, the normal pacemaker for the heart is the SAN, whereas an ectopic focus may arise as a result of a damaged area of muscle or due to the actions of drugs; for example, digoxin or catecholamines. A particular feature of an ectopic focus is an increased liability to depolarize during diastole so giving rise to enhanced automaticity.

Conduction abnormalities occur when some part of the conducting pathway is damaged, resulting in the formation of a unidirectional block. When this occurs in one branch of the bundle, the passage of impulses within it are blocked whereas those in the other branch progress normally; these may then travel via the ventricular muscle to excite that part of the damaged bundle distal to the block and so lead to retrograde impulse conduction. As a consequence, a re-entry or 'circus' mechanism is set up, which is self-perpetuating and so induces arrhythmias.

A large number of drugs can now be used as anti-arrhythmic agents and, whilst a particular drug may be very effective in a particular patient, we do not necessarily know which of the several actions possessed by that drug may be responsible for the beneficial effect. Nevertheless, as Krikler (1974) has pointed out, the target is to control the abnormal process or, in other words: (i) to diminish enhanced automaticity; or (ii) to interrupt a re-entry mechanism.

Enhanced automaticity may be diminished by:

(1) slowing the rate of rise of spontaneous diastolic (phase 4) depolarization

(2) increasing the threshold potential;

(3) lengthening the refractory period, especially in relation to the duration of AP;

(4) lowering the maximum repolarization potential at the end of phase 3.

Re-entry may be broken by prolonging the circuit-time until conduction is too slow to support it (it is only rarely possible to do this in the opposite way by speeding it up).

Classification of anti-arrhythmic agents

As a result of extensive electrophysiological studies carried out by a number of workers—see especially Vaughan Williams (1983), and also Weidmann (1955)—it is now possible to classify anti-arrhythmic agents. Vaughan Williams (1983) classification divides these drugs into four classes (I–IV) as follows:

Class I.　　This class is sub-divided into three sub-zones:
　　　　　　Ia: quinidine, procainamide, disopyramide.
　　　　　　　　These drugs inhibit pacemaker depolarization.
　　　　　　Ib: lignocaine, mexiletine, tocainide.
　　　　　　　　These drugs do not inhibit pacemaker depolarization but inhibit the inward sodium currents that are associated with the ectopic beats characteristic of ventricular arrhythmias.
　　　　　　Ic: flecainide, encainide (USA), proppafenone (Germany)
Main use: ventricular arrhythmias.

Class II.　　Antisympathetic, e.g. β-blockers, bretylium.
　　　　　　These drugs act on sinus nodal tissues.
Main use: supraventricular and ventricular arrhythmias.

Class III.　　Prolongation of AP, e.g. amiodarone, bretylium.
　　　　　　This group act on all cardiac tissues.
Main use: supraventricular and ventricular arrhythmias.

Class IV.　　Calcium entry blockers (also known as calcium antagonists), e.g. verapamil, diltiazem.
　　　　　　These drugs act on AV nodal conducting tissues.
Main use: supraventricular arrhythmias.

Class I drugs with a direct membrane action

Quinidine and procainamide

Class I drugs produce a slowing in the rate of rise of AP although they may produce other effects as well. One of the oldest anti-arrhythmic drugs is quinidine, which is the D-isomer of quinine, and is the prototype of Class I drugs. It causes decreased excitability, prolonged refractoriness, and decreased conduction velocity. All of these properties might be expected to suppress ectopic foci or 'circus' movements in the heart. The primary effect of quinidine is to slow the rate of rise of depolarization (phase 4); this results in a delay in the firing of an excitable ectopic focus and thus may abolish any arrhythmia due to it.

Procainamide has similar properties to quinidine; both have anticholinergic effects that antagonize vagal activity, thereby reducing their effects with consequent increased conduction and decreased atrial refractory period. Procainamide and quinidine also block conduction; they may therefore, cause conduction disturbances.

Pharmacodynamics

(a) Direct effects

These comprise reduced conduction velocity, prolonged refractory period (atrium greater than ventricle), and reduced excitability.

(b) Electrocardiograph (ECG) changes

Widening of QRS with prolonged PR and QT intervals.

Pharmacokinetics

After absorption, which is complete, distribution of procainamide is extensive with 15 per cent of the drug bound to plasma proteins. The drug is eliminated partly by metabolism (acetylation 30 to 60 per cent) and partly excreted by the kidney (30 to 60 per cent). The N-acetyl metabolite is as active pharmacologically as the parent compound. The half-life is two hours, and frequent four- to six-hourly doses are necessary to maintain adequate plasma concentrations. Slow release preparations may be given eight- to twelve-hourly.

Unwanted effects

Manifestations

Heart block (AV block)

Anorexia, nausea, vomiting, diarrhoea

Hallucinations

Agranulocytosis

Systemic lupus erythematosus-like syndromes with rash, fever, arthralgia, myalgia, pneumonitis, and a positive antinuclear factor (ANF).

Lignocaine

This well-known and versatile local anaesthetic is also a useful anti-arrhythmic agent belonging to Class I. It differs from quinidine and procainamide in that it does not have anticholinergic properties and neither does it affect (or possibly may even increase) conduction velocity. It has been tentatively suggested that the relative lack of toxicity of lignocaine is because, *in the doses used for anti-arrhythmic purposes* (and unlike quinidine and procainamide), it does not block conduction and is therefore less likely to produce conduction disturbances in therapeutic dosage.

Pharmacodynamics

Lignocaine reduces automaticity, modifies and may prevent re-entrant arrhythmias, and produces a slight negative inotropic effect.

Pharmacokinetics

Absorption is complete but the drug undergoes extensive first pass metabolism, which makes oral administration ineffective. After IV or IM administration, the drug is rapidly redistributed to muscle and fat.

Lignocaine is completely metabolized (oxidized) by the liver, where there is a high hepatic clearance of approximately 800 ml per minutes, which means that its elimination is dependent upon the liver blood flow. Impaired elimination is therefore seen in patients with cardiac failure or liver disease.

These pharmacokinetic properties mean that lignocaine must be administered by continuous IV infusion for its effect to be maintained and regulated. Therapeutic effects are observed at plasma concentrations of 2 to 4 μg/ml.

Unwanted effects

These are manifested by paraesthesia around the mouth, and convulsions may occur. Treatment is to stop the infusion and give midazolam for the fits if necessary.

Disopyramide

This is a much more recently introduced drug.

Pharmacodynamics

Conduction is slowed so influencing automatic and re-entrant arrhythmias. As a consequence of its mode of action the QRS interval on ECG is prolonged. It is particularly important for the treatment of a rare form of re-entry arrhythmia that occurs in the Wolff–Parkinson–White syndrome. In this condition, an anatomically abnormal bundle of cardiac muscle fibres joins the atria to the ventricles, thus bypassing the AVN. As a consequence, after normal excitation through the AVN–Purkinje pathway, impulses may pass retrogradely through the abnormal bundle back to the atria and thereby set up a 'circus' excitation.

Pharmacokinetics

Disopyramide is completely absorbed and converted to inactive metabolites. The therapeutic $T_{0.5}$ is 4 to 8 hours, with a therapeutic window in the range 3–6 mg/ml.

Unwanted effects

The drug may induce a metallic taste in the mouth; it may aggravate heart failure and is sometimes associated with arrhythmogenicity.

Class II drugs with antisympathetic effects

This group might be expected to protect against arrhythmias associated with increased sympathetic activity. Thus, the well-known sensitization of the heart to catecholamines, which can occur during anaesthesia with halogenated hydro-carbons (see Chapter 8), can be protected by agents with anti-sympathetic effects. However, this group will also protect against other types of arrhythmias, especially those induced by cardiac glycosides or by ischaemia. The main group of drugs with Class II properties are the β-adrenoceptor blocking agents (β-blockers) and these are dealt with elsewhere (see Chapter 13).

Class III drugs that prolong the duration of the AP

These agents, amiodarone and bretylium, are important because they are active against ventricular arrhythmias.

Amiodarone

This is a remarkable drug because it:

(1) prolongs the duration of the AP;

(2) increases the refractory period;

(3) is active against a variety of arrhythmias, including ventricular fibrillation;

(4) is safe in the presence of severe congestive heart failure;

(5) has a cumulative effect due to an exceptionally long half-life ($T_{0.5} = 4$ weeks).

Pharmacodynamics
(a) Direct effects

Amiodarone prolongs the duration of the AP by slow repolarization (phase 3). It has no effect on phases 4 or 0 and neither does it alter the threshold potential. Thus, it prolongs the refractory period in the SA node, atria, AVN, and conducting system. These effects are similar to those that occur in hypothyroidism.

(b) ECG changes

The QT interval is prolonged.

Pharmacokinetics

This drug has an exceptionally long half-life so that the $T_{0.5}$ is of the order of 4 weeks or longer; its effects thus continue for several weeks after it has been withdrawn. As would be anticipated of a drug with a long $T_{0.5}$, the therapeutic action takes several days to develop.

Unwanted effects

Amiodarone can cause a number of potentially serious unwanted effects. These include photosensitization (ranging from an increased tendency to sunburn to severe erythema); corneal microdeposits of lipofucsin, which are reversible on stopping the drug; interference with thyroid function (probably due to chemical similarity to thyroxine), decreasing the peripheral conversion of thyroxine (T4) to tri-iodothyronine (T3); and, in about 5 per cent of patients, actual hypothyroidism or hyperthyroidism. Other conditions attributed to this drug include a reversible peripheral neuropathy, pneumonitis, and also headache, nausea, vomiting, bradycardia, constipation, nightmares, and tremor.

Drug interactions produced by amiodarone include the potentiation of warfarin, and increase in the plasma concentration of digoxin with enhanced risk of toxicity.

Bretylium

This is an adrenergic neurone blocker, originally used for the treatment of hypertension (see later). After such use was abandoned (because it is poorly absorbed), it made a come back as an anti-arrhythmic drug because it was found to be effective for the treatment of ventricular fibrillation, including that refractory to lignocaine and multiple direct-current (DC) shocks. It is also used to treat other ventricular arrhythmias resistant to lignocaine or procainamide. However, it should be noted that the use of bretylium is steadily declining.

Pharmacodynamics

Bretylium accumulates in adrenergic nerve endings and depresses noradrenaline release thus accounting for its adrenergic neurone-blocking action (although initially it may cause a *release* of catecholamines). However, its anti-arrhythmic action is probably independent of this blocking property and may be due to lengthening of the ventricular (but not the atrial) AP. Although it acts slowly against some ventricular arrhythmias, fortunately it acts quickly against ventricular fibrillation. Experimentally it has been shown to raise the threshold to electrically-induced ventricular fibrillation. However, the initial release of catecholamine may *induce* ventricular arrhythmias, which therefore calls for careful ECG monitoring of therapy.

Pharmacokinetics

Bretylium contains a quaternary nitrogen atom ($-N^+R_4$), thus accounting for its poor absorption, lack of hepatic metabolism, and renal excretion with a $T_{0.5}$ of seven to eight hours.

Unwanted effects
Initial transient hypertension and increased arrhythmias may occur; also hypotension with continued treatment.

Class IV drugs

These are the calcium entry blockers (calcium antagonists; calcium channel blockers).

Calcium is a universal second (or intermediate) messenger responsible for regulating all forms of cellular activity (Berridge 1981; 1985). Intracellular calcium can be increased by one of two mechanisms: (i) extracellular calcium may enter the cell through specific calcium channels; or (ii) calcium may be released from intracellular stores, such as the sarcoplasmic reticulum of cardiac or skeletal muscle, or the endoplasmic reticulum of non-muscle cells. In cardiac muscle, membrane depolarization leads to opening of voltage-dependent calcium channels in the plasma membrane; it is these channels that can be blocked by calcium entry blockers such as nifedipine and verapamil.

Verapamil

This was originally used for the treatment of angina pectoris because of its vasodilator properties (see p. 332). However it has been found to be more useful for the treatment of supraventricular arrhythmias.

Pharmacodynamics
Verapamil blocks the transport of calcium across the cell membrane of cardiac and vascular smooth muscle, thus prolonging phase 2 of the AP (see Fig. 15.2 above) and increasing the effective refractory period. This effect is especially marked in the SAN and AVN so that conduction is slowed, thereby producing a negative inotropic effect. As verapamil also acts on vascular smooth muscle it produces peripheral vasodilatation. The combined effects on cardiac and smooth muscle result in reduced myocardial work and thus reduced myocardial oxygen demand.

Pharmacokinetics
After oral administration, verapamil is well-absorbed and undergoes extensive first pass metabolism. It takes two hours to act, with a peak action at about five hours. It is not clear whether hepatic metabolites are active, but excretion is mainly by the kidneys.

Unwanted effects
The negative inotropic and vasodilatory actions may produce hypotension and also worsen cardiac failure. Verapamil may interact with a β-blocker because both drugs possess negative inotropic and hypotensive actions. This interaction is particularly liable to occur when verapamil is administered intravenously to a patient already taking β-blockers, so this combination is not recommended.

Diltiazem

This recently introduced drug has both anti-arrhythmic and vasodilator effects.

Pharmacokinetics
It has a relative lack of first pass metabolism, which may well suit it better for long-term use than a drug like verapamil.

Cardiac glycosides (digitalis)

Digitalis was introduced into clinical medicine by William Withering over 200 years ago and is remarkable in that it remains the only drug that can be administered to patients over a long time in order to improve myocardial contractility. In addition, it has the important property of being able to control the ventricular rate in arrhythmias arising in the atria.

Pharmacodynamics

Various species of digitalis plant (e.g. foxglove) contain three cardiac glycosides of medicinal importance—digoxin, digitoxin, and ouabain. In the UK, digoxin is used most commonly whereas, in North America, digitoxin is more popular. Chemically, they all consist of an aglycone (or genin) ring structure, which determines their pharmacological activity, coupled to one to four molecules of a sugar, which influence their water solubility and hence determine their pharmacokinetic properties, including penetration into cells.

In essence, cardiac glycosides produce four main effects:

(i) increased force of myocardial contraction;
(ii) slowed conduction velocity in the AVN with subsequent increase in AV conduction time (thus lengthening the PR interval on the ECG);
(iii) decreased refractory period of the myocardium;
(iv) increased automaticity.

Improved contraction of the myocardium by digitalis leads to reflex vagal stimulation resulting in sinus bradycardia. The ECG reflects these effects so that the increase in AV conduction time produces a lengthening of the PR interval. Other ECG effects are depression of the ST segment followed by the development of a biphasic T wave. Ultimately, the T wave may become inverted whilst the QT interval is shortened by the shortened duration of ventricular systole.

The mechanism of action of cardiac glycosides is to inhibit the enzyme known as sodium–potassium ATPase, which resides in the sarcolemma of cardiac muscle. Sodium-potassium ATPase is responsible for the sodium pump; when this enzyme action is depressed the outcome is an accumulation of intracellular sodium ions, which in turn results in an increase in the concentration of free intracellular calcium ions. This increase leads to improved excitation–contraction coupling of the myocardial cells and thereby increased force of myocardial contraction.

Pharmacokinetics

These are different for digoxin and digitoxin. Digoxin is incompletely absorbed; bioavailability varies between about 65 per cent for tablets and 80 per cent for the elixir. Only about 25 per cent of digoxin is bound to plasma proteins and so the drug becomes widely distributed throughout the body. The concentration in cardiac tissue may reach 30 times that of the plasma concentration. Digoxin is primarily eliminated by the kidney unchanged, with a $T_{0.5}$ of about 40 hours. As a consequence, in renal failure and also in the elderly, renal excretion is slowed and this must be taken into account when calculating the appropriate dose. The therapeutic plasma concentration is in the range 0.8–1.6 μg/l and concentrations above 2.5 μg/l are usually associated with unwanted effects (see later). However, the correlation between plasma concentration and effect is variable.

Digitoxin is by contrast almost completely absorbed after oral administration and highly bound (90 per cent) to plasma proteins. Approximately 70 per cent of the drug is metabolized in the liver, where it undergoes extensive enterohepatic recirculation, with the result that it has a very long $T_{0.5}$ of about seven days.

Uses

Cardiac glycosides have two main uses:

1. The treatment of supraventricular arrhythmias, in which the aim is to slow the heart rate by virtue of the action of digitalis on the conduction system. In atrial fibrillation, digitalis slows the ventricular rate and very occasionally this is followed by restoration of normal rhythm.

2. The treatment of cardiac failure secondary to ischaemic and hypertensive heart disease and also that secondary to valvular disease.

It should be noted that these indications apply with or without the presence of an arrhythmia. By contrast, digitalis is of very limited value in the treatment of heart failure secondary to chronic pulmonary disease.

Unwanted effects

The therapeutic index (safety margin) of cardiac glycosides is very small, as intimated already when discussing the relationship between plasma concentration and therapeutic effect (see p. 28). The commonest signs of overdosage include anorexia, nausea, vomiting, and diarrhoea, and when these symptoms occur in any patient taking cardiac glycosides the possibility of overdose must be considered. Neurological and psychiatric symptoms may also arise; these include headache, confusion, depression, and insomnia. Rarely, visual disturbances including photophobia and disturbances of colour vision occur. Along with these unwanted non-cardiac effects there may be various cardiac ones, especially ventricular ectopic beats. With these there may be coupling so that an ectopic beat immediately follows on a normal contraction. In addition, varying degrees of heart block can occur due to the effect of digitalis on the conducting system. Elderly patients and those with electrolyte disturbances, particularly hypokalaemia, hypercalcaemia, or hypomagnesaemia, are more susceptible to these induced arrhythmias, as are patients already suffering from hypothyroidism. Any simultaneously administered drug that interferes with the renal clearance of digoxin also increases the risk of these unwanted effects. By contrast, those suffering from hyperthyroidism are more resistant to the actions of cardiac glycosides. When it is possible that there are unwanted effects due to cardiac glycosides, measurement of the plasma concentration may well prove helpful in providing diagnostic information, as well as in following the progress of treatment.

DRUGS ACTING ON THE CARDIOVASCULAR SYSTEM:
2. VASODILATORS

Any drug that causes relaxation of smooth muscle in the wall of a blood vessel, thereby increasing its cross-sectional area (and hence decreasing its peripheral resistance), may be called a vasodilator. In the past, the therapeutic approach to heart failure has been to try to 'flog a tired horse' or, in other words, to use drugs to increase the cardiac output. Recently the more logical approach of using vasodilators to reduce the load has gained ground, and this has been applied particularly to the treatment of hypertension and congestive cardiac failure.

Several groups of drugs acting in different ways can produce vasodilatation; these may act predominantly on the arterial (resistance) vessels or on the venous (capacitance) vessels, or on both. Arterial vasodilators, for example hydralazine, primarily lower diastolic blood pressure and are used for the treatment of hypertension. On the other hand, venous vasodilators, for example nitrites, lower systolic pressure but have only a small effect on diastolic pressure and are used therefore to treat congestive cardiac failure.

From Table 15.1 it can be seen that there are at least six mechanisms whereby a drug can produce vasodilatation. Thus it may act directly, via α- or β-adrenoceptors, by blocking the entry of calcium ions, by interference with angiotensin, or by way of diuretic therapy. Some of the groups of vasodilators listed in Table 15.1 are dealt with in this Chapter whilst others are discussed elsewhere in this book as follows:

	Chapter	Page
Direct vasodilators	This	332
α-adrenoceptor antagonists	13	275
β-adrenoceptor·agonists	13	270
Calcium entry blockers (calcium antagonists)	This	328
Angiotensin inhibitors	This	335
Diuretics	This	337

Table 15.1. The various groups of vasodilator drugs $\qquad$ (angina)

Group	Drug	Type of vasodilatation		Uses	
		Arterial	Venous	Hypertension	Refractory cardiac failure
1. Direct vasodilator	hydrallazine	++	−	√	√
	nitrites	+	++	0	√
	diazoxide	++	−	√(acute)	(√)
	minoxidil	++	−	√	(√)
	nitroprusside	++	++	√(acute)	
2. α-adrenoceptor antagonists					
(i) α₁ vascular receptors	prazosin	++	++	√	√
	indoramin			√	0
	labetalol (also β)			√	0
(ii) α₂ (presynaptic) receptors	phentolamine	++	−	(√)	√
	phenoxybenzamine	++	−	(√)	0
3. β-adrenoceptor agonists	isoprenaline dopamine dobutamine salbutamol	++	++	0	√
4. calcium antagonists	nifedipine	++	+	√	√
	verapamil			(√)	
	diltiazem			?	?
5. angiotensin II inhibitors					
(i) inhibit angiotensin converting enzyme	captopril teprotide			√	√
(ii) inhibit angiotensin effect on vessel wall	saralasin			√	√
6. diuretics	frusemide			√	√

Key: + mild effect, + + strong effect, 0 not used, √ used, − insignificant effect (√) used infrequently, ? may be useful

Direct vasodilators are agents that act through some direct mechanism that varies according to the substance involved. These are exemplified by hydralazine and the nitrates/nitrites.

Hydralazine

This was first introduced many years ago and then abandoned because it induced a reflex tachycardia and rapid tolerance. In some it leads to a condition resembling systemic lupus erythematosus (SLE), now known to occur in those who metabolize (acetylate) the drug slowly. However, it has been introduced successfully in combination with β-blockers, which reduce the reflex tachycardia, so that a maximum daily dose of 200 mg becomes not only an effective hypotensive dose but one at which the likelihood of SLE is greatly reduced. The vascular effects outlast the $T_{0.5}$ of two to four hours, probably due to binding of the drug to vascular tissue.

The commonest adverse effects of hydralazine are nausea, anorexia, headache, palpitations, flushing, sweating, and rarely, peripheral neuropathy and drug fever. As mentioned above, SLE is likely to occur in 10 to 20 per cent of those patients who acetylate the drug slowly but is reversible on withdrawal.

Nitrates and nitrites

It has long been known that inorganic nitrate is pharmacologically inactive whereas organic nitrates, and both inorganic and organic nitrites, are effective direct-acting relaxants of smooth muscle. Thus the vascular smooth muscle of both arteries and veins is relaxed by these agents; the mode of action is direct and does not involve the usual receptor mechanisms, such as those of acetylcholine, histamine, noradrenaline, or 5-HT. The mechanism of action is not yet fully elucidated but two possibilities have been considered. The first is that the compounds are converted into nitric oxide (NO), which interacts with a specific receptor containing a sulphydryl group. The second is that the compounds act by virtue of the nitrite ion, the nitrites acting directly and the nitrates after conversion to nitrites in the tissues.

Organic nitrates, and inorganic and organic nitrites, are predominantly venodilators resulting in venous pooling with consequent reduction in both venous return, and left ventricular and diastolic pressure. The reduction in ventricular-wall tension and consequent reduced oxygen demand lead to the relief of angina.

Nitrates/nitrites are conveniently divided into short- and long-acting.

Short-acting

Amyl nitrite

This volatile liquid is administered from crushable glass ampoules (vitrellae) each containing 0.1 to 0.3 ml. On inhalation, rapid arteriolar dilatation is produced and this leads to a compensatory tachycardia and venoconstriction. This reduces left ventricular afterload. However, amyl nitrite is rarely used now because it is inconvenient and unpleasant, produces a short-lived effect, and is also expensive. Today its main use is for the management of cyanide poisoning.

Glyceryl trinitrate (nitroglycerine, TNT).

This is inactive when swallowed because it undergoes almost complete first pass metabolism. A tablet is therefore placed under the tongue when required. It is rapidly metabolized in the liver to inorganic nitrate; it acts within 2 minutes and lasts up to about 30 minutes.

Patients need to be warned that these tablets may cause headache or a fall of blood pressure and should therefore be taken whilst sitting down.

Unwanted effects are flushing, palpitations, dizziness, headaches, and collapse. Tolerance to the headache may develop but is apparently not associated with loss of circulatory effect.

Long-acting

Several longer-acting preparations of nitrates are available; these include pentaerythritol tetranitrate, isosorbide dinitrate, and also slow-release formulations of glyceryl trinitrate, including Nitrocontin Continus, Suscard, Sustac, and Transiderm-Nitro. The last named is a self-adhesive skin dressing that contains glyceryl trinitrate. The response to these long-acting preparations varies and must be determined by trial and error. Their unwanted effects are similar to those of glyceryl trinitrate.

Diazoxide

This is related chemically to the thiazide diuretics but differs radically from them in that it has sodium-retaining properties, and also hypotensive and hyperglycaemic effects.

Pharmacodynamics

Diazoxide is a direct arterial vasodilator and does not affect venous (capacitance) vessels; neither does it affect cardiovascular reflexes. It is normally employed to treat acute hypertensive emergencies, when it is given intravenously, producing a marked fall in blood pressure, followed by a reflex tachycardia and increased cardiac output. The fall of blood pressure also induces a reflex sympathetic discharge of catecholamines.

In patients with cardiac failure the sodium retention caused by diazoxide may obviously worsen their condition and so a loop diuretic, for example, frusemide, should be given along with the diazoxide. The hyperglycaemic effect is due to (i) a direct inhibitory effect on the release of insulin from the β-cells in the pancreas, and (ii) the release of adrenaline (see above) resulting in an increase in the release of glucose.

Pharmacokinetics

Diazoxide is highly protein-bound (about 90 per cent) and eventually undergoes mainly renal excretion with a long $T_{0.5}$ of about 25 hours.

Uses

Diazoxide is used almost exclusively for the emergency reduction of acute hypertension (intravenous injection). Naturally, once the hypertension has been brought under control it is essential to institute effective oral medication with other appropriate hypotensive drugs (see treatment of hypertension, pp. 352–3).

Unwanted effects

The undesirable effects of sodium retention have been mentioned earlier. The hyperglycaemic effect may produce problems where the ability to excrete excess glucose is impaired, such as in renal failure. Although diazoxide has different pharmacological actions from other thiazides, its close chemical similarity is responsible for hypersensitivity reactions similar to those caused by other thiazides. Furthermore, if a patient is known to be hypersensitive to thiazide diuretics there is likely to be a cross-reaction with diazoxide, which is therefore contra-indicated. As diazoxide is highly bound to plasma proteins it can displace other highly bound drugs from these sites, such as oral anticoagulants, the dose of which may therefore need to be adjusted appropriately.

Nifedipine

Pharmacodynamics

This is a calcium entry blocker and relaxes vascular smooth muscle, resulting in peripheral vasodilatation. It also dilates coronary arteries. However, unlike verapamil (see Section on anti-arrhythmic drugs, p. 322), it does not affect the conducting system in man (Rowland *et al.* 1979) although it does in animals (Endo *et al.* 1978). Thus it is used to treat coronary artery spasm but not supraventricular arrhythmias.

Pharmacokinetics

It is well-absorbed after oral administration (and also sublingually); it undergoes extensive metabolism and has a $T_{0.5}$ of about 5 hours.

Unwanted effects

Headache and flushing, due to vasodilatation, are the main complaints. It has been reported to increase the plasma concentration of digoxin (by some unknown mechanism), and this interaction must therefore be anticipated if these two drugs are used concomitantly. It is of significance to the dental surgeon that patients on nifedipine may experience gingival hyperplasia (Jones 1986).

Angiotensin and its inhibitors

Several polypeptides produce powerful effects on vascular and other smooth muscles and thereby play important roles in the control of local or general blood flow and blood pressure. Thus, vasoconstrictors include angiotensin II and vasopressin, whilst vasodilators include bradykinin, vasoactive intestinal peptide (VIP), substance P, and neurotensin.

Formation of angiotensin

The active form is known as angiotensin II and is formed from the precursor angiotensin I, which is itself formed by the action of the enzyme renin on angiotensinogen, a circulatory protein substance (see Fig. 15.3). Renin is synthesized and stored in the juxtaglomerular apparatus of the kidney and its

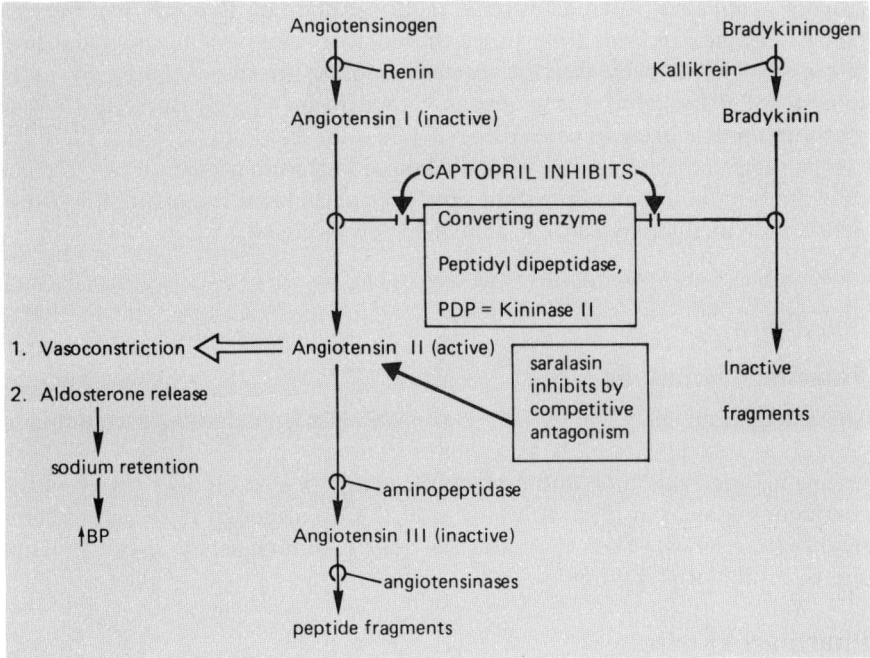

Fig. 15.3. The formation and activation of angiotensin.

release appears to depend upon a number of factors, particularly a vascular stretch receptor in the afferent arteriole of the glomerulus. When this receptor is stretched it leads to a decrease in renin release and vice versa. The sympathetic nervous system also stimulates renin secretion via the release of noradrenaline, which acts on β-adrenoceptors ($?\beta_1$ or β_2).

Relationship to kinins

As the converting enzyme, peptidyl dipeptidase (PDP), is identical with kininase II, which inactivates bradykinin, it is clear that any factors affecting the enzyme will simultaneously affect the production of angiotensin II and the destruction of bradykinin (see Fig. 15.3).

Angiotensin-converting enzyme inhibitors (ACE inhibitors)

Pharmacodynamics

Captopril, a typical ACE inhibitor, is a competitive inhibitor of PDP, so leading to a decrease in the production of angiotensin II (and secondarily, of aldosterone), and also to an accumulation of bradykinin, a vasodilator. These effects are responsible for the therapeutic actions of captopril.

Pharmacokinetics

Captopril is well-absorbed on oral administration but seriously affected by the presence of food, which reduces absorption to 50 per cent. About half of the dose is metabolized in the liver to inactive metabolites, and the $T_{0.5}$ is about two hours.

Therapeutic uses

Until recently, captopril was reserved for the treatment of severe hypertension and severe congestive cardiac failure that had failed to respond to other antihypertensive therapy. However, there is now a move to use captopril for the treatment of patients with lesser degrees of hypertension. Newer ACE inhibitors, such as enalapril, with a smoother action are also now available and others are likely to follow.

Unwanted effects

Captopril is a potentially toxic drug. Rashes are common (10 per cent), and may be associated with pyrexia and eosinophilia. Loss of taste, usually transient, occurs in five per cent of patients. Occasionally, there may be proteinuria and haematuria, as also neutropenia, which may progress to agranulocytosis.

DIURETICS

A diuretic is, strictly speaking, any agent that produces an increased output of urine. This can be useful when it is necessary to (i) flush out poisons from the body, (ii) to dilute drug metabolites that might injure the kidney during excretion e.g. cyclophosphamide, or (iii) to prevent the crystallization of substances of low solubility in urine; for example, certain sulphonamides, or uric acid during the treatment of gout.

However, the most important and common use of a diuretic is in order to increase the excretion of sodium, usually with chloride, together with water. A drug with this property is strictly speaking a saluretic but this term is not used as much as it ought to be and, instead, drugs that are saluretics are simply referred to as diuretics, imprecise as this may be.

Normal renal physiology

In order to understand how diuretics (saluretics) work and how they can be used selectively in the treatment of disease, a brief review of normal renal function will be presented first (see Fig. 15.4).

Urine secretion is a two-stage process involving glomerular filtration followed by tubular reabsorption and/or tubular secretion. Thus:

urinary excretion =
    glomerular filtration − amount reabsorbed in tubules + tubular secretion.

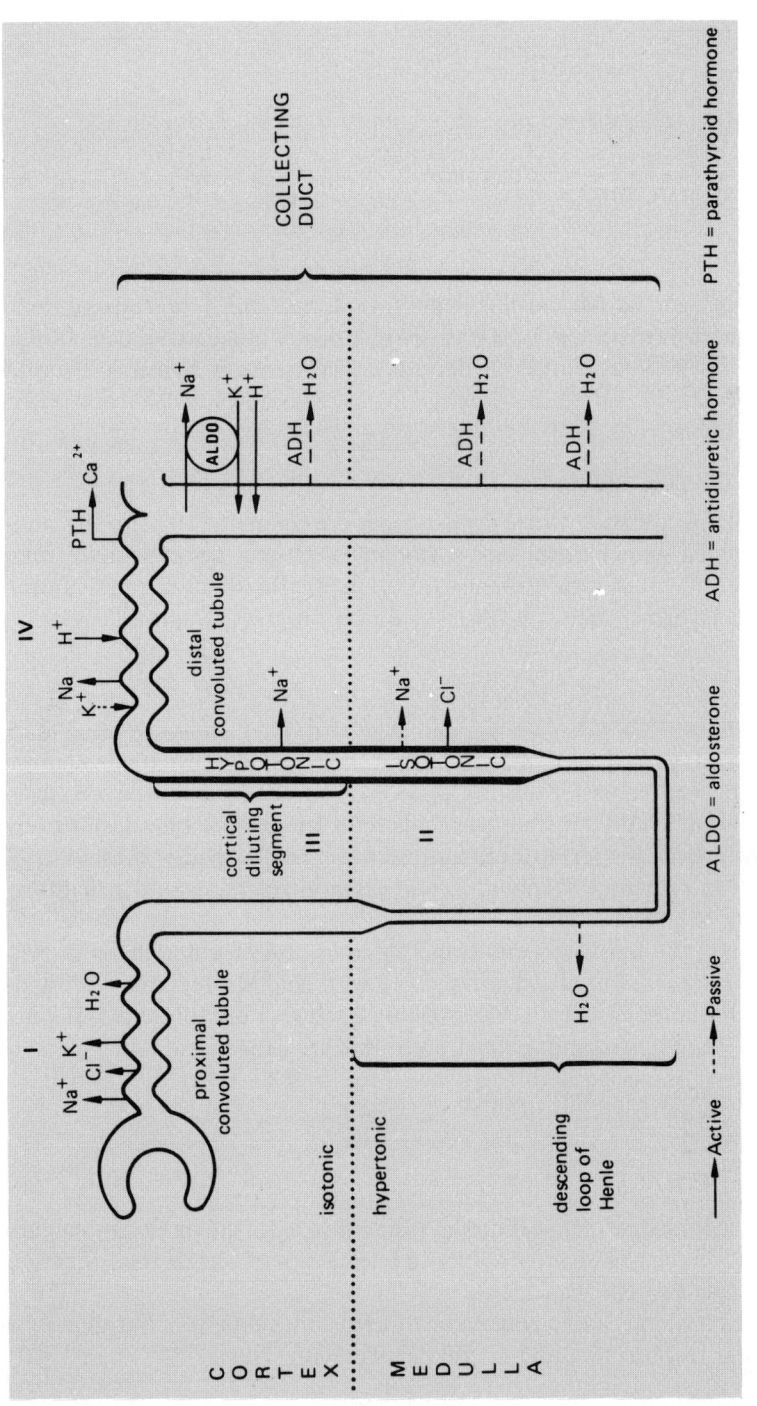

Fig. 15.4. Renal tubular transport systems.

ALDO = aldosterone   ADH = antidiuretic hormone   PTH = parathyroid hormone

1. The glomerular filtration, which depends on the hydrostatic pressure of the arterial circulation, is normally produced at the rate of 125 ml/min, so that in 24 hours, $125 \times 60 \times 24 = 180\,000$ ml $= 180$ l will be formed, and this contains 25 000 mmol of sodium. However, in 24 hours, only about 1.5 l of urine containing approximately 100 mmol of sodium is voided. This means that $180\,000 - 1500 = 178\,500$ ml or 99.2 per cent of the glomerular filtrate, containing $25\,000 - 100 = 24\,900$ mmol of sodium or 99.6 per cent of sodium is reabsorbed.

2. The reabsorption of water and electrolytes takes place as the result of a number of energy-requiring mechanisms, and these are modified by diuretics. The renal tubule can be divided up into four sites, each of which has its own pattern of reabsorption, and is selectively modified by diuretics (see Fig. 15.5).

Site 1: proximal tubule
At this site about 60 per cent of filtered sodium (Na^+) is actively absorbed accompanied by anions of chloride (Cl^-), two-thirds, and bicarbonate (HCO_3^-), one-third. All filtered potassium (K^+) is absorbed, and the proximal tubule fluid is isosmotic with peritubular fluid.

Site 2: ascending limb of Henle
Here chloride ions are actively reabsorbed together with 25 per cent of filtered sodium (25 per cent of $25\,000 = 6250$ mmol Na^+), which moves passively. This part of the tubule is impermeable to water, as a result of which the concentration of sodium and chloride in the tubular fluid falls whilst *pari passu*, the

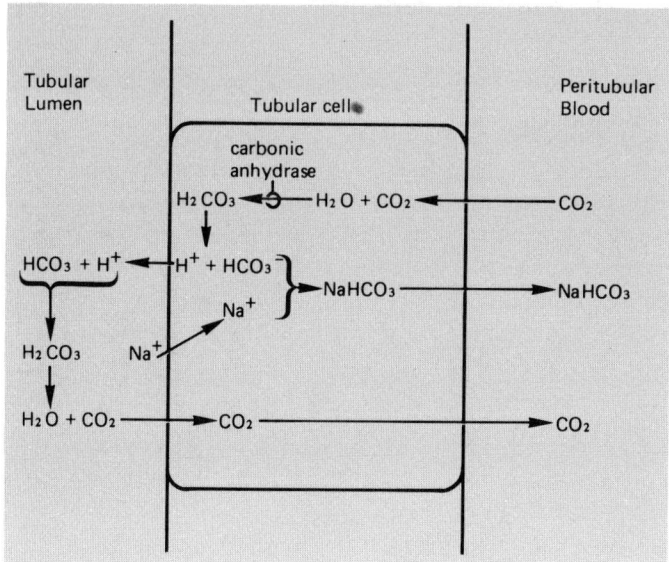

Fig. 15.5. The mechanism of bicarbonate reabsorption in the renal tubule.

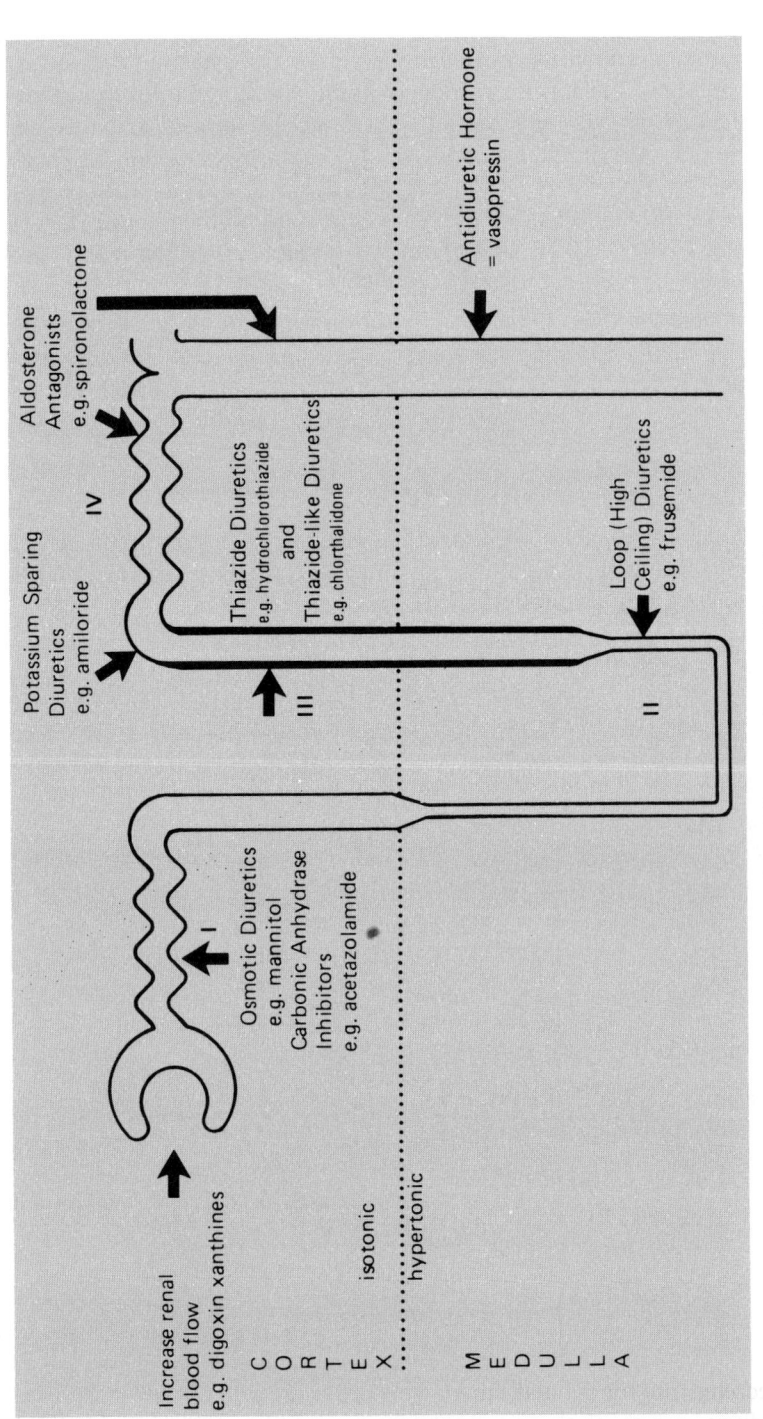

Fig. 15.6. The sites of action of diuretics.

concentration of sodium and chloride ions in the interstitial fluid rises to become hypertonic. The generation of the hypertonic milieu of the interstitium is fundamental in providing the osmotic force needed to produce hypertonic urine in the collecting ducts of the nephron.

Site 3: the cortical segment of the ascending loop of Henle

This is often called the cortical diluting segment, and differs from sites 1 and 2 in that 5 per cent sodium (5 per cent of $25\,000 = 1250$ mmol Na^+) is absorbed *without* water, with the result that the tubular fluid becomes hypotonic. It is important to note that because the reabsorption of sodium from this site takes place within the cortical region (and therefore outside the medullary region) drugs that act on site 3 can reduce cortical diluting ability without affecting the subsequent concentration of urine, which takes place in the collecting duct and depends upon the hypertonic medullary zone (see above).

Site 4: distal convoluted tubule and collecting duct

At this site some additional sodium and chloride reabsorption takes place. In addition, potassium and hydrogen ions are secreted in exchange for sodium ions, the exchange depending upon the amount of sodium delivered to the site and also upon the amount of aldosterone secreted. A diuretic that reduces the amount of sodium reabsorption proximal to Site 4 will result in an increased load of sodium ions being presented to Site 4. As a consequence there will be an increased exchange of sodium ions for potassium and thus an increased loss of potassium ions in the urine.

Site 4 is also important for the reabsorption of water (as mentioned earlier), which takes place under the control of antidiuretic hormone (ADH; vasopressin) and which renders the collecting ducts permeable to water so that it then moves down the osmotic gradient into the interstitium of the medulla. As a result the urine becomes hypertonic.

Control of acid–base balance by the kidney

A major function of the kidney is to control the acid–base balance of the body. The kidney achieves this by:

(1) the tubular reabsorption of bicarbonate ion;

(2) the excretion of hydrogen ions with regeneration of bicarbonate.

These processes, which are illustrated above in Fig. 15.5, operate as follows. Carbon dioxide enters the renal cell from the blood and is hydrated in a reaction that is catalysed by carbonic anhydrase. The carbonic acid so formed then dissociates to form hydrogen ions and bicarbonate ions. The hydrogen ions are then secreted into the tubular lumen where they are exchanged for sodium ions. The sodium ions are then reabsorbed into the tubular cell where they combine with bicarbonate ions (formed from dissociation of carbonic acid) to form sodium bicarbonate, which is reabsorbed into the peritubular blood. At the same time, the hydrogen ions, which were secreted into the lumen and which were exchanged for sodium ions, combine with luminal bicarbonate ions to form carbonic acid, which then dissociates into water and carbon dioxide. The carbon dioxide diffuses back first into the tubular cell and ultimately into the peritubular blood. Thus any drug that is able to inhibit the enzyme, carbonic anhydrase, will interfere with bicarbonate reabsorption and hence acid–base balance (see under carbonic anhydrase).

Mechanism of excretion of organic acids and bases

Secretory systems for naturally occurring organic acids (e.g. uric acid) and organic bases (e.g. creatinine) exist in the proximal tubule. As many drugs are weak organic acids (e.g. aspirin) or weak organic bases (e.g. amitriptyline) (see Chapter 1), they are secreted by these active transport systems. As a consequence, a drug so transported may interact with one of the natural substances, for example, uric acid, being secreted by the same transport system. Furthermore it is possible to block the secretion of a drug that utilizes such a transport system with another that has a high affinity for the same system, e.g. probenecid blocks the secretion of benzylpenicillin (see Chapter 1).

Some drugs are partially reabsorbed from the tubules by non-ionic diffusion and, as the tubule cells are only permeable to the un-ionized fraction, reabsorption is dependent on the pK_a of the drug and the pH of the tubular urine (see Chapter 1). Thus, in the treatment of salicylate poisoning, the urine is made alkaline so that the salicylate will be highly ionized (pK_a of aspirin = 3.5) with the result that the amount of diffusion back into the tubular cell, and thence to the circulation via the peritubular blood, will be very small.

Classification of commonly used diuretics (saluretics)

It has already been seen that urinary excretion depends ultimately upon the difference between the amount of glomerular filtrate formed and the amount of the filtrate that is reabsorbed by the tubules. Again, this may be expressed in the form of a simple equation:

urinary excretion = glomerular filtrate − amount reabsorbed in the tubules.

It therefore follows that urinary excretion can be increased either by (i) *increasing* the glomerular filtrate, or (ii) by *decreasing* the reabsorption of the filtered load by the tubules. Diuretics can thus be classified into two groups:

(1) those that act by increasing renal blood flow and glomerular filtration rate;

(2) those that act by inhibiting the reabsorption of sodium by the renal tubules.

Drugs that increase renal blood flow

Digitalis glycosides

Digoxin (and other cardiac glycosides) increase the output of the failing heart (see p. 329) and thereby increase glomerular blood flow. As a consequence glomerular filtration is increased, leading to increased urine production. Digitalis glycosides may therefore be considered to have diuretic activity.

Xanthines

It is a matter of common knowledge that tea, coffee, and other beverages have a diuretic action; this is due to the xanthines (caffeine, theophylline, and theobromine) that they contain. These drugs increase cardiac output by inhibition of the enzyme phosphodiesterase that normally destroys cylicAMP, and hence increase renal blood flow; in addition, they dilate blood vessels in the renal medulla. However, the most potent drug in this group, aminophylline, is not a naturally occurring compound but is made in the laboratory by combining theophylline with ethylene diamine in order to produce a more soluble form of theophylline, suitable for slow intravenous injection.

Drugs that inhibit the reabsorption of sodium

Excess water retention is commonly due to associated sodium retention. It therefore follows that an effective way to reduce an excess of body water should be to increase the excretion of sodium, and this has proved to be the case. As shown earlier (see p. 339), sodium reabsorption takes place along the length of the renal tubule but the major part is reabsorbed in the proximal tubule, whilst sodium is actively reabsorbed without water in the ascending limb of the loop of Henle. In the distal tubule, sodium is exchanged for potassium under the control of aldosterone; as water passes down the collecting tubules it is reabsorbed under the control of ADH.

Diuretics in this group may be divided into several clinically useful classes based on their mode and/or site of action, and their chemical group. They are listed here in descending order of frequency of use, and then described in turn.

   I Thiazides
  II Loop (high-ceiling)
 III Potassium-sparing
 IV Aldosterone antagonists
  V Osmotic diuretics
 VI Carbonic anhydrase inhibitors

I Thiazides (benzothiadiazines)

These agents were introduced in the mid-1950s and represented a great step forward, being the first orally active diuretics that were effective. They are derived from the sulphonamide structure of carbonic anhydrase inhibitors. The drugs that they replaced were the mercurial diuretics and, whilst they are weaker than these predecessors, they have the great advantage that they are active by mouth. Over 10 thiazide and thiazide-like drugs are now available: bendrofluazide, chlorothiazide, chlorthalidone, clopamide, cyclopenthiazide, hydrochlorothiazide, hydroflumethiazide, mefruside, methylclothiazide, polythiazide, xipamide. No one drug is outstandingly superior to the others.

Pharmacodynamics

1. Diuretic action: they act at site III in the cortical diluting segment and also at site IV, producing an increased output of sodium and water. The increased concentration of sodium ions presented to the distal tubule results in the secondary loss of potassium ions by increased secretion in exchange for the sodium ions.

2. Hypotensive action: thiazides and related compounds produce an antihypertensive effect that is independent of their diuretic action and probably due to a direct action on vascular smooth muscle, possibly by modulating its response to various pressor agents, including catecholamines and angiotensin. The initial reduction of blood volume caused by the diuretic cannot be the primary hypotensive mechanism because the fall in blood pressure continues after homeostatic mechanisms have led to a rise in the blood volume.

Uses

These compounds are used to counter oedema caused by cardiac failure, nephrotic syndrome, and drugs; and to treat hypertension and diabetes insipidus.

Pharmacokinetics

All these drugs are well absorbed by mouth and excreted unchanged in the urine. The $T_{0.5}$ is about four hours, although they act for about three times as long and must therefore be taken in the morning to avoid a disturbed night.

Unwanted effects

All thiazides tend to exhibit the following several unwanted effects. Potassium loss causing hypokalaemia will occur when they are given for a prolonged period. For this reason, potassium supplements should always be taken by those who are on thiazides indefinitely. There may be hyperglycaemia but this is not usually of clinical significance; however, occasionally diabetes mellitus is precipitated in a susceptible patient. In established diabetics being treated with oral hypoglycaemic drugs, increased doses may be needed. Hyperuricaemia occurs due to reduced excretion of uric acid, and this may precipitate an acute attack of gout. Hypercalcaemia may arise due to decreased urinary excretion of calcium. There may be reduced urinary output in patients with nephrogenic diabetes insipidus.

II Loop (high-ceiling) diuretics

This group of drugs includes frusemide, bumetanide, and ethacrynic acid.

Pharmacodynamics

These drugs inhibit sodium and chloride reabsorption in the ascending limb of the loop of Henle and, as a consequence, are much more potent than the thiazides. Because of this action they are also called 'loop diuretics' and 'high-ceiling' diuretics. Although the degree of potassium loss is less than that produced by the thiazides for an equivalent diuresis, they are potent enough to produce substantial potassium loss, so that it is important to administer potassium supplements to patients receiving them. They are readily absorbed from the gut, but can be given intravenously. Their actions persist up to about six hours.

Pharmacokinetics

Frusemide is only 50 per cent absorbed, whereas bumetanide and ethacrynic acid are well absorbed. The $T_{0.5}$ of these drugs are short (1–1.5 hours), and they are mainly secreted unchanged in the urine.

Uses

They are used to treat systemic oedema due to cardiac failure, hepatic disease, and nephrotic syndrome; and acute pulmonary oedema.

Unwanted effects

Their powerful diuretic action can lead to hypokalaemia, hyponatraemia, and dehydration. Hypokalaemia must be prevented by giving adequate potassium supplements (see Pharmacodynamics) or, if appropriate, giving potassium-sparing diuretics, such as spironolactone, triamterene, or amiloride. As hypokalaemia potentiates the effects of cardiac glycosides, particular care must be taken when loop diuretics are given to patients already taking digoxin, Magnesium excretion may also be excessive and result in hypomagnesaemia.

Hyperglycaemia may occur but is not usually of clinical significance except in those suffering from diabetes mellitus, whose dose of oral hypoglycaemic drugs may need to be increased.

There may be hyperuricaemia but it is uncommon for it to precipitate an attack of acute gout. However, the powerful diuretic action of these drugs may precipitate acute urinary retention in those already suffering from prostatic hypertrophy.

III Potassium-sparing diuretics

Pharmacodynamics

Triamterene and amiloride are chemically similar diuretics that act upon the distal convoluted tubule. They cause an increase in sodium and chloride excretion but, in contrast to the diuretics mentioned earlier, they inhibit the exchange of sodium for potassium by an unknown mechanism, which is independent of aldosterone. Consequently, their use is associated with retention of potassium and may thus result in hyperkalaemia.

Pharmacokinetics

Triamterene and amiloride are poorly absorbed by mouth, and almost completely excreted unchanged in the urine with a $T_{0.5}$ of about six hours.

Uses

These drugs are used in combination with other diuretics that cause depletion of potassium; for example, thiazides, frusemide. Moduretic, a proprietary preparation consisting of a combination of hydrochlorothiazide and amiloride, is used when it is necessary to give a diuretic but minimize the risk of hypokalaemia.

Unwanted effects

Hyperkalaemia, dehydration, and hyponatraemia may occur. Both drugs can cause nausea, vomiting, and diarrhoea.

IV Aldosterone antagonists

Pharmacodynamics

Spironolactone is a synthetic steroid that has a structural formula similar to that of aldosterone. It is metabolized to canrenone, which is a competitive antagonist to aldosterone on the distal convoluted tubule. Its effects will clearly depend upon the amount of aldosterone with which it can compete; such competition will cause increased sodium and water excretion, and potassium retention. Furthermore, spironolactone is a weak diuretic because the reabsorption of sodium in the distal convoluted tubule accounts for only a relatively small proportion of the total amount of sodium reabsorbed.

Pharmacokinetics

Spironolactone is absorbed well after oral administration and, although its $T_{0.5}$ is only about 10 minutes, the active metabolite, canrenone, has a much longer half-life ($T_{0.5} = 16$ hours) and, as a consequence, its onset of action is slow.

Uses

Naturally, it is particularly effective when circulating levels of aldosterone are high as may occur in the nephrotic syndrome, hepatic failure, or as a result of intensive diuretic therapy.

Spironolactone can also be used to treat oedema due to cardiac failure, nephrotic syndrome, and liver disease. For reasons given above, it is usually prescribed in combination with a thiazide or one of the high-ceiling diuretics.

Unwanted effects

There may be nausea and vomiting with high doses. Hyperkalaemia may occur even when spironolactone is used in combination with a potassium-losing diuretic, and it is therefore important to be alert to this possibility.

There is chemical similarity between spironolactone (and its active metabolite, canrenone) and the sex hormones, so the drug may act as an agonist at sex hormone receptors. Thus gynaecomastia is common (and often painful); of less frequent occurrence are impotence, testicular atrophy, and menstrual disturbances. For similar reasons the peptic ulcer-healing properties of carbenoxolone may be reversed by spironolactone so that these two drugs should not be given concurrently.

V Osmotic diuretics

Pharmacodynamics

Mannitol is the most important drug in this group; it is a sugar alcohol, which is not metabolized by the body. Under normal circumstances (as has been described earlier) the major reabsorption of sodium from the glomerular filtrate takes place in the proximal convoluted tubule. As the proximal tubule is freely permeable to water, the reabsorption of sodium and water can take place together, with the result that the contents of the tubule remain isosmotic. However, when a substance such as mannitol, which is not reabsorbed by the tubule, is present, this impedes the reabsorption of water in order that the osmotic pressure of the tubular fluid shall remain the same as that of the plasma. As a consequence, the reabsorption of water and, secondarily, of sodium is reduced and a diuresis results. As with other diuretics, the increased sodium load presented to the distal tubule results in an increased exchange of sodium for potassium with consequent increased potassium loss in the urine. It should be noted that for a substance to act as an osmotic diuretic it must (i) enter the glomerular filtrate from the plasma, and (ii) fail either completely or partially to be reabsorbed by the tubule.

Pharmacokinetics

Mannitol is, as might be expected, very poorly absorbed and must therefore be given parenterally. After parenteral administration it remains in the extracellular compartment and depends upon renal excretion for its removal from the body, which takes place rapidly. The intravenous administration of mannitol must be carried out with great care because it can lead to an increase in the circulating volume of blood with a consequent rise in central venous pressure, which in turn may lead to cardiac failure. Furthermore, the increased osmolality of the plasma may then lead to hyponatraemia. It should be noted that if it is given by mouth it will remain within the gastro-intestinal tract and behave as an osmotic laxative.

Uses

Mannitol is used when oedema becomes refractory to other diuretics. It will also improve renal blood flow in certain forms of renal failure (e.g. shock). It may also be employed to produce a forced diuresis in drug poisoning, so as to increase the rate of drug eliminations.

VI Carbonic anhydrase inhibitors

The role of the enzyme carbonic anhydrase has been discussed earlier (see p. 341). Before the advent of the thiazides and the loop diuretics, carbonic anhydrase inhibitors represented a group of orally active but weak diuretic agents. They have since been superseded by the much more potent agents but are occasionally used for special purposes, for example, in the treatment of glaucoma.

Pharmacodynamics

Inhibition of carbonic anhydrase will reduce the supply of hydrogen ions available for exchange with sodium ions (together with bicarbonate ions) with the result that there is an increased excretion of an alkaline urine containing sodium bicarbonate. If this is maintained, the increase in bicarbonate excretion leads to a metabolic acidosis, which unfortunately reduces the further efficacy of the drug. As a consequence the response to subsequent doses rapidly falls off and alternative methods of diuresis must be considered.

Pharmacokinetics

Acetazolamide is well adsorbed after oral administration and is excreted by tubular secretion with a half-life of 2.5–6 hours.

Uses

The increased intra-ocular pressure in chronic glaucoma can be reduced by carbonic anhydrase inhibitors. The enzyme inhibition results in a diminished secretion of aqueous humor into the anterior chamber of the eye, and also a reduced formation of cerebrospinal fluid. Thus, as well as being used for the treatment of glaucoma, carbonic anhydrase inhibitors have also been used as adjuvant therapy for the treatment of epilepsy.

TREATMENT OF SOME CARDIOVASCULAR DISEASES

Treatment of cardiac arrhythmias

The treatment of all but the simplest forms of cardiac arrhythmia fall within the province of the cardiologist. Therefore, the following account attempts only an outline of this complex problem in which it is vital for accurate diagnosis to precede treatment. Furthermore, with the large and bewildering number of anti-arrhythmic drugs now available the selection of the appropriate drug or drugs for a particular patient requires (i) specialized knowledge and experience of this branch of cardiology, and (ii) understanding of the pharmacology of the drugs to be employed. Only an overview of this problem can be given.

Causes of cardiac arrhythmias

There are six main causes of cardiac arrhythmias:

(1) ischaemic heart disease;

(2) valvular heart disease;

(3) cardiomyopathies;

(4) congenital heart disease;

(5) drug induced e.g. cardiac glycosides and other anti-arrhythmic drugs;

(6) metabolic disturbances e.g. hypokalaemia.

When a patient presents with an arrhythmia it is necessary not only to find out the type but also the factor responsible for it. It is not possible to put into reverse changes due to ischaemic heart disease or due to congenital conduction abnormalities. On the other hand, it should be possible to correct drug-induced abnormalities and also to correct metabolic disturbances.

Classification of cardiac arrhythmias

These may arise within the ventricle, above it in the atrium, or in the nodal tissue. Arrhythmias may also be induced by digitalis. It is therefore convenient to consider them under four headings as follows:

(1) sinus node arrhythmias;

(2) supraventricular arrhythmias;

(3) ventricular arrhythmias;

(4) drug-induced arrhythmias.

Some of the more common arrhythmias within each of these groups will now be discussed briefly.

Sinus node arrhythmias

These comprise either sinus tachycardia, in which the heart rate is greater than 100 per minute, or sinus bradycardia, in which the rate is less than 60 per minute. Sinus tachycardia does not require specific treatment, but the underlying cause should be investigated; anxiety or hyperthyroidism are two possible causes.

Chronic sinus bradycardia can be caused by any drug that (i) reduces sympathetic drive to the heart (b-adrenoceptor antagonists); (ii) drugs that increase vagal tone (e.g. acetylcholinesterase inhibitors); (iii) cardiac glycosides. It is also a feature of hypothyroidism. After an acute myocardial infarction, bradycardia is common but does not need treatment unless it results in an unacceptable reduction of cardiac output, in which case the antimuscarinic drug, atropine, is used to antagonize this vagal effect. It should be remembered that sinus bradycardia is a normal occurrence in highly trained athletes. Thus, whilst the cause of sinus bradycardia should always be sought, usually it does not need treatment.

Supraventricular arrhythmias

These comprise (i) atrial flutter, (ii) atrial fibrillation, and (iii) paroxysmal tachycardia.

Atrial flutter

In this condition the atria beat regularly at a rate of 250 to 350 per minute. The precise mechanism is not clear; it may be due to a 'circus movement' in which a self-perpetuating wave of excitation moves in a circle around the orifices of the superior and inferior vena cavae. An alternative view is that it is due to a single, rapidly firing ectopic atrial focus from which impulses spread out over the atrium. However, the high rate of atrial impulses is not usually conducted to the ventricles due to varying degrees of atrioventricular block. Thus, there is usually a 2:1, 3:1, or 4:1 atrioventricular block present, with the result that the ventricular rate is a sub-multiple of the atrial rate; the commonest situation is a 2:1 block with a ventricular rate of 140 to 160 beats per minute. Digitalis (digoxin or digitoxin) is the drug of first choice, with a β-blocker or calcium entry blocker as a second choice. Disopyramide is also useful and should be given in combination with digoxin. However, if digoxin fails it is then usual to attempt direct-current (DC) cardioversion.

Atrial fibrillation

This condition is usually due to acute or chronic myocardial ischaemia, mitral stenosis, or hyperthyroidism, but other less common causes may be responsible. If it is of recent origin an attempt is usually made to convert this completely irregular rhythm to normal rhythm by means of DC cardioversion. However, if the fibrillation has been present for some time then restoration of regular sinus rhythm is unlikely, and the aim then is to use drugs to slow the ventricular rate to the normal range. Once again, digitalis is the drug of first choice but, if this is ineffective on its own, then it may become effective with the addition of a β-adrenoceptor antagonist or calcium entry blocker. Disopyramide is also a useful drug for this problem. Amiodarone, though very effective, should only be considered as a last resort.

Paroxysmal supraventricular tachycardia

This consists of paroxysms of sudden onset during which the heart rate is found to be 140 to 220 per minute although regular in rhythm. Three forms can be identified by means of specialist techniques (Kulbertus 1986; true atrial tachycardia, nodal tachycardia, and pre-excitation tachycardia). The duration of the attacks may be only seconds but, more often they persist for minutes or hours, and occasionally for days. Precipitating factors should be sought (and avoided), and these include dietary (coffee, tobacco, alcohol), psychological (anxiety), or physical (exercise).

During an acute attack, measures designed to increase vagal tone, such as carrying out the Valsalva manoeuvre (see p. 322), swallowing cold water, facial massage, or carotid sinus massage, may be effective. If drug treatment is required, verapamil 10 mg IV slowly (or one of the other calcium entry blockers) is often effective. Alternatively, a β-adrenoceptor blocker can be tried. If these measures fail the patient should be referred to a specialist.

A wide variety of treatments are used in prophylaxis; these include digoxin and/or calcium entry blockers; disopyramide (for true atrial tachycardia or for nodal tachycardia); flecainide, disopyramide, or amiodarone (for pre-excitation tachycardias)

Ventricular arrhythmias

These are most commonly ventricular extrasystoles (premature beats), ventricular tachycardia, and ventricular fibrillation. They are most likely to occur after acute myocardial infarction; they may, however, occur in otherwise healthy individuals, or be caused by ischaemic heart disease or by any drug that has arrhythmogenic properties; for example, digitalis or tricyclic antidepressants.

Ventricular extrasystoles (premature beats) often arise after myocardial infarction and may need treatment. However, the indications for treatment and the best drug for this purpose remain a controversial subject. If treatment is indicated then all anti-arrhythmic drugs (except calcium entry blockers) can be useful and the potential of β-blockers should not be overlooked. For ventricular tachycardia, lignocaine is also considered to be the drug of choice.

Drug-induced arrhythmias

Digitalis is the most likely culprit and commonly produces supraventricular arrhythmias, ectopic ventricular arrhythmias, or heart block, or a combination of these. Sinus bradycardia can be the result of excessive medication with digitalis but only needs treating if it is causing hypotension. As noted earlier, atropine is an effective way of reducing vagal tone and would be an appropriate treatment here if required. The occurrence of atrial tachycardia with heart block might call for treatment with lignocaine or phenytoin, or possibly a combination of a β-adrenoceptor antagonist and the insertion of a cardiac pacemaker. Ventricular arrhythmias would also call for treatment with phenytoin, lignocaine, or a β-adrenoceptor antagonist. It might also be necessary to insert a pacemaker, and DC cardioversion may need to be considered. It should be noted that arrhythmias can be induced by all anti-arrhythmic drugs.

Heart failure and its treatment

There are several different types of heart failure, of which the commonest is due to inadequate contraction of either the right or the left ventricle, or both. If contraction of the right ventricle is inadequate this leads to systemic venous congestion, whilst if the contraction of the left ventricle is inadequate this leads to pulmonary oedema; or there may be a mixture of both. Treatment aims to remove the cause, if this is possible, and to control the signs and symptoms by means of appropriate drugs.

If the underlying cause of heart failure can be removed or modified then this should be done. Thus, if cardiac failure is secondary to valvular disease of the heart it may be possible to deal with this surgically. If the cause is hypertension then this can be treated (see below). Likewise, if cardiac failure is secondary to anaemia or hyperthyroidism these conditions must also be treated (see Chapters 18 and 19). Drugs with negative inotropic properties, such as Class I and Class II anti-arrhythmic agents (see above), may also precipitate cardiac failure, and appropriate modification of the dose or withdrawal of the drug (and possibly replacement by another) would be appropriate treatment here.

When the cause of cardiac failure cannot be removed then drug therapy becomes mandatory and, from earlier sections in this chapter, it will be evident that there are three groups of drugs that can be used to treat the condition.

1. Diuretics are the first drugs of choice because they remove the excess sodium and water that occurs in cardiac failure. Furthermore, if the failure is secondary to hypertension then many of the diuretic agents appear to have an additional and direct action on vascular smooth muscle, which lowers the blood pressure and thereby assists treatment. Thiazides and loop diuretics are most commonly used for this purpose.

2. Digitalis glycosides, which have a positive inotropic action, are also important, and commonly form the mainstay of therapy in patients with congestive cardiac failure.

3. Vasodilators are also important because, as discussed earlier (see p. 331), they reduce the load on the heart and thereby assist it to work more within its reduced capabilities.

The appropriate combination of drugs and their doses calls for careful clinical judgement and continuous review in order that changes in the condition of the patient may be monitored and appropriate modification of drug therapy made.

Treatment of hypertension

Hypertension is a persistently raised blood pressure and, in the early stages, is unlikely to be recognized as it is asymptomatic. Symptomatic recognition may only occur after some considerable time, when damage has already been done to the cardiovascular system. The lesson to be learned from this observation is that regular screening of blood pressure may well be desirable, particularly in patients with a family history of cardiovascular disease.

In the vast majority of patients the reason for the raised blood pressure is unknown, and this is called 'essential' hypertension. Essential hypertension is probably multifactorial in its causation. There is another form of hypertension that arises from a known disorder, such as kidney malfunction, and this is known as 'secondary' hypertension. The discussion here will deal solely with the problem of essential hypertension.

The blood pressure varies as the product of the cardiac output and the resistance to the flow of blood in the peripheral circulation (peripheral resistance).

The smooth muscle in the arteriolar wall is constantly in a state of partial contraction and this state is modified by the vasomotor centre acting by way of the sympathetic nervous system. Increased sympathetic activity causes arteriolar vasoconstriction with a rise in blood pressure, and vice versa. Although many of the drugs used to treat hypertension do so by blocking sympathetic outflow, it is unlikely that excessive activity of the sympathetic nervous system is the sole mechanism causing a raised blood pressure. In recent years, the role played by renin in hypertension has exercized some interest. Renin, as outlined earlier and shown in Fig. 15.3, splits the protein angiotensin to form the peptide angiotensin I, the angiotensin being found in the blood. Angiotensin I is converted to angiotensin II and this, in its turn, is metabolized to angiotensin III. Both angiotensin II and angiotensin III are vasoconstrictors of peripheral arterioles and this can lead to hypertension. Any increased renin activity will lead to excessive production of these angiotensins.

Whatever the cause, essential hypertension is a progressive disease and it will eventually cause damage to the entire cardiovascular system. Treatment is necessary in many instances in order to avoid the consequences of the pressure, e.g. stroke, renal damage, and ischaemic heart disease.

Essential hypertension is an age-related disease, and a pressure in the range 140–150/90 is usually regarded as hypertension in the average patient (Neidle, et al. 1985). There is a wide variety of drugs available for the treatment of essential hypertension and, in general, patients whose average diastolic pressure exceeds 100 should receive antihypertensive treatment. Diuretics are often the first choice of drug for the treatment of hypertension and may suffice in themselves. They will often be quite adequate to control a mild hypertension (Ramsay 1987). Other drugs can be added to diuretics as required in order to produce a satisfactory anyihypertensive effect. It seems that the diuretics potentiate the effects of most other antihypertensive drugs.

The β-adrenoceptor blocking drugs (see Chapter 13) are sometimes used alone to control the blood pressure, and they are also used together with diuretics when either, used separately, have proved inadequate. In more severe hypertension, a third drug, such as a vasodilator, may have to be added, hydralazine being the one normally advocated.

Apart from the use of drugs other remedial factors must be considered. If the patient is overweight, there should be an attempt to reduce this; those who smoke should be encouraged to stop. Alcohol consumption should be moderate.

Treatment of angina pectoris

Angina pectoris is manifested by a sudden and severe pain occurring substernally and this pain often radiates to the left shoulder and arm and, less frequently, to the left mandible and teeth. The pain is typically brought on by exercize, emotion, and cold. This type of angina is referred to as angina of effort and it is a manifestation of myocardial ischaemia, which in itself is caused by atherosclerosis producing narrowing of the coronary arteries. The drugs available for treatment have been considered above; one mainly used to treat an anginal attack is glyceryl trinitrate. The treatment of an acute attack should be prompt and this is best done by placing a tablet of the drug under the tongue from where it is rapidly absorbed. The effects start within about 2 minutes and last up to 30 minutes. Unwanted effects include flushing, headache, and postural hypotension. Glyceryl trinitrate can also be used as a prophylaxis prior to exercize or other factors that tend to bring on an attack.

Amyl nitrite was used at one time but it causes marked vasodilatation of all arterioles with a considerable fall in blood pressure.

Pentaerythritol tetranitrate is a drug that is swallowed; it takes about 10 minutes to become effective and its effects are prolonged over several hours. The drug is used as a prophylactic agent, rather than to treat an acute attack.

Many situations will stimulate the sympathetic nervous system and precipitate an attack of angina, e.g. fear or anxiety. The β-adrenergic antagonists block sympathetic activity to the heart and are effective in reducing the frequency and severity of attacks of angina of effort. They lessen the myocardial oxygen consumption. Beta blockers are taken prophylactically, that is they are taken regularly, and are not used to treat an acute attack of angina. These drugs are not useful if the angina is due to vasospasm.

Calcium entry blockers, e.g. verapamil, nifedipine, are useful in the treatment of angina of effort and of atypical angina. In exertional angina they may produce their effect by reducing myocardial oxygen demands and this, in itself, may be due to the decrease in cardiac contractility produced by these drugs. On the other hand, calcium entry blockers are likely to be effective in the treatment of angina due to vasospasm because they produce vasodilatation in non-atherosclerotic coronary arteries. Nifedipine is particularly valuable in this respect as it is a more potent coronary vasodilator than verapamil.

REFERENCES

Berridge, M. J. (1981). Receptors and calcium signalling. In *Towards understanding receptors* (ed. J. W. Lamble), p. 122. Elsevier, Oxford.

Berridge, M. J. (1985). The molecular basis of communication within the cell. *Scientific American*, **253**, 142–52.

Endo, M., Yanagisawa, T., and Taira, N. (1978). Effects of calcium-antagonist coronary vasodilators, nifedipine and verapamil, on ventricular automaticity of the dog. *Nawnyn-Schimiedeberg's Archiv für Pharmakologie*, **302**: 235–38.

Jones, C. M. (1986). Gingival hyperplasia associated with nifedipine. *British Dental Journal*, **160**, 416–7.

Krikler, D. M. (1974). A fresh look at cardiac arrhythmias IV Theory. *Lancet*, i, 1034–7.

Kulbertus, H. E. (ed.) (1986). Management of cardiac arrhythmias. Churchill Livingstone, Edinburgh.

Neidle, A., Kroeger, D. G., and Yagiela, J. A. (1985). *Pharmacology and therapeutics for dentistry*, (2nd ed). Mosby, St. Louis.

Noble, D. (1979). *The initiation of the heart-beat* (2nd edn). Clarendon Press, Oxford.

Noble, D. (1984). The surprising heart: a review of recent progress in cardiac electrophysiology. *Journal of Physiology*, **353**, 1–50.

Ramsay, L. E. (1987). The management of mild hypertension. *Prescribers' Journal*, **27**(2), 1–8.

Rowland, E., Evans, T., and Krikler, D. (1979). Effect of nifedipine on atrioventricular conduction as compared with verapamil. Intracardiac electrophysiological study. *British Heart Journal*, **42**, 124–7.

Vaughan Williams, E. M. (1983). *Antiarrhythmic actions*. Academic Press, London.

Weidmann, S. (1955). The effect of the cardiac membrane potential on the rapid availability of the sodium carrying system. *Journal of Physiology*, **127**, 213–24.

16

Drugs acting on the respiratory system and the gastro-intestinal tract

RESPIRATORY SYSTEM

THIS section will limit itself to those drugs that are used to treat asthma, and that provide some symptomatic relief in respiratory infections, with a brief consideration of respiratory stimulants.

Drugs used to treat bronchial asthma

Bronchial asthma is commonly due to an allergy to some extrinsic factor. Infection may be a precipitating factor and sometimes emotional distress is an important element. The management of acute asthma occurring in an adverse drug reaction is considered in Chapter 21. The asthmatic attack is characterized by acute airway obstruction due to spasm of the bronchiolar smooth muscle (bronchoconstriction). At the same time the bronchial mucosa is oedematous and the lumen contains many mucus plugs. Fortunately the airway obstruction is reversible by certain drugs.

The mechanism of bronchoconstriction is seemingly through release of mediators from sensitized mast cells in the lungs. The substances so released include histamine, slow reacting substance (SRS-A) (now known to be a mixture of leukotrienes C_4 and D_4), 5-hydroxytryptamine (5-HT), and prostaglandins. Although these substances cause bronchoconstriction, histamine is probably little involved for certainly antihistamines (H_1-blockers) are not effective in the management of the disease.

The drugs used in the management of asthma include:

(1) sympathomimetic drugs;

(2) xanthine derivatives;

(3) sodium cromoglycate and ketotifen (mast cell stabilizers);

(4) corticosteroids.

Sympathomimetic drugs

Directly acting sympathomimetic drugs, such as adrenaline and isoprenaline, which stimulate β_2-receptors in the bronchi, will bring about relaxation of the bronchial smooth muscle. Unfortunately, both of these drugs are somewhat unselective and stimulate β_1-receptors in the heart with possible production of tachycardia at the least. Newer drugs are now available, e.g. salbutamol and terbutaline, which are also β_2-stimulants in the bronchi producing relaxation, but which are relatively selective. These drugs have much less effect on cardiac receptors and are to be preferred.

This group has been considered in more detail in Chapter 13.

Xanthine bronchodilators

Theophylline is a xanthine derivative, as is caffeine. Both are CNS stimulants, but caffeine more so. Theophylline is a mild diuretic (see Chapter 15); it also stimulates β_2-receptors in the bronchi, relaxes bronchial smooth muscle, and relieves the bronchospasm of asthma. The mast cell has β_2-adrenergic receptors that are stimulated by the appropriate agonists. The stimulation of the receptor causes an increase of intracellular cyclic adenosine monophosphate (cAMP). This accumulation of cAMP relaxes bronchial smooth muscle and to some extent decreases the release of the mediators from the mast cells.

Over the years theophylline has proved a very useful drug in relieving bronchial asthma. When administered by mouth it is a gastric irritant. A widely used theophylline compound is called aminophylline; this drug also causes gastric irritation when given orally. Attempts to overcome this problem have been made by various pharmaceutical firms: for instance, aminophylline has been combined with the antacid aluminium hydroxide (aminophylline 195 mg, dried aluminium hydroxide gel 260 mg in each tablet), a preparation which counteracts the gastric acidity so that larger doses of aminophylline can be given with less risk of causing nausea and vomiting. Aminophylline and theophylline are also available as sustained-release preparations that are administered every 12 hours and are thought to cause less gastric irritation.

Aminophylline is also given by slow intravenous injection over a period of at least 10 to 15 minutes, with later maintenance if necessary—by slow intravenous infusion. This regimen is useful in terminating an attack of acute asthma.

The exact place of these xanthine derivatives in the treatment of asthma is somewhat uncertain, and has varied from time to time. However, there is no doubt they are effective in acute asthmas. They do have a stimulant action on the heart and this should add a cautionary note.

Sodium cromoglycate

This is a prophylactic drug and is of no use in the treatment of an acute attack of asthma (see Chapter 21). It is administered by inhalation as it is poorly absorbed when given by mouth. It seems to work by stabilizing the mast cell membranes, so preventing the release of the pharmacologically active mediators that cause the bronchospasm. Children seem to respond to the drug better than the older patient. Some patients find that the dry powder inhalations of sodium cromoglycate actually precipitate bronchospasm, although this is usually transient.

Ketotifen, a relatively new drug, is administered orally. Although it is thought to act in the same way as sodium cromoglycate, it is not as effective.

Corticosteroids

The mechanism of action of the corticosteroids in asthma is somewhat uncertain. They are not the first choice of drugs for the treatment of bronchial asthma when the attack can be brought under control by other means. Steroids may occasionally be required when other remedies have failed, and a relatively short course may re-establish the patient's response to drugs such as salbutamol.

Some patients find the use of a steroid inhalant satisfactory. Seemingly the best of the corticosteroids for inhalation is beclomethasone dipropionate. After the inhalation (by aerosol) the drug is deposited in the mouth, nasal passages, and bronchi. In therapeutic doses this steroid does not appear to cause suppression of adrenal function. Such an inhalant can be useful in controlling asthma prophylactically. It must be taken regularly for a prescribed time, and it is not suitable for the treatment of an acute attack. The use of the aerosol inhalant is directed to less severe and more chronic asthma.

One unfortunate, unwanted effect of the use of beclomethasone inhalant is the occurrence of candidiasis of the mouth or throat. This is unlikely to happen unless large doses are used and is rarely seen. A preventitive measure is to rinse the mouth out with water after inhalation of a dose of the steroid.

Patients with severe bronchospasm may be treated with short courses of oral corticosteroids, e.g. prednisolone, for a few days. This dosage is gradually reduced over a week; the regimen may be useful when other remedies have temporarily failed.

In the treatment of an emergency, hydrocortisone is administered intravenously in large doses together with β_β-receptor stimulants.

Nasal decongestants

Ephedrine

This is both a directly and indirectly acting sympathomimetic drug. On the one hand it acts directly on α- and β-receptors and, on the other, it displaces noradrenaline from sympathetic nerve endings, which then acts on the appropriate receptors. Its pharmacological action differs from that of adrenaline in a number of ways: (a) it is absorbed from the intestinal tract after oral administration; (b) its effects are weaker but more prolonged; and (c) it has quite a marked stimulating effect on the CNS.

Ephedrine nasal drops may provide symptomatic relief from the nasal congestion associated with the common cold. The effect is produced by vasoconstriction of the mucosal blood vessels, which reduces the thickness of the nasal mucosa. The use of decongestants should be confined to short periods. All can cause what is termed a 'rebound phenomenon', in this instance, a secondary vasodilation, which occurs as the effects wear off and which, temporarily at least, increases the nasal congestion. This is much less likely to happen with ephedrine than with the more potent sympathomimetic drugs used for the purpose, such as phenylephrine. It should be remembered that indirectly acting sympathomimetics may produce a hypertensive crisis if given to a patient taking a monoamine oxidase inhibitor (see Chapter 13).

Ephedrine also has a mild bronchodilatory effect so ephedrine hydrochloride tablets have been used in the treatment of mild chronic asthma. It produces a more sustained effect than adrenaline. Because of its stimulant effect on the CNS, using it to treat the mild asthmatic may have the disadvantage that it keeps them awake at night.

Steam inhalations

These are useful in the symptomatic treatment of acute infective conditions, e.g. a cold. Volatile substances, such as menthol and eucalyptus, are used for such a purpose. For example, menthol and benzoin inhalation consists of menthol 2 per cent in benzoin inhalation; one teaspoonful of the substance is added to a pint of hot water and the vapour inhaled.

Cough suppressants

These antitussive drugs should be used with discrimination. Coughing is the way of getting rid of excessive secretions and foreign matter and, when the cough is productive, it would be wrong to suppress it. However, the hard non-productive, painful cough is another matter altogether. The opioids (Chapter 6) are cough suppressants and the most commonly used for this purpose is codeine as a linctus. Pholcodine is also a popular preparation. More potent preparations, such as diamorphine hydrochloride linctus, are available for the management of dry or painful cough in terminal illness. All of these drugs are centrally acting.

Expectorants

These are drugs that promote the ejection by spitting of mucus or other fluids from the lungs and trachea. It is very doubtful whether any drug will facilitate the expectoration of bronchial secretions. Ammonium chloride, ipecacuanha, and squill are all used in near emetic doses to promote expectoration. Any effect is probably more that of a placebo than anything else. Expectorants are to be found in compound preparations, with sedatives, for example. One such popular mixture is Benylin Expectorant containing ammonium chloride and the antihistamine sedative, diphenhydramine. There is little evidence of the value of expectorants.

Respiratory stimulants (analeptics)
(e.g. doxapram and nikethamide)

These two respiratory stimulants have a limited use in the treatment of acute respiratory failure in those with chronic obstructive airways disease. Respiratory stimulants are of no value whatsoever in respiratory failure due to drug overdosage. For instance, if the respiratory problem is due to opioid overdosage, a specific antagonist should be given and naloxone is the drug of choice (see Chapter 6). Respiratory depression due to an overdosage of barbiturates will not respond to the respiratory stimulants, nor is naloxone an antidote to such poisoning.

Chronic bronchitis

Respiratory insufficiency may occur due to infection. In some instances, broad-spectrum antimicrobials should be prescribed (tetracyclines, amoxycillin, or co-trimoxazole) although a specimen of sputum should be taken and the organism typed.

THE ALIMENTARY TRACT

This section will contain a brief review of drugs commonly used in treating gastro-intestinal disorders.

Anti-emetic drugs

Anti-emetic drugs can act at the following sites:

(1) vomiting centre in the brain, e.g. hyoscine and some antihistamines;

(2) chemoreceptor trigger zone (CTZ), e.g. metoclopramide, and some phenothiazines, such as chlorpromazine;

(3) stomach, e.g. metoclopramide.

Certain H_1 blockers, such as diphenhydramine and cyclizine, have the ability to counter motion sickness.

Chlorpromazine (see Chapter 14) is a potent anti-emetic under certain circumstances. It does not seem to control motion sickness but is very useful in the treatment of vomiting caused by carcinoma, radiation sickness, and uraemia. The major tranquillizers prevent stimulation of the CTZ by such drugs as morphine, a drug that may well be used in the management of terminal illness.

Metoclopramide acts peripherally to enhance the action of acetylcholine at muscarinic synapses. In the CNS it has an inhibitory effect on the CTZ in the brain, acting in a similar way to the phenothiazines. The CTZ is situated adjacent to and connected with the vomiting centre and so stimulation of the CTZ produces vomiting. Metoclopramide prevents vomiting caused by various agents but is not effective in motion sickness.

The phenothiazine derivatives and metoclopramide occasionally cause dystonic reactions like smacking of lips and even spontaneous temporo-mandibular joint dislocations.

Peptic ulceration

Very often the gastro-duodenal mucosa is subject to erosions rather than to frank ulcerations. Both are caused by the over-production of acid (hyperacidity) secreted by the gastric mucosal cells. Peptic ulceration or erosions may cause a lot of gastric pain, there may be gastro-intestinal bleeding, and there may even be a gastric perforation.

Apart from rest, proper attention to diet, stopping smoking and alcohol, a number of drugs have been used to treat these conditions.

Antacids

The action of these is to neutralize the hydrochloric acid secreted by the stomach. They are effective in many dyspepsias and provide pain relief in conditions such as peptic ulcer. The antacids do not accelerate healing.

Sodium bicarbonate has been used for many years as an antacid; it leaves the stomach quickly so that its action is short-lived. If given in large quantities the excess is absorbed from the intestine and may produce alkalosis. It is not a good antacid because of this problem, but it acts quickly to relieve pain.

Aluminium hydroxide is one of the best antacids. It is usually given as a gel or as a tablet to suck. It combines slowly with the gastric acid to form aluminium chloride and water. After leaving the stomach, aluminium salts are not absorbed and do not lead to alkalosis.

There are other antacids, such as calcium, magnesium, and bismuth salts.

Liquorice derivatives

Liquorice has been a favourite remedy for many years and the older generation will certainly recall liquorice root. However, folk-lore has been translated into two medical preparations containing liquorice, namely carbenoxolone and deglycyrrhizinized liquorice. The use of these substances does seem to promote the healing of gastric ulcers, even without the patient being confined to rest. Carbenoxolone has anti-inflammatory activity and it probably increases the amount of adherent mucus on the gastric mucosa thus providing it with protection. It does not appear to produce any real change in gastric acid secretion.

Carbenoxolone has a number of unwanted effects as it causes sodium retention and oedema, together with hypokalaemia. The potassium depletion leading to hypokalaemia may produce muscle weakness.

Cimetidine and ranitidine

These are histamine- (H_2-)receptor blockers, and they promote the healing of peptic ulcers by a reduction of gastric acid output. These drugs should only be used after a definitive diagnosis of erosions or ulcerations, not simply on a clinical suspicion of their existence. It has been suggested that H_2-receptor blockers allow nitrosamine formation in the stomach and so predispose to gastric carcinoma, but there is no real evidence to suggest that there is such a hazard. These blockers, particularly ranitidine, are relatively free from unwanted effects. Both drugs have revolutionized the management of peptic ulcerations (see Chapter 4).

Pirenzepine

This is an anticholinergic and seems to inhibit gastric acid and pepsin secretion. It is a relatively new drug and requires a long-term assessment.

Diarrhoea

Antidiarrhoeal drugs can be divided into antidiarrhoeal adsorbent mixtures, antidiarrhoeal drugs that reduce motility, and a miscellaneous group of other preparations. Adsorbent mixtures include mixtures of chalk and kaolin. Methylcellulose is also adsorbent.

Diarrhoeas not controlled by an adsorbent mixture may be treated with drugs that reduce motility, such as diphenoxylate, loperamide, or a kaolin and morphine mixture.

Other preparations are used for particular conditions, for instance, sulphasalazine in the treatment of ulcerative colitis, or even the topical use of corticosteroids.

Diarrhoea due to specific infections is treated by the appropriate antimicrobial.

Laxatives

These should be avoided wherever possible, and usually an increase of dietary fibre (bran) will suffice to relieve mild constipation. Laxatives are useful when straining is likely to cause a problem, e.g. in patients with haemorrhoids, and where there has been drug-induced constipation, e.g. with drugs such as codeine or the opioids.

17

Chemotherapeutic agents in neoplastic disease

INTRODUCTION

Chemotherapeutic agents are widely used in the treatment of cancer and other neoplastic conditions. They are often the treatment of choice for some types of neoplasia, such as Hogdkin's disease and acute leukaemia. These agents are either used on their own, or as an adjunct to surgery or radiotherapy. The precise treatment will depend upon the type of neoplasia, its rate of growth, and capacity to metastasize. All chemotherapeutic agents block various stages in the cell cycle through inhibition or blockade of a biochemical or metabolic pathway essential for cell division. Therefore, knowledge of the normal cell-growth cycle is necessary for an understanding of their mechanism of action.

THE CELL CYCLE

Cells progress through stages of development while they are synthesizing, growing, and dividing. However, most cells in the body are fully developed and differentiated, and are no longer cycling or replicating. A portion of normal cells in tissues undergoing cellular turnover are in the process of controlling growth and division (for example, skin, bone marrow, and the lining of the gastro-intestinal tract). In contrast, tumour cells continue to grow and divide beyond the normal control of the host.

The stages of cell growth and division are called the cell cycle. Cells begin the cycle in the intermitotic phase (G_1). Substances necessary for cell growth and division are produced in the synthetic phase (S), during which DNA, RNA, and major protein synthesis occurs. At the cessation of S phase, the pre-mitotic or G_2 phase occurs, followed by mitosis (M phase). Cells that are not in the replicating cycle move into the non-proliferating phase (G_0), from which they may return to the active proliferating phase. As the S phase is the period when the cell carries out intensive metabolic and synthetic activities, it is also the phase when it may be most sensitive to agents that interfere with DNA, RNA, and protein synthesis.

PRINCIPLES OF CHEMOTHERAPY

The following factors will govern the success or otherwise of chemotherapy in the treatment of neoplastic disease.

1. *Tumour susceptibility.*   Different tumours will respond to different drugs at varying rates. To achieve optimal results, the tumour cells must be susceptible to the chemotherapeutic agent.

2. *Drug/tumour contact.*   It is essential that the drug comes into contact with the tumour cells, not only in sufficient concentrations, but also during the critical period of cell division.

3. *Size of tumour.*   Chemotherapeutic agents destroy a constant percentage of cells, rather than a constant number. This is referred to as first-order kinetics (see Chapter 1). If a drug destroys 99.99 per cent of tumour cells, this will still leave a substantial numbers of cells especially if the initial tumour mass was large. Even if a few tumour cells remain, there is the possibility of relapse and metastasis.

4. *Tumour cell resistance.*   If a tumour becomes unresponsive to a chemotherapeutic agent, it may be due to a build-up of tumour cell resistance. A number of factors can cause this resistance; for example, poor penetration of the tumour due to an impaired blood supply, enzyme alteration, and tumour cell mutation.

5. *Immunotherapy.*   The host tissues will possess some measure of defence against the tumour cells. Appropriate immunotherapy may enhance this defence mechanism and, given in conjunction with chemotherapy, may increase the tumour-killing potential of the drugs.

6. *Combination therapy.*   Various chemotherapeutic agents act at different stages in the cell cycle. The administration of different drugs will increase their range of activity against the tumour. Furthermore, when combination therapy is used, lower doses are given, which will reduce the incidence of unwanted effects.

7. *Unwanted effects.*   The drugs chosen should not cause severe unwanted effects that may prevent the completion of treatment. For a given drug, altering the route of administration may reduce the incidence of these effects.

CLASSIFICATION OF CHEMOTHERAPEUTIC AGENTS

Chemotherapeutic agents can be conveniently divided into five groups:

1. Alkylating agents: these release alkyl radicals that react with organic compounds essential for cell metabolism; they also prevent cell division by cross-linking strands of DNA.

2. Antimetabolites: these act as competitive antagonists for folic acid, purine, and for pyramidine bases, which are essential for the synthesis of DNA, RNA, and certain co-enzymes.

3. Natural products: this group comprises the vinca alkaloids, certain antibiotics, and enzymes.

4. Hormones: those used in the treatment of neoplasia include oestrogen, progesterone, and adrenocorticosteroids.

5. Radioactive isotopes and implants.

Alkylating agents

These were the first drugs to be used in the treatment of neoplastic disease. All alkylating agents are based on the chemical structure of nitrogen mustard, a compound used in chemical warfare; examples include cyclophosphamide, chlorambucil, and mechlorethamine.

Pharmacodynamics and pharmacological properties

Alkylating agents disrupt mitotic activity, cell growth, differentiation, and function. Their primary target is the DNA molecule (Price 1975). They are particularly effective if the tumour cells are rapidly proliferating, but they can also affect tissues with low mitotic activity. Tumour cell resistance can develop against an alkylating agent, which would impart cross-resistance to other drugs in this category.

Unwanted effects

Bone marrow suppression is of rapid onset after administration of an alkylating agent. Lymphocytopenia and thrombocytopenia occur at six to eight days after the start of therapy. Amenorrhoea and impairment of spermatogenesis usually follow a course of treatment. Alopecia, due to damage of the hair follicles, and damage to the epithelial lining of the gastro-intestinal mucosa, are common unwanted effects. Alkylating agents are potent stimulants of the CNS, and nausea and vomiting frequently accompany therapy.

Specific alkylating agents

Mechlorethamine is a nitrogen mustard that can only be given intravenously as it produces local tissue necrosis if given intramuscularly. The drug is mainly used in the treatment of Hodgkin's disease and other lymphomas.

Cyclophosphamide is a cyclic mustard that can be given orally or parenterally. It is probably the most widely used chemotherapeutic agent, either solely or in combination with other drugs. Cyclophosphamide has achieved good results in Hodgkin's disease, lymphosarcoma, leukaemia, and Burkitt's lymphoma.

Chlorambucil is a derivative of mechlorethamine; it is well-absorbed when given orally. The drug is useful in the treatment of chronic lymphocytic leukaemia, Hodgkin's disease, and malignant lymphomas.

Bisulphan an alkyl sulphonate, is the treatment of choice in chronic granulocytic leukaemia.

Nitrosureas are alkylating agents that have attracted special interest because of their high lipid solubility, and hence their ability to cross the blood–brain barrier. These drugs are useful in the treatment of brain tumours and the infiltration of leukaemic cells into the meninges (meningeal leukaemia).

Antimetabolites

These can be calssified according to the substrate they antagonize, i.e. folic acid, pyrimidine, and purine.

Folic acid analogues

Methotrexate is the principal folic acid analogue. *In vivo*, folic acid is metabolized to tetrahydrofolic acid by the enzyme, dihydrofolate reductase. Tetrahydrofolic acid is essential for the synthesis of purines, pyrimides, and nucleic acids. Methotrexate binds irreversibly to dihydrofolate reductase (Osborn *et al.* 1958), and this binding indirectly inhibits such synthesis.

Pharmacological properties and uses

Methotrexate destroys cells during the S phase of the cell cycle. The drug can be given orally, and about 50 per cent is bound to plasma proteins (albumin). Hence other drugs that also bind to albumin, such as salicylates, tetracyclines, and sulphonamides, should be avoided in those already receiving methotrexate therapy.

The binding of methotrexate can be reversed by folinic acid, and normal tissues can be protected from methotrexate by thymidine. Such findings have led to the introduction of 'rescue techniques', which allow the use of very high doses of methotrexate that can subsequently be reversed by folinic acid. These techniques have enabled methotrexate to be used against very resistant tumours.

Methotrexate is useful in the treatment of acute lymphoblastic leukaemia. Other tumours that show a good response are carcinoma of the breast, tongue, and pharynx. The 'rescue technique' has produced effective results in carcinoma of the lung and in osteosarcoma. Methotrexate is also used in the treatment of severe psoriasis (McDonald 1981), Wegener's granulomatosis, hydatidiform moles, and mycosis fungoides.

Unwanted effects

Leukopenia and thrombocytopenia due to aplasia of the bone marrow are the serious unwanted effects associated with methotrexate therapy. Troublesome oral ulceration and diarrhoea may occur in some patients, and often requires an alteration or interruption of dose regimes.

Pyrimidine analogues

These analogues, such as fluorouracil and cytarabine, affect the synthesis of pyrimidine nucleotides and other nucleic acids. Both drugs are usually administered intravenously and are of palliative value in the treatment of a variety of malignant conditions. Topical application of fluorouracil has been shown to be effective in the treatment of both premalignant keratosis and basal cell carcinoma of skin (Klien *et al.* 1972).

Unwanted effects of pyrimidine analogues include anorexia, nausea, diarrhoea, and a severe stomatitis with sloughing and ulceration of the oral mucous membrane. Suppression of bone marrow activity is also very common and produces a neutropenia and thrombocytopenia.

Purine analogues

These are widely used, either as chemotherapeutic agents or as immunosuppressants; examples include mercaptopurine and azathioprine. Their precise mechanism of action in producing cell death is not clearly established. It is suggested that they inhibit purine nucleotide synthesis and alter the synthesis of both DNA and RNA (Elion and Hitchings 1965).

Mercaptopurine is effective when given orally, and is useful in treating most types of leukaemia. It does cause bone marrow suppression, but the onset is gradual.

Azathioprine is widely used as an immunosuppressant in kidney transplant, idiopathic thrombocytopenic purpura, and systemic lupus erythematosus. Infection is a common complication associated with immunosuppressant therapy (see Chapter 10).

Natural products

Vinca alkaloids

These are derived from the periwinkle plant (*Vinca rosea*); examples include vincristine and vinblastine.

Pharmacological properties and uses

Vinca alkaloids block mitosis at the metaphase by binding to tubulin, an essential protein component of cellular microtubules (George *et al.* 1965). Vincristine and vinblastine are given intravenously and, in certain circumstances, they can be infused into the arterial blood supply of a tumour.

These alkaloids are used in a variety of neoplastic conditions, such as Hodgkin's disease, leukaemias, carcinoma of the breast, and tumours of the reproductive system. Vinblastine is also used to treat neuroblastomas and Letterer–Siwe disease (histiocytosis X).

Unwanted effects

Leukopenia is the most serious unwanted effect associated with the vinca alkaloids. Vincristine therapy is accompanied by a high incidence of neurological disturbances, which include muscular weakness, tremors, numbness, and tingling of the extremities. Mood changes can occur on the second or third day of therapy.

Antibiotics

These interfere with bacterial cell division, cell wall synthesis, or intracellular protein synthesis (see Chapter 10); and some have been shown to have antineoplastic properties.

Actinomycin D

This antibiotic is obtained from streptomyces; it binds with DNA, which in turn prevents RNA synthesis (Franklin 1963). It can only be given intravenously and is probably the most potent chemotherapeutic agent in use today. Actinomycin D is used in the treatment of rhabdomyosarcoma, Wilm's tumour, Ewing's sarcoma, and Kaposi's sarcoma.

Unwanted effects include nausea, vomiting, and pancytopenia. Glossitis, cheilitis, and oral ulceration commonly occur one to seven days after completion of treatment.

Bleomycin

This is a fermentation product of *Streptomyces vorticillus*; several different congeners have been prepared. The cytotoxic properties of bleomycin are through its ability to fragment the DNA molecule by chain scission (Suzuki *et al.* 1969). It is usually administered intravenously as oral absorption is poor. This antibiotic is useful in the treatment of squamous cell carcinoma of the head and neck, oesophagus, skin, and genito-urinary tract.

In contrast to other chemotherapeutic agents, bleomycin causes minimal depression of bone marrow activity. Unwanted effects include stomatitis, alopecia, and ulceration and vesiculation of the skin. Pulmonary toxicity, which can be fatal, occurs in five to ten per cent of patients receiving this drug.

Mithramycin

This antibiotic is isolated from *Streptomyces tanashiensis*, it inhibits the synthesis of RNA. Mithramycin has a specific effect on osteoclasts and lowers plasma calcium concentrations (Robins and Jowsey 1973); hence, its main use is in the treatment of bone metastases. Mithramycin has also been used in the treatment of Paget's disease of bone. Haemorrhagic diatheses are the serious unwanted effects associated with this drug, which may limit its use.

Enzymes

The only enzyme that is used as a chemotherapeutic agent is L-asparaginase, which is produced by the bacterium *E. coli*.

L-*Asparaginase.*

L-Asparagine is an amino acid that is essential for cell protein synthesis. The enzyme, L-asparaginase, catalyses the hydrolysis of L-asparagine into aspartic acid and ammonia. Hence, malignant cells are unable to synthesize proteins and die. The main advantage of L-asparaginase is its minimal effect on bone marrow and epithelial tissue, such as the oral mucosa, hair follicles, and the lining of the gut. However, it has unwanted effects on the liver, kidneys, pancreas, and clotting mechanisms, which may limit its use. L-asparaginase is solely used in the treatment of acute lymphoblastic leukaemia.

Hormones

The pharmacological properties of the various hormones are dealt with in Chapter 18; only the use of hormones in the treatment of neoplastic disease will be considered in this section. Adrenocorticosteroids. oestrogen, progesterone, and testosterone are the principal hormones so used.

Adrenocorticosteroids

Of the several synthetic adrenocorticosteroids used to treat neoplastic disease, prednisolone is the most widely deployed. This drug is usually given orally up to dosages of 100 mg/day. Adrenocorticosteroids suppress mitosis in lymphocytes; hence they are extensively used in the treatment of acute leukaemia, particularly in children. These drugs are also used to suppress some of the unwanted effects that accompany other types of cancer therapy. For example, they will suppress oedema associated with radiotherapy, and will reduce pain and fever, and restore appetite. They also produce a feeling of well-being, which is beneficial in the critically ill patient. Unwanted effects of steroid therapy are discussed in Chapter 18.

Progestogens

Progestogens are used for the treatment of carcinoma of the breast in post-menopausal women. If given to women who are still able to menstruate, progestogens may accelerate the neoplastic process. They can be administered orally, and have a slow onset of action. Nausea, vomiting, and diarrhoea are the common unwanted effects; hypercalcaemia and ectopic calcification can occur if progestogens are given together with an adrenocorticosteroid.

Oestrogen

Oestrogen therapy is mainly associated with the treatment of carcinoma of the prostate. Diethylstilboestrol is the oestrogen widely used in this condition, and this drug has greatly improved the life expectancy of patients with this disease. Like adrenocorticosteroids, oestrogen also causes an increase in appetite, weight gain, and an improvement in well-being. Sexual impotence and gynaecomastia are the main unwanted effects.

Radioactive isotopes

Radioactive iodine (^{131}I) and sodium phosphate (^{32}P) are the main isotopes used in the treatment of neoplastic disease.

Radioactive iodine

The half-life of ^{131}I is eight days; the isotope emits both X-rays and β-particles. It is used for a variety of diagnostic procedures related to thyroid function, and also to treat metastatic thyroid cancer. If thyroid metastases accumulate iodine, then therapy with large doses of ^{131}I may prolong life. It is particularly effective in young children (Leeper 1973).

Sodium phosphate

This has a half-life of 14 days, and emits β-particles. The isotope can be given orally or parenterally; ^{32}P will enter those tissues with a high metabolic turnover of phosphate, as in neoplastic cells, bone marrow, spleen, lymph nodes, and bone. However, it has been replaced by other chemotherapeutic agents for, in some instances, the isotope has induced malignant change in bone marrow tissues.

ORAL AND DENTAL PROBLEMS ASSOCIATED WITH CHEMOTHERAPY

Many of the chemotherapeutic agents cause unwanted effects that manifest themselves in the mouth and related structures. The oral epithelium has a rapid cell turnover and is therefore very susceptible to the cell destructive properties of these drugs (Guggenheimer *et al.* 1977). In addition, the oral bacterial flora is large, and the mouth is important as a potential portal of entry for infective agents in those with suppressed bone-marrow activity.

Common problems that accompany chemotherapy are oral ulceration and stomatitis (due to an atrophic thinning of the oral mucosa), xerostomia, infection, gingivitis, pain, and haemorrhage (Sonis *et al.* 1978).

Management

Many of these oral and dental problems can be reduced or alleviated by certain pre-treatment measures. Oral hygiene should be meticulous in these patients, which will reduce the incidence of gingival problems (Beck 1979). All potential sources of infection, such as periapical inflammatory lesions, impacted third molars, periodontal pockets, and carious cavities, should be treated. Sharp cusps or restorations should be smoothed to avoid trauma to the oral mucosa.

Stomatitis and oral ulceration

Benzocaine lozenges or lignocaine gel may provide sufficient surface analgesia to make eating more comfortable Secondary infection of the ulcers can be reduced by using a chlorhexidine mouthwash 0.2 per cent. If the ulcers become infected, a tetracycline mouthwash together with an antifungal agent should be used both topically and then swallowed.

Xerostomia

Saliva substitutes (such as carboxymethylcellulose) may be of some use in those with xerostomia, or regular use of lemon drops may encourage salivary flow. There should be treatment with a topical fluoride to prevent xerostomia-induced dental caries. Angular cheilitis often accompanies xerostomia and should be treated with an appropriate anti-fungal agent, such as nystatin ointment or miconazole cream.

Oral infection

Chemotherapeutic agents used in the treatment of neoplastic disease often produce a neutropenia and subsequent oral infections are common. Candidiasis and herpes labialis are the most frequent of these. Candidiasis should be treated with an antifungal agent, and herpes labialis should respond to an antiviral agent, such as idoxuridine or acyclovir (see Chapter 10).

Gingival and mucosal bleeding

Haemorrhage associated with chemotherapy is invariably due to bone marrow suppression and the resultant thrombocytopenia. Mild cases of bleeding may respond to systemic aminocaproic acid. Severe haemorrhage should be treated by platelet transfusion (Lockhart 1983).

Pain

Patients on chemotherapy often complain of pain in the teeth and jaws. It is essential to eliminate any causative dental factors; if there is no dental cause, the pain will resolve on cessation of treatment. Pain associated with chemotherapy may respond to a peripherally acting analgesic, the type and dosage of which should be tailored to the individual patient.

REFERENCES

Beck, S. (1979). Impact of a systematic oral care protocol on stomatitis after chemotherapy. *Cancer Nursing*, **2**, 185–99.

Elion, G. B. and Hitchings, G. H. (1985). Metabolic basis for the actions of analogs of purines and pyrimidines. *Advances in Chemotherapy*, **2**, 91–177.

Franklin, R. M. (1963). The inhibition of ribonucleic acid synthesis in mammalian cells by actinomycin D. *Biochemica et Biophysica Acta*, **72**, 555–65.

George, P., Journey, L. J., and Goldstein, M. N. (1965). Effects of vincristine on the fine structure of Hela cells during mitosis. *Journal of the National Cancer Institute*, **35**, 355–75.

Guggenheimer, J., Verbin, R. S., Appel, B. N., and Schmitz, J. (1977). Clinicopathological effects of cancer chemotherapeutic agents on human buccal mucosa. *Oral Surgery*, **44**, 58–63.

Klein, E., Milgrom, H., Stoll, H. L., Helm, F., Walker, H. J., and Holtermann, O. A. (1972). Topical 5-fluorouracil chemotherapy and malignant epidermal neoplasia. In *Cancer chemotherapy*, II (ed. I. Brodsky and S. G. Kahn), pp. 146–66. Grune and Stratton, New York.

Leeper, R. D. (1973). The effect of ^{131}I therapy on survival of patients with metastatic pupillary or follicular thyroid carcinoma. *Journal of Clinical and Endocrinological Medicine*, **36**, 1143–52.

Lockhart, P. G. (1983). Dental management of patients receiving chemotherapy. In *Oral complications of cancer chemotherapy* (ed. D. E. Peterson and S. T. Sonis), pp. 113–49. Martinus Nijhoff, The Hague.

McDonald, C. J. (1981). The uses of systemic chemotherapeutic agents in psoriasis. *Pharmacology and Therapeutics*, **14**, 1–24.

Osborn, M. J., Freeman, M., and Heunnekens, F. M. (1958). Inhibition of dihydrofolic reductase by aminopterin and amethopterin. *Proceedings of the Society for Experimental Biology and Medicine*, **97**, 429–31.

Price, C. C. (1975). Chemistry of alkylation. In *Antineoplastic and immunosuppressive agents*, part II, (ed. A. C. Sartorelli and D. G. Johns), pp. 1–5. Springer–Verlag, Berlin.

Robins, P. R. and Jowsey, J. (1973). The effect of mithramycin on normal and abnormal bone turnover. *Journal of Laboratory and Clinical Medicine*, **82**, 576–86.

Sonis, S. T., Sonis, A. L., and Lieberman, A. (1978). Oral complications in patients receiving treatment for malignancies other than of the head and neck. *Journal of the American Dental Association*, **97**, 468–72.

Suzuki, H., Nagai, K. Yamaki, H., Tanaka, N., and Umezewa, H. (1969). On the mechanism of action of bleomycin: scission of D.N.A. steroids *in vitro* and *in vivo*. *Journal of Antibiotics*, **22**, 446–8.

18

The endocrine system

INTRODUCTION

Endocrine glands secrete hormones, which regulate cellular metabolism and maintain homeostatis. Hormones are defined as substances secreted by specific tissues and transported to a distant tissue where they exert their effect. The endocrine system is mostly regulated by the pituitary gland, which comprises a glandular component (adenohypophysis) and a neural component (neurohypophysis). Trophic hormones are produced by the adenohypophysis, which in turn regulates the activity of other endocrine glands. The secretion of trophic hormones is controlled by specific releasing factors from the hypothalamus. Production of these factors and of trophic hormones is controlled by a feedback mechanism from circulating hormones. The neurohypophysis stores and releases hormones that are produced in the hypothalamus.

NEUROHYPOPHYSEAL HORMONES

The neurohypophysis secretes two hormones, antidiuretic hormones (ADH; vasopressin) and oxytocin. Both are synthesized in the hypothalamus and transported along nerve fibres to be stored in the posterior lobe of the pituitary gland.

Antidiuretic hormone (ADH)

This affects the distal tubules and collecting ducts of the kidney, and increases water absorption. Secretion of ADH is controlled by hypothalamic neurones that act as osmoreceptors. A high plasma osmotic pressure and a low blood volume stimulate secretion of ADH. Nicotine, alcohol, morphine and physical and emotional stress also influence ADH secretion.

This hormone is used to treat diabetes insipidus. It cannot be given orally because it is destroyed by trypsin in the alimentary tract. It is a potent vasoconstrictor and, at high dose, ADH is sometimes used to arrest haemorrhage from oesophageal varices. A derivative of vasopressin is felypressin, which is used as a vasoconstrictor with the local anaesthetic agent, prilocaine (see Chapter 7).

Oxytocin

This octapeptide is synthesized in the paraventricular nucleus of the hypothalamus. It is released from the posterior pituitary gland following suckling of the breast or uterine stretching. Oxytocin acts on the myoepithelial cells of the mammary glands, causing contraction and milk ejection. The hormone also acts on the smooth muscle of the uterus, initiating contraction; it is widely believed that oxytocin initiates labour and parturition. The main therapeutic use of oxytocin is in obstetrics to stimulate contraction of the uterus and induce labour.

ADENOHYPOPHYSEAL HORMONES

The anterior pituitary gland secretes the following trophic hormones: adrenocorticotrophic hormone (ACTH), thyroid-stimulating hormone (TSH), follicle-stimulating hormone (FSH), and leutenizing hormone (LH). These trophic hormones are discussed under the sections relating to the various glands upon which they act.

   Prolactin and growth hormone are also secreted by the anterior pituitary and are discussed now.

Growth hormone

Growth hormone is a peptide that is synthesized and stored in specific cells, known as somatotrophs, in the anterior pituitary gland. The secretion of growth hormone is controlled by two regulating factors produced in the hypothalamus— growth hormone releasing factor and growth hormone inhibiting factor (somatostatin). Plasma concentrations of growth hormone are reduced by food, and increased by fasting, during sleep and physical exercise, and at times of stress and emotional excitement.

Pharmacological and physiological actions

Growth hormone affects growth, protein synthesis, and carbohydrate metabolism.

Growth

The hormone is essential for normal growth and development. A lack of production during the growth period will cause dwarfism; excessive production in a child will cause gigantism and, in an adult, acromegaly. Many of the actions of growth hormone on tissue size are mediated by its effects on sulphation factors or somatomedins. Somatomedins are growth-promoting factors produced by the liver and kidneys. They occur in serum and are activated by growth hormone. Examples of somatomedins are nerve growth factor, epidermal growth factor, fibroblast growth factor, and erythropoietin.

Protein synthesis
Growth hormone increases the transport of amino acids into tissues, and accelerates their incorporation into proteins. This action results in a reduction of blood urea levels due to a diversion of amino acids into anabolic pathways.

Carbohydrate and lipid metabolism
Growth hormone, insulin and, to a lesser extent, corticosteroids, glucagon, and catecholamines, play important roles in carbohydrate and lipid metabolism. Insulin and growth hormone have opposite effects, with insulin utilizing glucose as a source of energy and growth hormone utilizing fat. Hence it may appear that growth hormone has an antagonistic effect with insulin. The increased production of growth hormone during fasting may be an adaptation to lack of food. Growth hormone causes an increase in free fatty acids in the blood due to its lipolytic action on adipose tissue. This action may explain the increased secretion of the hormone that occurs during exercize, which will utilize fat deposits as an alternative source of energy.

Uses
Growth hormone is used to correct pituitary dwarfism.

Prolactin

This has a similar structure to growth hormone and is synthesized, stored, and secreted by lactotrophic cells in the anterior pituitary gland. Its principal action is on the development of the mammary glands and the production of milk. Prolactin is also produced by the placenta. The plasma concentration of prolactin increases throughout pregnancy. During breast feeding, prolactin production is controlled by the sucking stimulus.

Pharmacological and physiological properties
Prolactin is essential for the development of the mammary glands and their preparation for milk production. The hormone promotes proliferation and subsequent differentiation of mammary ductal and alveolar epithelium. In preparation for milk production, prolactin increases the synthesis of RNA, milk proteins, and enzymes necessary for lactose synthesis. Like growth hormone, production of prolactin is influenced by sleep, fasting, and stress.

THYROID HORMONES

The thyroid gland secretes three hormones, thyroxine, tri-iodothyroxine, and calcitonin, which is dealt with in Chapter 20. Secretion of thyroxine and tri-iodothyroxine are under the control of the anterior pituitary peptide, thyroid-stimulating hormone (TSH). Secretion of TSH is stimulated by the hypothalamic peptide, thyrotrophin-releasing hormone (TRH). The pituitary TSH increases the vascularity, cellularity, and size of the thyroid gland, and accelerates the synthesis and release of thyroid hormones. The production of TSH is inhibited by circulating levels of thyroxine and tri-iodothyroxine.

Thyroxine and tri-iodothyroxine

These two thyroid hormones are synthesized and stored as thyroglobulin in the thyroid gland. Synthesis and release of thyroid hormones involve the following processes:

(1) uptake of iodide ions by the gland;

(2) oxidation of iodide and iodination of *p*-tyrosyl groups of thyroglobulin;

(3) conversion of iodotyrosil to iodothyronyl;

(4) proteolysis of thyroglobulin and release of thyroxine and tri-iodothyronine into the blood stream;

(5) conversion of thyroxine to tri-iodothyronine in the tissues.

Thyroid hormones are strongly bound to plasma proteins (globulin and albumin). They are broken down in the liver, conjugated with glucuronic acid and sulphate, and excreted in the bile. In health, these hormones are slowly eliminated from the body and have a half-life of six to seven days.

Physiological and pharmacological properties

Thyroid hormones have three main functions: they regulate growth and development; they have a calorigenic and a metabolic effect.

Growth and development
They exert their effect on growth and development by controlling protein synthesis. They are also essential for the development of the nervous system, in particular, cell differentiation and proliferation.

Calorigenic effects
Thyroid hormones regulate body temperature (calorigenic effect) by controlling basal metabolic rate. They have a particular effect on the heart, lungs, liver, and kidneys. It is suggested that they exert their calorigenic effect by an action on the enzymes that control the sodium pump.

Metabolic effect

These hormones stimulate the metabolism of cholesterol to bile salts, and accelerate the utilization of carbohydrate for increased calorific demand.

Iodine

This element is essential for the formation of the thyroid hormones. Dietary iodine, in the form of iodide, is absorbed from the stomach and small intestine, transported in the blood, and taken up by the thyroid gland. Within the gland, iodide is oxidized to iodine and utilized to form thyroxine and tri-iodothyroxine. A deficiency of iodine causes non-toxic goitre, which usually responds to potassium iodide. Iodized salt is used to prevent this type of goitre, especially in areas of iodine deficiency.

Disorders of thyroid gland function

Hypofunction of the thyroid gland at birth results in cretinism and, in adults, causes myxoedema. Hypothyroidism is often associated with impairment of the normal immune response and those affected may be susceptible to oral candidiasis. Both cretinism and myxoedema are treated with thyroxine.

Hyperfunction of the thyroid gland (hyperthyroidism) can take the form of a diffuse toxic goitre (Graves' disease) or toxic nodular goitre (Plummer's disease). Signs and symptoms of hyperthyroidism include an intolerance to heat, muscle weakness, tremor, insomnia, anxiety, and an increased heart rate. The cardiovascular changes in hyperthyroidism may be due to an increased sensitivity of the heart to catecholamines. However, the small amount of adrenaline in local anaesthetic solutions is unlikely to cause a problem in those with hyperthyroidism.

Antithyroid drugs

These are used to treat hyperthyroidism; they inhibit the formation of the thyroid hormones by interfering with the incorporation of iodine into thyroxine and tri-iodothyroxine. Examples include carbimazole and propylthiouracil: both drugs can cause a leucopenia, so monitoring of white blood cells is important during therapy.

Potassium perchlorate is also used to treat hyperthyroidism by preventing the uptake and storage of iodine in the thyroid gland.

THE ADRENAL CORTEX

This part of the adrenal gland synthesizes and secretes mainly glucocorticoids and mineralocorticoids, together with small amounts of testosterone, oestrogen, and progesterone. Secretion of glucocorticoids is under the control of ACTH, whereas secretion of mineralocorticoids is controlled by the renin–angiotensin system.

Adrenocorticotrophic hormone (ACTH)

This peptide, secreted by the anterior pituitary gland (adenohypophysis), stimulates the adrenal cortex to secrete glucocorticoids (cortisol and corticosterone). It also stimulates the synthesis of adrenocortical hormones through the agency of the cyclic AMP. The release of ACTH is under dual control. One controlling element is the hypothalamus, which produces a peptide known as corticotrophin-releasing factor (CRF). This travels via the hypophyseal-portal vessel to the anterior pituitary and there stimulates the production of ACTH. The release of CRF is under neural control.

The second element controlling production and secretion of ACTH and CRF is a negative feedback regulatory influence from cortisol and other glucocorticoids. High levels of glucocorticoids suppress the secretion of ACTH and the converse applies with low levels. Production of ACTH also shows diurnal variation, with maximum levels occurring in the early morning and minimal levels at midnight.

This hormone is mainly used as a diagnostic agent in adrenal insufficiency.

Physiological and pharmacological properties of corticosteroids

Two types of steroids are synthesized in the adrenal cortex, the 19-carbon androgens and the 21-carbon corticosteroids; both are derived from cholesterol. The 21-carbon corticosteroids can be further classified into glucocorticoids (cortisol), because of their action on carbohydrate metabolism, and mineralocorticoids (aldosterone), because of their effect on sodium retention. However, the two types of corticosteroids possess both actions.

Aldosterone production is under the control of angiotensin acting on the adrenal cortex. The synthesis and secretion of all other corticosteroids is under control of ACTH. The corticosteroids are continuously synthesized and secreted, hence there is minimal storage in the adrenal cortex.

Corticosteroids have a diverse range of properties and functions. They are involved in carbohydrate, fat, and protein metabolism; they affect electrolyte and water balance; and they are essential for the normal function of the cardiovascular system, kidney, skeletal muscle, and nervous system. They also enable the organism to withstand changes in environment and cope with stressful events. The many different properties of the corticosteroids are due to their action on protein synthesis, especially RNA transcription and the production of specific proteins.

Carbohydrate and protein metabolism

Corticosteroids have the following effect on carbohydrate metabolism: they stimulate the formation of glucose; reduce the utilization of glucose in the peripheral tissues (perhaps by antagonizing the action of insulin); and promote the storage of glucose as glycogen. These actions ensure that the brain always has sufficient glucose for the essential glucose-dependent functions. Corticosteroids act on the liver and stimulate the synthesis of glucose from amino acids. They also inhibit protein synthesis in muscles and connective tissue, thus mobilizing additional amino acids. Therefore, the overall effect of corticosteroids is to cause an increase in blood sugar and liver glycogen content, and an increase in urinary nitrogen excretion. Hence long-term corticosteroid administration (see Other unwanted effects below) or high output from the adrenal cortex will cause protein wasting, resulting in an increase in capillary fragility, muscle wasting, and a reduction in the protein matrix of bone (osteoporosis).

Lipid metabolism

Corticosteroids have several actions on lipid metabolism. They inhibit fatty acid synthesis, but facilitate the mobilization of fatty acids from adipose tissue by lipolytic enzymes. They also have an effect on the distribution of body fat, with excessive production causing an increase in fatty acid deposits in the face (moon face) and on the back of the neck (buffalo hump).

Electrolyte and water balance

Corticosteroids affect this balance through a direct action on the kidney. They cause an increase in the urinary excretion of potassium and hydrogen ions, and enhanced reabsorption of sodium ions from the tubular fluid. These actions result in an increase in sodium retention, hypokalaemia, alkalosis, and an increase in extracellular fluid. Hence, excessive corticosteroid production or long-term use will cause oedema and hypertension. In patients with a pre-existing cardiac problem, long-term corticosteroid therapy will increase the incidence of left ventricular hypertrophy and congestive heart failure. Conversely, a deficiency of endogenous corticosteroids will cause sodium loss, a reduction in extracellular fluid, and cellular hydration.

Effects on blood

Excess corticosteroids cause an increase in red blood cells and their haemoglobin content, and an increase in polymorphs, whereas other white blood cells are reduced in number. A reduction in corticosteroid production will cause a normochromic, normocytic anaemia.

Immune system

Corticosteroids suppress immune reactions (Parillo and Fauci 1979) and are widely used in organ transplants to suppress graft rejection. The precise mechanism of corticosteroid immunosuppression is unknown. Possible modes of action may be an impairment of white blood-cell production and migration, or a reduction in lymphokine production from sensitized T-lymphocytes (see Chapter

21). Alternatively, corticosteroids may act on macrophages by inhibiting their ability to process antigens. The immunosuppressant properties of corticosteroids may also be closely linked to their anti-inflammatory actions (see Chapter 4).

Pharmacokinetics

Synthetic corticosteroids can be administered orally, topically, parenterally, and rectally. Some preparations are given into the synovial fluid. Corticosteroids are well-absorbed from any site of administration, and are transported in the plasma extensively bound to plasma protein. Most are broken down in the liver, conjugated with glucuronic acid, and excreted in the urine as the metabolites, 17-hydroxycorticosteroid and 17-ketohydroxycorticosteroid.

Unwanted effects of corticosteroids

Adrenocortical suppression

Long-term administration of corticosteroids causes suppression of the adeno-hypophysis–adrenal cortex axis, with a reduction in the production and release of ACTH. As a result, there is atrophy of the adrenal cortex, and the cortex cannot produce endogenous corticosteroids to cope with stress, so an adrenal crisis may develop. After cessation of corticosteroids, the return of adrenal function may take nine months (Graber *et al.* 1965). During this recovery period, and for an additional one to two years, patients with adrenocortical suppression will need to be protected with supplementary corticosteroids during stressful situations, such as dental surgical procedures and severe infections. The features and treatment of an adrenal crisis are dealt with in Chapter 24.

The extent of adrenocortical suppression will depend upon the type of steroid, its potency, dose, and duration of treatment. Adrenocortical suppression is not observed when corticosteroids are used for just a few weeks (Livanou *et al.* 1967).

Abrupt cessation of corticosteroid therapy can result in acute adrenal insufficiency, characterized by fever, joint and muscle pain, and malaise. Therefore, corticosteroid therapy should be slowly reduced over a long time.

Other unwanted effects

Alterations in carbohydrate metabolism can cause glycosuria, but this is usually controlled by diet. Altered protein metabolism may lead to an increase in capillary fragility causing ecchymosis, muscle wasting, and poor wound healing. Osteoporosis is a common unwanted effect of long-term corticosteroid therapy, especially in the elderly. Steroids produce hypocalcaemia by inhibiting calcium absorption and increasing urinary calcium excretion. The hypocalcaemia causes an increase in parathyroid hormone secretion, which in turn stimulates osteoclastic activity. Thus, there is both an increased resorption and decreased formation of bone (Hahn 1978). Steroid-induced osteoporosis commonly affects the spinal column and sometimes the mandible; spontaneous fractures of these and other bones may occur. The actions of corticosteroids on lipid metabolism will cause the characteristic 'moon face' and 'buffalo hump' (see Lipid metabolism above). Disturbances in electrolyte and water balance will cause hypokalaemia, oedema formation, hypertension, and alkalosis.

Immunosuppressive effects render the patient more susceptible to opportunistic infections, such as candidiasis, and to postoperative infections, the incidence of which can be reduced by prophylactic antibiotic cover prior to surgery. Topical or systemic corticosteroids should not be used for their anti-inflammatory properties if the underlying cause of the inflammation is infective. If corticosteroids are erroneously used in the presence of infection, they will mask its signs and permit it to spread.

Peptic ulceration is an occasional complication of corticosteroid therapy; it may be due to alterations in the mucosal cell's defence mechanisms.

Administration of corticosteroids can cause a feeling of well-being; however, long-term corticosteroid administration can cause certain behavioural disturbances, including insomnia, anxiety, mood changes, and even suicidal tendencies, the mechanisms of which are unknown.

Corticosteroids cause inhibition or arrest of growth in children because these drugs inhibit DNA synthesis and cell division.

Uses

They are particularly used for their anti-inflammatory and anti-allergic properties in various medical conditions exemplified by rheumatoid arthritis, nephrotic syndrome, collagen diseases, allergic states, ocular disease, skin disease, ulcerative colitis, and certain malignancies. Corticosteroids are also for substitution therapy in patients with adrenal insufficiency. Their use in dentistry is discussed in Chapter 4.

PANCREATIC HORMONES

The islets of the pancreas produce two hormones that are essential for glucose metabolism; the β-cells synthesize and secrete insulin, and the α-cells synthesize and secrete glucagon. The secretion of insulin and glucagon is controlled by blood glucose levels. A high glucose concentration stimulates the secretion of insulin, whereas a low concentration stimulates the release of glucagon. Thus both hormones control blood glucose levels and maintain a concentration of 100 mg/ml.

Insulin

This was first isolated in 1921 and used to treat diabetes (see below) in the following year. The insulin molecule is made up of two chains of amino acids, an acidic or A-chain, and a basic or B-chain. Insulin is synthesized in β-islet cells from the precursor, pro-insulin, which in turn is derived from prepro-insulin. Proteolytic enzymes convert the pro-insulin to insulin, which is then released from the Golgi complex together with any unconverted pro-insulin and a superfluous C-peptide. Insulin secretion is stimulated by many factors including carbohydrates, fatty acids, amino acids, growth hormone, ACTH, thyroxine, and glucagon. Secretion of insulin is inhibited by insulin itself, somatostatin, α-adrenergic antagonists, and β-adrenergic blockers.

Pharmacokinetics

Insulin is broken down in the gastro-intestinal tract and hence can only be given parenterally. The hormone has a half-life of six to nine minutes, and is metabolized in both the liver and kidney to inactive peptides. The commercially available insulins show different pharmacokinetic properties, as listed below. All insulin preparations are available in different concentrations.

Soluble insuline   This has a short duration of action and is mainly used to treat diabetic emergencies; for example, ketoacidosis and hyperglycaemia.

Protamine zinc insulin   A long-acting insulin, which in some diabetics needs only to be administered once a day. However, the long duration of action may have an accumulative effect that could cause hypoglycaemia, especially at night.

Biphasic insulin   This contains porcine soluble insulin for an immediate effect, and slow-release bovine insulin, which increases the duration of action. Biphasic insulin is usually given twice a day, but can produce hyperglycaemia because of insufficient amounts of porcine soluble insulin.

Insulin zinc suspension   This is prepared either in the amorphous form, which is rapidly absorbed, or the crystalline form, which is slowly absorbed from the site of injection.

Pharmacological and physiological properties

Insulin controls the blood concentration of glucose by acting via receptors on cell membranes. Activation of receptors causes the following:

(1) an increase in the diffusion of glucose through cell membranes;

(2) an increase in the rate of glucose utilization;

(3) an increase in the rate of glycogen deposition;

(4) inhibition of hepatic gluconeogenesis.

Insulin also causes increases in cellular amino acid uptake, DNA and RNA synthesis, and oxidative phosphorylation.

Insulin requirements increase during pregnancy, prolonged exercize, severe infections, and stress.

Unwanted effects of insulin

The most serious of these is hypoglycaemia, which can be fatal if not promptly recognized and treated. The clinical features and management of hypoglycaemia are discussed in Chapter 24.

Insulin is a protein and so antibodies can develop against it, which will give rise to local or systemic allergic reactions. However, the incidence of such reactions is falling due to the development of very pure insulin preparations.

Repeated insulin injections at the same site can cause lipodystrophy and swelling. This problem can be overcome by regularly changing the site of injection.

Diabetes mellitus

This disorder of glucose metabolism is due to insufficient production of insulin or glucagon or both. A lack of insulin will cause a rise in blood glucose levels due to increased gluconeogenesis and decreased glucose uptake. Fat metabolism is also altered with an increase in lipase activity and a decrease in triglyceride synthetase activity. Both altered enzyme activities result in an increase in blood levels of unesterified fatty acids. The excess fatty acids are metabolized by acetyl coenzyme A, which results in the formation of ketone bodies, so causing the metabolic acidosis that often accompanies hyperglycaemia. The increase in blood glucose, fatty acids, and their metabolites contributes to the polyuria and dehydration that is so often an early sign of the disease.

Diabetes, depending upon the severity, can be controlled by diet alone, diet and insulin, or diet and oral hypoglycaemic drugs.

Dental problems associated with diabetic patients

Patients with diabetes are more susceptible to periodontal disease and excessive periodontal destruction (Cohen *et al.* 1970). White blood cells (especially polymorphs) from diabetics show impaired chemotactic and phagocytic activities, which may enhance periodontal breakdown (McCullen *et al.* 1981). Poorly controlled diabetics may suffer from xerostomia and candidiasis. Diabetics are more prone to infections and should perhaps receive prophylactic antibiotics prior to a dental surgical procedure.

The main problem with diabetics in dentistry is that dental treatment may interrupt their food intake and insulin requirements, especially if a general anaesthetic is to be administered. Several dental infections may also cause hazards with the insulin-controlled diabetic; such infections should be treated promptly. Monitoring of blood sugar and urine is essential to ensure that diabetics do not become hypo- or hyperglycaemic as a consequence of the infection.

Dental procedures and simple oral surgical procedures under local anaesthesia are usually well-tolerated by diabetic patients. Treatment should ideally be in the morning and not interfere with meal times. Management of diabetic patients prior to a general anaesthetic will depend upon their current therapy. Those controlled by diet alone can usually tolerate a general anaesthetic for minor oral surgical procedures. Regular monitoring of their urine and blood sugar levels is essential, and soluble insulin should be available if hyperglycaemia develops. If the diabetic is controlled by oral hypoglycaemic drugs (see below), they should be admitted to hospital two days before the procedure and placed on insulin. Those on insulin therapy should also be admitted to hospital two days before the procedure and placed on soluble insulin. During surgery, patients are infused with 3 units of soluble insulin per hour and glucose solution at the rate of 6 g/hour. This regime is continued until normal feeding and soluble insulin control can be resumed.

All diabetic patients must be treated in a hospital environment if general anaesthetics are being administered. Changes in their insulin regime should only be made in consultation with their physician. Because diabetics are more prone to infection they should receive prophylactic antibiotic cover for minor oral surgical procedures.

Oral hypoglycaemic drugs

Oral drugs used to control hypoglycaemia are of two types, sulphonylureas and biguanides.

Sulphonylureas

These stimulate islet tissues to secrete insulin by causing degranulation of the β-cells. Their action therefore depends upon the pancreas having some ability to synthesize and secrete insulin. Examples of sulphonylureas are tolbutamide, tolazamide, and chlorpropamide.

Pharmacokinetics

All sulphonylureas are well-absorbed from the gastro-intestinal tract and differences between individual drugs relate to their duration of action. Tolbutamide is taken every six to eight hours whereas chlorpropamide is given only once a day.

Unwanted effects

There is a high incidence of these, the most serious being hypoglycaemia. Other unwanted effects include skin rashes, gastro-intestinal disturbances, jaundice, and haemopoietic changes. Alcohol interacts with the sulphonylureas causing an enhancement of their hypoglycaemic effect. Aspirin reduces the urinary excretion of chlorpropamide and so increases plasma levels, which in turn would enhance the hypoglycaemic effect. Because aspirin also has an effect on blood sugar levels, this analgesic should not be given to patients on chlorpropamide.

Biguanides

It is not clearly established how the biguanides exert their hypoglycaemic effect. They may reduce glucose absorption from the gastro-intestinal tract or facilitate glucose entry into tissues, thus increasing glucose uptake by the peripheral tissues. The biguanides are rarely used as hypoglycaemic agents because of their high incidence of unwanted effects. These include nausea, vomiting, anorexia, and a metallic taste in the mouth. Examples of biguanides include metformin.

Glucagon

This is a single-chain polypeptide secreted by the α-cells of the islets. Secretion is mainly controlled by plasma glucose concentration, with a rise in plasma glucose inhibiting secretion and a fall facilitating secretion. Glucagon is broken down in the plasma, liver, and kidney; it has a plasma half-life of three to six minutes.

Physiological and pharmacological properties

Glucagon antagonizes the actions of insulin: whereas insulin acts as a hormone of glucose storage, glucagon is a hormone of glucose utilization. During fasting or starvation, there is an increase in glucagon secretion and an inhibition of insulin secretion. Glucagon breaks down food substances, which are then stored intracellularly for energy requirements of the brain and other essential tissues. Glucagon secretion is also increased after severe trauma and injury (for example, after burns). In such instances, glucagon stimulates gluconeogenesis and provides an essential supply of glucose.

SEX HORMONES

Hormonal production from the ovaries and testes is under the control of gonadotrophic hormones synthesized and secreted by the adenohypophysis. The gonadotrophic hormones are follicle-stimulating hormone (FSH) and luteinizing hormone (LH). The placenta also produces two gonadotrophins, chorionic gonadotrophin (CG) and chorionic follicle-stimulating hormone (CFSH). The function of CFSH is unknown.

Properties of FSH and LH

These are glycoproteins produced and secreted by cells in the adenohypophysis. The plasma concentrations of these hormones are low in infancy, but increase at puberty. Postpubertal concentrations of gonadotrophins vary in women according to the phase of their menstrual cycle. Gonadotrophins are mainly used for the treatment of infertility.

Action on the ovary

The FSH controls the development of ovarian follicles, stimulates granulosa cell proliferation, and increases oestrogen production; LH induces ovulation and initiates and maintains the corpus luteum.

Action on the testes

The FSH is responsible for spermatogenesis, whereas LH acts on Leydig calls to produce the hormone, testosterone, which is essential for the maturation of spermatocytes and the development of male secondary sexual characteristics.

Chorionic gonadotrophin (CG)

This is produced by syncytiotrophic cells of the placenta shortly after implantation; it maintains the corpus-luteum phase of the ovary, which forestalls the next menstrual cycle.

Female sex hormones

These are produced by the ovaries, and comprise the oestrogens (oestradiol-17β, oestrone, and oestriol) and progesterone. The production and excretion of the female sex hormones is under the control of the gonadotrophins, FSH and LH, with oestrogens exerting a negative feedback control on both these adenohypophyseal hormones.

Oestrogens

These steroids are synthesized in the ovary from acetate and cholesterol. There are three types of oestrogens, oestradiol-17β, oestrone and oestriol. The oestrogens are metabolized in the liver, and excreted as glucuronide and sulphate conjugates in the bile and urine. Oestrone and oestriol are derived from the potent oestradiol-17β by oxidation and hydration respectively.

Physiological and pharmacological properties
Oestrogens control the secondary female sexual characteristics, which occur from puberty onwards. Oestrogen production also plays an essential role in the menstrual cycle, with the cyclic decline in production bringing about menstruation.

High concentrations of oestrogens can cause bone resorption. The osteoporosis sometimes seen in post-menopausal women may be partly due to reduced oestrogen levels.

Many of the actions of oestrogens in the development of secondary sexual characteristics, the menstrual cycle, and pregnancy are often complementary with those of progesterone.

Progesterone

This is structurally similar to oestrogen; it is secreted by the ovary, mainly from the corpus luteum, during the second half of the menstrual cycle. Production of progesterone is under the control of LH.

Properties
Progesterone secretion causes the development of the secretory endometrium; abrupt cessation of progesterone from the corpus luteum determines the onset of menstruation. Progesterone is also important for the maintenance of pregnancy and in preparing the breast for milk production.

Uses

The main use of oestrogens and progesterone is the oral contraceptive pill (see below). Oestrogen is also used for replacement therapy where there is hypofunction of the ovaries. It is also used to treat certain neoplastic conditions, such as carcinoma of the prostate and breast (see Chapter 17). Progesterone is used for certain gynaecological conditions, which are beyond the scope of this book.

Women suffering from menstrually related oral aphthous ulceration have shown an improvement in their symptoms when treated with the contraceptive pill (Carruthers 1977) or progesterone (Ferguson et al. 1978).

The contraceptive pill

These usually contain a mixture of an oestrogen (ethinyloestradiol) and a progesterone (norethisterone). The oestrogen component suppresses ovulation by preventing the mid-cycle rise in LH (the trigger of ovulation). Progesterone produces changes in the endometrium that discourage implantation, and has a thickening effect on cervical mucus, thus making it impenetrable to sperm.

The combined pill is taken daily for 21 days, medication is then stopped for 7 days and the withdrawal of oestrogen produces uterine bleeding; the pill is restarted on day 28.

Unwanted effects
It is estimated that some 20 million women take the contraceptive pill, and many epidemiological studies have outlined the risks associated with this very effective method of contraception. The incidence of unwanted effects increases with age (especially in women over the age of 35), the length of time on the pill, and whether there is a history of smoking. Unwanted effects include:

(1) an increased risk of myocardial infarction and cerebral arterial thrombosis (Kaplan 1978; Mann et al. 1975);

(2) an increase in blood pressure by increasing renin substrate;

(3) an increase in the incidence of venous thrombosis and thromboembolism, due to an increase in blood clotting factors (Meade 1982);

(4) an increase in migraine attacks;

(5) precipitation of diabetes mellitus;

(6) cancer of the endometrium—this may increase in pill takers (Weiss and Sayvetz 1980; Vessey *et al.* 1983) but there is a decrease in breast lesions and ovarian cysts—however, the mortality associated with pregnancy and childbirth is greater than the risk of endometrial cancer.

Of dental significance is the effect of the contraceptive pill on the gingival tissues, which causes an enhancement of plaque-induced inflammation and an increase in gingival crevicular fluid (Lindhe and Attstrom 1967; Lindhe and Bjorn 1967). It has also been reported that women taking the contraceptive pill are more susceptible to 'dry socket' after tooth extraction (Catellani *et al.* 1980). They also have an increased incidence of radiopacities in the mandible (Darzenta and Giunta 1977).

Drug interactions
The widespread use of the contraceptive pill has implicated this drug in a number of interactions. Of concern to the dental surgeon is that between the pill and antibiotics, although there is recent evidence, detailed in Chapter 22, that suggests the problem has been over-stated. Oestrogen and progesterone are conjugated with glucuronide and extensively excreted in the bile. Once excreted, they may in part undergo entero-hepatic circulation, whereby the conjugates are broken down (hydrolyzed) by bacteria in the gut. Oestrogen and progesterone are released from the conjugate and absorbed through the bowel wall. Any antibiotic therapy that destroys the gut flora will subsequently impair the breakdown of the conjugated hormone; hence they will not be absorbed and the conjugate will be excreted in the faeces. Plasma levels of oestrogen and progesterone may be considerably reduced and the pill may be ineffective as a contraceptive.

Those antibiotics implicated in destruction of the gut flora and reduction of the pill's effectiveness include penicillin, ampicillin, co-trimoxazole, and the tetracyclines (Dossetor 1975; Bacon and Shenfield 1980). Thus, when these are prescribed to those on the contraceptive pill, they should be warned of the reduced efficacy of their oral contraceptive and additional alternative forms of contraception should be used.

Rifampicin and anticonvulsants also cause failure of oral contraceptives; both drugs induce hepatic microsomal enzymes, thereby decreasing the plasma concentration of the steroids (Back *et al.* 1980; Coulam and Annegers 1979).

Other drug interactions associated with the contraceptive pill are between it and coumarin anticoagulants. The pill increases levels of factor VII and reduces the efficacy of this group of anticoagulants. Also, anti-hypertensive and antidepressant therapy becomes less effective in pill takers; the mechanism for this interaction is uncertain.

The effect of female sex hormones on the oral mucosa

It is well-documented that puberty and pregnancy are associated with an increase in the incidence of gingival inflammation (Loe and Silness 1963; Cohen *et al.* 1969). Also, menopausal women frequently complain of sore mouths, which may be due to thinning (atrophy) of the epithelial lining of the oral mucosa.

The gingival changes in puberty and pregnancy may be due to progesterone causing an increase in vascular permeability (Hugoson 1970). The action of progesterone on vessel walls is uncertain. It has been suggested that this hormone affects the nature of the carbohydrate fraction associated with the vessel wall and ground substance. Alternatively, progesterone may enhance pore formation in the vessel wall, causing an increase in permeability and oedema formation. These gingival changes usually resolve after puberty and parturition.

Male sex hormones

The principal male sex hormone is testosterone, produced by the Leydig cells of the testes (90 per cent) and, to a lesser extent, by the adrenal cortex (10 per cent). Secretion of testosterone is stimulated by LH. Testosterone acts on a variety of tissues and, in most target tissues, is converted by the enzyme 5α-reductase to the more active hormone, dihydrotestosterone. Both testosterone and dihydrotestosterone are extensively bound to plasma protein and are inactivated in the liver.

Properties

Testosterone is essential for the development of the male secondary sexual characteristics. The hormone is also required for spermatogenesis, the maturation of sperm, and the production of seminal fluid. Testosterone has marked anabolic effects by causing the retention of nitrogen and an increase in protein synthesis. Hence, this hormone has been used in some sporting activities to encourage muscle development.

Uses

Testosterone is used in replacement therapy in cases of hypogonadism and to initiate puberty in those with a delayed onset of this state. When used injudiciously in women, testosterone will cause the development of male characteristics.

REFERENCES

Back, D. J. *et al.* (1980). The effect of rifampicin on the pharmacokinetics of ethinyloestradiol in women. *Contraception*, **21**, 135–43.

Bacon, J. F. and Shenfield, G. M. (1980). Pregnancy attributable to interaction between tetracycline and oral contraceptive. *British Medical Journal*, **1**, 293.

Carruthers, R. (1979). Recurrent aphthous ulcers. *Lancet*, **ii**, 259.

Catellani, J. E., Harvey, S., Erickson, S. H., and Cherkin, D. (1980). Effect of oral contraceptive cycle on dry socket (local alveolar osteitis). *Journal of the American Dental Association*, **101**, 777–80.

Cohen, D. W., Friedman, L., Shapiro, J., and Kyle, G. C. (1969). A longitudinal investigation of the periodontal changes during pregnancy. *Journal of Periodontology*, **40**, 563–70.

Cohen, W. D., Friedman, L. A., Shapiro, J., Kyle, C. G. and Franklin, S. (1970). Diabetes mellitus and periodontal disease: two year longitudinal observations. *Journal of Periodontology*, **41**, 709–12.

Coulam, C. B. and Annegers, J. F. (1979). Do anticonvulsants reduce the efficacy of oral contraceptives. *Epilepsia*, **20**, 519–26.

Darzenta, N. C. and Giunta, J. L. (1977). Radiographic changes of the mandible related to oral contraceptives. *Oral Surgery*, **43**, 478–81.

Dossetor, J. (1975). Drug interactions with oral contraceptives. *British Medical Journal*, **4**, 467–8.

Ferguson, M. M., McKay, H. D., Lindsay, R., and Stephen, K. W. (1978). Progesterone therapy for menstrually related aphthae. *International Journal of Oral Surgery*, **7**, 463–70.

Graber, A. L., Ney, R. L., Nicholson, W. E., Island, D. P., and Liddle, G. W. (1965). Natural history of pituitary-adrenal suppression with corticosteroids. *Journal of Clinical Endocrinology and Metabolism*, **25**, 11–6.

Hahn, T. J. (1978). Corticosteroid-induced osteopenia. *Archives of Internal Medicine*, **138**, 882–5.

Hugoson, A. (1970). Gingival inflammation and female sex hormones. A clinical investigation of pregnant women and experimental studies in dogs. *Journal of Periodontal Research*, **5** (suppl), 1–18.

Kaplan, N. M. (1978). Cardiovascular complications of oral contraceptives. *Annual Review of Medicine*, **29**, 245–76.

Lindhe, J. and Attstrom, R. (1967). Gingival exudation during the menstrual cycle. *Journal of Periodontal Research*, **2**, 194–8.

Lindhe, J. and Bjorn, A. L. (1967). Influence of hormonal contraceptives on the gingiva of women. *Journal of Periodontal Research*, **2**, 1–6.

Livanou, T., Ferriman, D., and James, V. H. T. (1967). Recovery of hypothalamic pituitary adrenal function after corticosteroid therapy. *Lancet*, **ii**, 856–9.

Loe, H. and Silness, J. (1963). Periodontal disease in pregnancy. I. Prevalence and severity. *Acta Odontologica Scandinavica*, **21**. 533–51.

Mann, J. I., Vessey, M. P., Thorogood, M., and Doll, R. (1975). Myocardial infarction in young women with special reference to oral contraceptive practice. *British Medical Journal*, **ii**, 241–5.

McCullen, J. A., Van Dyke, T. E., Horoszewicz, H., and Genco, R. J. (1981). Neutrophil chemotaxis in individuals with advanced periodontal disease and a genetic predisposition to diabetes mellitus. *Journal of Periodontology*, **52**, 167–73.

Meade, T. W. (1982). Oral contraceptives, clotting factors and thrombosis. *American Journal of Obstetrics and Gynecology*, **142**, 758–61.

Parillo, J. E. and Fauci, A. C. (1979). Mechanism of glucocorticoid action on immune processes. *Annual Review of Pharmacology and Toxicology*, **19**, 179–201.

Vessey, M. P., Lawless, M., McPherson, K., and Yeates, D. (1983). Neoplasia of the cervix uteri and contraception: a possible adverse effect of the pill. *Lancet*, **ii**, 930–4.

Weiss, N. S. and Sayvetz, T. A. (1980). Incidence of endometrial cancer in relation to the use of oral contraceptives. *New England Journal of Medicine*, **302**, 551–4.

19

Vitamins and minerals

INTRODUCTION

Vitamins are organic substances that must be provided in small quantities in the diet for the synthesis, by tissues, of co-factors essential for a variety of metabolic reactions. Vitamins can be classified as either water-soluble (B and C) or fat-soluble (A, D, E and K). Normal human requirements and sources of the various vitamins are shown in Table 19.1. Vitamin D is considered in Chapter 20.

Iron is essential for many of the body's functions and occurs in a variety of forms in the earth's crust.

Table 19.1. Daily requirements and food sources of the various vitamins

Vitamin	Daily requirements	Food sources
A	2 mg	Dairy products, fish liver oils,
B$_1$ (thiamine)	2 mg	Cereals, meat, kidneys, eggs
B$_2$ (riboflavin)	3 mg	Cereal germ, meat, liver, kidney, milk
Nicotinic acid	20 mg	Liver, yeast
B$_6$ (pyridoxine)		Cereals, liver
Folic acid	5 mg	Green vegetables, salad, yeast
B$_{12}$	1 μg	Liver, lean meat
C	10–30 mg	Citrus fruits, potatoes, green vegetables
D	500 i.u.	Dairy products. Action of sunlight on skin.
K	Adequate supply from gut bacterial flora	Green vegetables, salads

VITAMIN A

A night blindness that could be corrected by diet was first described about 1500 BC; however, it was not until 1923 that this type of night blindness was associated with a deficiency of vitamin A. There are several variants and sources of vitamin A. Vitamin A$_1$ (retinol) is present in fish and meat. The plant pigment, carotene, is a pro-vitamin that is rapidly converted to vitamin A in the body.

Properties and functions

Vitamin A has many important properties: it is essential for the normal function of the retina; for the growth and differentiation of epithelial tissues; and for bone growth and embryonic development. These different functions are mediated by different forms of the vitamin A molecule, which are collectively known as the retinoids (e.g. retinal, retinol, and retonic acid). Retinal is essential for normal vision, whereas retinol is important in the reproductive process. There has been considerable interest in the apparent ability of the retinoids to interfere with carcinogenesis. Animal experiments have shown that a deficiency of vitamin A can result in marked epithelial hyperplasia and reduced cellular differentiation, changes that may be associated with premalignancy. These changes are reversed when vitamin A is restored to the diet. However, in man, severe toxicity is associated with excessive use of this vitamin.

A variety of food substances contain vitamin A, and ideal sources are shown in Table 19.1. Supplementary doses of vitamin A are given orally in the form of halibut liver-oil capsules. The vitamin is well absorbed from the gastro-intestinal tract, and any excess is stored in the liver. The storage of vitamin A is enhanced by vitamin E.

Deficiency

Dietary deficiency of vitamin A leads to retarded growth and development. The first sign of this is often impaired vision in dim light, a condition known as nyctalopia (night blindness). Other signs include hyperkeratosis of the skin, impaired renal function, and urinary calculi. Severe deficiency results in faulty modelling of bone; diarrhoea also occurs due to alteration in the epithelial lining of the gastro-intestinal tract.

Deficiency of vitamin A is commonly seen in undernourished populations from the Third World. Deficiency also occurs in patients with chronic diseases that affect fat absorption, such as colitis, sprue, and diseases of the biliary tract.

Hypervitaminosis A

Acute poisoning with vitamin A has been reported following consumption of polar bear liver, but is more commonly associated with accidental overdose in children. Signs and symptoms include drowsiness, headache, vomiting, papilloe-dema, and peeling of the skin. Chronic overdose can result in vomiting, loss of appetite, dryness of the skin, gingivitis, and angular cheilitis. Hyperostoses of the skull can occur with long-term consumption of excess vitamin A. Hypervitamino-sis A can be overcome by increasing the intake of vitamin E.

Uses

Vitamin A is used to correct deficiency states and as a prophylaxis during periods of increased requirements, which may occur in pregnancy, lactation, and infancy. Topical retinoic acid is used in the treatment of acne to promote healing.

Large single doses of vitamin A are used to treat certain skin diseases, such as psoriasis and Darier's disease.

THE VITAMIN B COMPLEX

This comprises 11 different chemical compounds, all of which are found in yeast and liver. Dietary deficiency often involves several components of the B complex in the same patient.

Thiamine (vitamin B$_1$)

This occurs in numerous plants and animal foods (Table 19.1), especially in the husks and coatings of many grain cereals. In the body, thiamine is converted to thiamine pyrophosphate, which then acts as an important co-enzyme in carbohydrate metabolism. Thiamine requirements are directly related to carbohydrate utilization and metabolic rate. The body is unable to store thiamine and a poor diet will lead to signs of deficiency within two weeks.

Deficiency

Thiamine deficiency causes beri-beri, a disease mainly confined to the Far East, where it is due to consumption of polished rice. In Western countries, thiamine deficiency is often seen in alcoholics and, occasionally, in pregnancy and infancy. Early signs of deficiency include a peripheral neuritis with areas of hyperaesthesia and anaesthesia, and a reduction in muscle strength. Severe deficiency will lead to cardiovascular changes, which include dyspnoea on exertion, palpitations, and tachycardia.

Uses

Thiamine is only used to correct deficiency states. If the deficiency is severe, then it should be given intravenously; however most cases can be corrected by giving the vitamin orally.

Riboflavin (vitamin B$_2$)

This occurs naturally as the yellow respiratory enzyme found in yeast. In the body, riboflavin is converted into two co-enzymes, flavine mononucleotide and flavine dinucleotide, both of which are essential for the respiratory electron transport of protein.

Deficiency

Early signs of riboflavin deficiency include sore throats and angular cheilitis. These are followed by a glossitis and cheilosis (sore and red lips). In extreme cases there is a generalized dermatitis, anaemia, and neuropathy. Deficiency states can be corrected by an oral dose of 5 to 10 mg daily.

Nicotinic acid

This is found mainly in liver and yeast, and functions in the body after conversion to the co-enzymes, nicotinamide adenine dinucleotide or nicotinamide adenine dinucleotide phosphate. Both co-enzymes catalyse a variety of oxidation–reduction reactions that are essential for respiration.

Deficiency

Lack of nicotinic acid causes pellagra, a disease found in countries where large quantities of maize are eaten. Early signs of deficiency include a generalized dermatitis and stomatitis; severe deficiency causes an enteritis and dementia. Deficiency states can be corrected by a daily oral dose of 50 mg of nicotinic acid.

Pyridoxine (vitamin B_6)

Pyridoxine, pyridoxal, and pyridoxamine are the three naturally occurring forms of vitamin B_6. All three forms are converted in the body to pyridoxal phosphate, which acts as a co-enzyme in the various stages of amino acid metabolism. Pyridoxine occurs naturally in various cereals and liver.

Deficiency

Vitamin B_6 deficiency is common in alcoholics, and produces a glossitis, seborrhoea, fits, and peripheral neuropathy. Signs of deficiency can also occur in tuberculosis patients taking isoniazid, and patients taking hydralizine, as both drugs interfere with the pyridoxine metabolism.

Biotin

This organic acid is found in egg yolk and yeast. Like most of the vitamins in the B complex, biotin is also a co-enzyme and catalyses several carboxylation reactions. The co-enzyme also plays an important role in carbon dioxide fixation. Hence biotin is essential for carbohydrate and fat metabolism.

Deficiency

Signs of biotin deficiency include dermatitis, an atrophic glossitis, hyperaesthesia, and muscle pain. Biotin deficiency can occur in new-born babies, and is readily corrected by daily oral doses of 5 to 10 mg.

Vitamin B$_{12}$ and folic acid

These two dietary components are essential for the synthesis of DNA and hence for chromosomal replication and cell division. Tissues with a high cellular turnover, such as haematopoietic tissue, are very sensitive to a deficiency of these two substances.

Vitamin B$_{12}$ represents a group of compounds known as the cobalamins in which the cobalt ion is linked to either cyanide (cyanocobalamin), a hydroxyl group (hydroxycobalamin), or a methyl group (methylcobalamin). Cobalamins are synthesized by micro-organisms in the intestines, but in man they are not absorbed. Hence man depends upon a dietary source of B$_{12}$ to meet requirements. Foods rich in vitamin B$_{12}$ include liver, kidneys, and shell fish.

Properties and functions

Vitamin B$_{12}$ is essential for cell growth and division, and for the normal myelination of nerve fibres. It is necessary for folic acid metabolism, and is also involved in the metabolism of lipids and carbohydrates. Deficiency of vitamin B$_{12}$ causes pernicious anaemia.

Absorption of vitamin B$_{12}$ from dietary sources is dependent upon an intrinsic factor (a glycoprotein) produced by the parietal cells of the stomach. Gastric acid causes the release of dietary B$_{12}$ from proteins. The released vitamin is immediately bound to intrinsic factor, and the combination reaches the ileum, where it combines with specific receptors on the ileal mucosal cell. The vitamin B$_{12}$ and intrinsic factor are then transported into the circulation. Total body stores of vitamin B$_{12}$ are approximately 3 mg.

Deficiency

This affects both the haematopoietic system and the nervous system. Vitamin B$_{12}$ is essential for cell growth and replication, so the high rate of cell turnover in the bone marrow makes it very susceptible to deficiency states of vitamin B$_{12}$. The result is pernicious anaemia, which is characterized by a hypochromic, macrocytic anaemia. Clinical signs of pernicious anaemia include a sore red tongue, angular cheilitis, and premature greying of the hair. Severe vitamin B$_{12}$ deficiency can result in irreversible damage to the nervous system due to demyelination of neurones. Early signs of such changes are paraesthesia of the extremities and decreased tendon reflexes. Those affected can become confused, disorientated, and suffer visual disturbances.

Vitamin B$_{12}$ deficiency can result from poor intake, as could occur in strict vegetarians. More commonly, the deficiency arises in those who lack intrinsic factor, including patients with gastritis or who have undergone gastric surgery. Various types of ileal disease (i.e. Crohn's disease and coeliac disease) can affect the absorption of the vitamin B$_{12}$–intrinsic factor complex, and result in signs and symptoms of deficiency. Certain drugs, for example para-aminosalicylic acid and neomycin, will affect the absorption of vitamin B_{12}. If these drugs are used for prolonged periods, a deficiency state can arise.

Uses

Vitamin B_{12} is used to treat pernicious anaemia and other signs of deficiency. It is usually given by injection, and mild forms of pernicious anaemia usually respond to 500 μg every two months.

Folic acid

This is a weak organic acid (pteroylglutamic acid) that occurs in yeast, liver, and green vegetables. Folic acid is essential for normal production of red blood cells, and a deficiency results in a megaloblastic anaemia. In the body, folic acid is reduced to tetrahydrofolate by the enzyme, dihydrofolate reductase. This enzyme is inhibited by various chemotherapeutic agents (see Chapter 17). Dietary folic acid is absorbed in the small intestines and mainly stored in the liver. These stores will last for about four months.

Deficiency

Folic acid deficiency is a common occurrence in patients with disease of the gastro-intestinal tract, where there is impaired absorption. Deficiency is also found in alcoholics, in pregnancy, and in patients taking phenytoin and phenobarbitone—drugs that affect the absorption of folic acid. Folic acid deficiency causes a megaloblastic anaemia identical to that produced by vitamin B_{12}. However, unlike vitamin B_{12} deficiency, there are no neurological symptoms with folic acid deficiency.

VITAMIN C (ASCORBIC ACID)

The dietary value of fresh lemons in the prevention of scurvy was first established by Lind in 1747. However, the identification of vitamin C and its link with scurvy did not occur until 1907.

Ascorbic acid is structurally related to glucose, and some species can synthesize their own vitamin C from this carbohydrate. Vitamin C is involved in a number of body functions, including the synthesis of collagen, corticosteroids, and lysine chains in certain proteins. The major function of vitamin C is in the synthesis of intercellular substances, including collagen, the matrices of teeth and bone, and the intercellular cement of the capillary endothelium. Vitamin C is well-absorbed when taken orally, and widely distributed throughout all tissues in the body.

Deficiency

This causes scurvy, which is associated with a defect in collagen synthesis. Clinical features include poor healing of wounds, rupture of capillaries leading to petechiae and ecchymoses, loosening of the teeth, and bleeding from the gingival tissues. Scurvy is sometimes seen in alcoholics, drug addicts, children, and the elderly.

Uses

Vitamin C is used in the treatment of scurvy. It is also widely used as a prophylaxis against the common cold. There is no firm evidence to suggest that vitamin C reduces either the chances of catching a cold or shortens its course. Indeed, excessive use of vitamin C can predispose the individual to oxalate renal calculi.

VITAMIN E

This vitamin, which occurs in wheat-germ oil, was first isolated in 1936. Its pharmacological and physiological functions in man are not established. Animal experiments have shown that deficiency of vitamin E causes spontaneous abortion and impaired spermatogenesis. The role of vitamin E in the reproduction system of man is uncertain. Evidence suggests that vitamin E may protect the red blood cell against haemolysis. This vitamin is widely consumed as part of multiple vitamin therapy; fortunately, large doses of vitamin E have no serious unwanted effects.

VITAMIN K

This is essential for the synthesis of several factors required for blood clotting (II, VII, IX, and X). The vitamin is concentrated in chloroplasts and in vegetable oils.

Deficiency of vitamin K causes hypoprothrombinaemia and hence an increased tendency to bleed. Patients will suffer from ecchymoses, epistaxis, haematuria, and gastro-intestinal bleeding. Vitamin K is used to treat symptoms of deficiency, drug-induced hypoprothrombinaemia, and the hypoprothrombinaemia of the new-born (see Chapter 12).

IRON

This is the fourth most abundant element in the earth's crust and is essential for the normal function of many living species. In man, iron is used for the synthesis of haemoglobin, myoglobin, and certain enzymes. Iron not utilized for these purposes is stored as ferretin or haemosiderin. Shortage of iron results in iron-deficiency anaemia.

Pharmacokinetics

Although iron is absorbed throughout the small intestine, the main site of absorption is the duodenum. Absorption of iron, either in the diet or from a variety of iron preparations, can be affected by many factors. Certain foods, particularly cereals, reduce iron absorption. Certain drugs, such as tetracyclines, chelate iron and there is impaired absorption of the chelate. Thus, patients on iron therapy should not be prescribed tetracyclines. Similarly, antacids reduce iron absorption. Iron in the ferrous form is more readily absorbed than ferric iron. In addition, vitamin C and intrinsic factor facilitate iron absorption. Control of absorption appears to be related to the capacity of the intestinal mucosa to transport iron into the blood stream.

On absorption into the mucosal cell, iron combines with the protein apoferritin to form ferritin. However, in patients with iron deficiency the formation of ferritin does not occur and the iron passes straight into the plasma. Free iron in the plasma, or iron released from ferritin, is transported in the bloodstream attached to the glycoprotein, transferrin, from where it is delivered and stored in the bone marrow. Total body stores of iron are 3 to 4 g.

Small quantities of iron are lost via shedding of the mucosal cell in the small intestine, from the bile, and via the kidneys. Iron requirements increase during pregnancy and lactation.

Uses

Iron is given to correct or prevent iron-deficiency anaemia (see below). Usually it is given orally in the form of either ferrous sulphate, gluconate, or fumarate. The response to iron replacement therapy usually occurs 5 to 10 days after commencement of dosage, and treatment should continue for six months after haemoglobin levels have reached the normal range.

Iron can also be given via the parenteral route (in the form of iron dextran), if iron stores are to be rapidly and completely replenished.

Unwanted effects of iron replacement therapy

When given orally, ferrous salts can produce nausea, epigastric pain, constipation, and diarrhoea. Iron dextran can produce staining of the skin.

Iron-deficiency anaemia

This is a common disease, and especially prevalent in the Third World. The incidence is higher in menstruating and pregnant women. The anaemia is either due to an inadequate diet, impaired iron absorption, or chronic blood loss. Thorough investigation of those with iron deficiency is essential in order to elucidate the underlying cause. Early signs of iron deficiency often occur in the mouth; these include ulceration, angular cheilitis, candidiasis, and glossitis. The patients may have cardiovascular problems, such as dyspnoea and angina, and they will appear pale. Their nails may be brittle and spoon-shaped (koilonychia).

Examination of the blood film is a useful diagnostic procedure for confirming iron-deficiency anaemia; the red blood cells are microcytic and hypochromic. The mean corpuscular volume (MCV), mean corpuscular haemoglobin concentration (MCHC), and serum ferritin levels are also significantly reduced.

20

Calcification

SALTS of calcium and phosphate comprise the major inorganic portion of bone. Also both types of compound have several important physiological roles in normal body function. This Chapter deals with the pharmacological and physiological properties of calcium and phosphate, together with the endocrine factors (parathyroid hormone, calcitonin, and vitamin D) that control their metabolism.

CALCIUM

Nearly all the body's calcium is found in the skeletal tissues; small quantities occur in cell cytoplasm and in the extracellular fluid. Ionized calcium is involved in nerve conduction, muscle contraction, cardiac function, and blood clotting. The body's calcium requirements vary with the demands of age, growth spurts, pregnancy, and lactation (dietary requirements are in the range 360–1200 mg/ daily).

Pharmacokinetics

Soluble, ionized calcium is mainly absorbed in the proximal segment of the small bowel; absorption is augmented by vitamin D and parathyroid hormone. Transport of calcium across the gut mucosal cells is probably by means of a calcium-binding protein. Glucocorticoids will depress this transport system. Absorption of calcium is also affected by phytate, oxalate, and phosphate ions in the bowel, which form insoluble salts with calcium. Patients with chronic diarrhoea and steatorrhoea suffer from decreased calcium absorption. Calcium ions are excreted into the gastro-intestinal tract, bile, saliva, and pancreatic juices; calcium is also lost in sweat, and in significant amounts during lactation. Calcium is excreted via the kidney under the control of parathyroid hormone and vitamin D. Parathyroid hormone stimulates calcium reabsorption by an action on the distal tubule, whereas vitamin D stimulates reabsorption from the proximal tubule. Calcitonin inhibits the proximal tubular reabsorption of calcium and thus facilitates excretion.

Pharmacological and physiological properties

Calcium is essential for normal function of the neuromuscular system. A rise in extracellular calcium concentration will cause a rise in the threshold for excitation of nerve fibres and muscle. This will result in muscle weakness, lethargy, and eventually coma. Calcium is involved in the activation of muscle contraction, both in skeletal and cardiac muscle. It is also involved in the release of catecholamines from the adrenal medulla. In addition, calcium ions are essential both for the release of neurotransmitters from synapses and of autocoids from various sites and tissues in the body.

In blood coagulation, Ca^{2+} (Factor V) are essential for the action of thromboplastin on prothrombin to form thrombin (see Chapter 12). Calcium salts, especially calcium chloride, cause irritation and sloughing of tissues if given subcutaneously. Hence this drug should only be given intravenously.

Abnormalities of calcium metabolism

Blood calcium levels can be affected by a variety of factors; these can give rise to either a hypocalcaemic or hypercalcaemic state.

Hypocalcaemia

The signs and symptoms of this include tetany, paraesthesia, laryngospasm, muscle cramps, and convulsions. Hypocalcaemia is associated with the following:

1. Poor intake of calcium and vitamin D: the resultant hypocalcaemia gives rise to an increased production of parathyroid hormone, which mobilizes Ca^{2+} from bone; in adults, this leads to osteomalacia, whereas in infants it causes rickets.
2. Hypoparathyroidism.
3. Renal insufficiency accompanied by hyperphosphatasia: the high plasma concentrations of phosphate inhibit the conversion, in the kidney, of 25-hydroxycholecalciferol to 1,25-dihydroxycholecalciferol.
4. Overdose of sodium fluoride: the fluoride forms a complex with calcium ions thus leading to reduced absorption of them.
5. Massive transfusions with citrated blood: the citrate ions will chelate calcium to form an insoluble complex, thus reducing plasma concentrations of calcium ions.

Hypocalcaemic states are corrected by a dietary increase in calcium. In severe cases of tetany associated with hypocalcaemia, treatment is with intravenous calcium chloride.

Hypercalcaemia

High plasma concentrations of calcium will principally affect the kidney, causing pathological changes in the collecting ducts and distal tubules. The net result is a reduction in renal function if left untreated, and hypercalcaemia will cause renal failure. Hypercalcaemia is associated with the following conditions:

1. Diet, especially the milk-alkali syndrome caused by excessive consumption of milk and antacids, which contain soluble calcium salts—massive amounts of antacids need to be regularly consumed to produce this syndrome.
2. Excessive intake of vitamin D_3.
3. Hyperparathyroidism
4. Sarcoidosis: patients with this granulomatous disorder may have a hypersensitivity to vitamin D.
5. Neoplasms: metastatic deposits in bone can secrete osteoclast activating factor and prostaglandins, which both stimulate bone resorption.
6. Disuse atrophy: as occurs when a limb has been immobilized for a long time.

Hypercalcaemia is usually corrected by the body's homeostatic mechanism. If very severe, it is treated with steroids such as prednisolone.

PHOSPHATE

Phosphate is present in extracellular fluids, collagen, and bone. A balance exists between plasma concentrations of calcium and phosphate. There is also an inverse relationship between plasma phosphate concentration and the rate of renal hydroxylation of 25-hydroxycholecalciferol. Thus, a reduction in plasma phosphate leads to an increase of calcium in the blood, which in turn inhibits the deposition of new bone salts. An increase in plasma phosphate facilitates the effect of calcitonin on the deposition of calcium in bone.

Phosphate ions are absorbed from the bowel, and absorption is enhanced by vitamin D. Large quantities of calcium and aluminium in the bowel will reduce the absorption of phosphate. Like calcium, phosphate requirements vary with age, growth, pregnancy, and lactation.

VITAMIN D (CALCIFEROL)

Although referred to as a vitamin, calciferol (or more precisely the metabolite of 1,25-dihydroxycholecalciferol) is now considered a hormone secreted by the kidney. The metabolism of vitamin D is shown in Fig. 20.1. The precursor of vitamin D is 7-dehydrocholesterol, which is synthesized in the skin. The action of ultraviolet light converts this precursor to cholecalciferol (vitamin D_3). Further

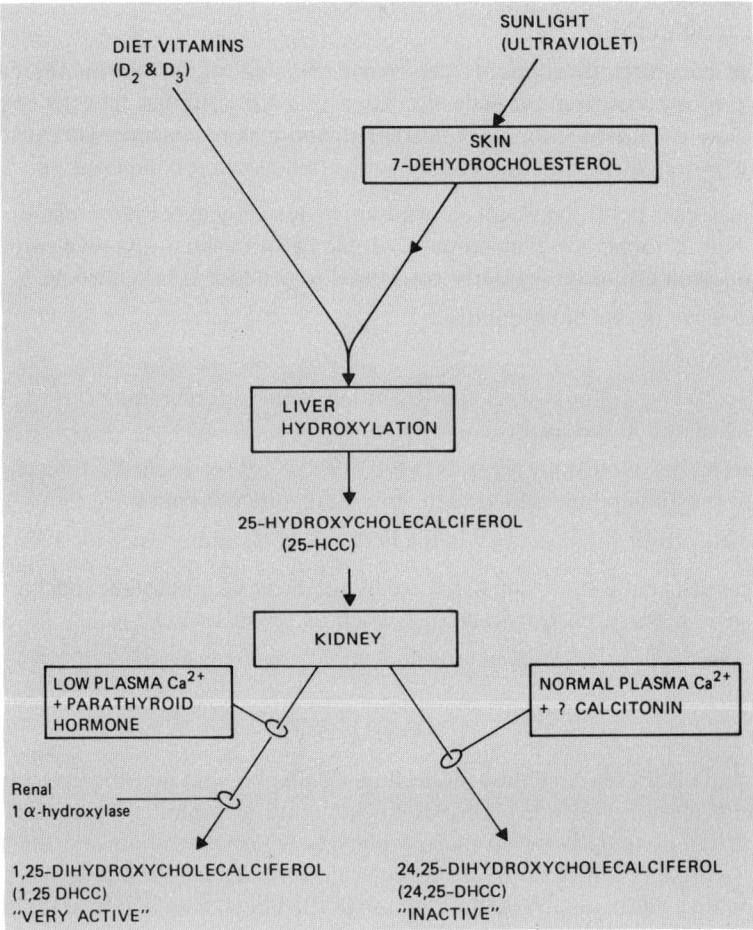

Fig. 20.1. Vitamin D synthesis.

hydroxylation of cholecalciferol occurs in the liver to form the compound 25-hydroxycholecalciferol (25-HCC). This hydroxylation process is controlled by circulating levels of cholecalciferol, with high levels inhibiting the hydroxylation. The 25-HCC is finally activated in the kidneys by the enzyme, renal 1α-hydroxylase, and the product depends upon the calcium needs.

In the presence of low calcium concentrations, 25-HCC is hydroxylated to 1,25-dihydroxycholecalciferol (1,25-DHCC), and the hydroxylation is facilitated by parathyroid hormone. The 1,25-DHCC is highly active, and acts on the intestine to increase the formation of calcium-binding proteins that augment calcium absorption. With normal or high calcium concentrations, 25-HCC is hydroxylated to the relatively inactive 24,25-dihydroxycholecalciferol. This hydroxylation may be facilitated by calcitonin.

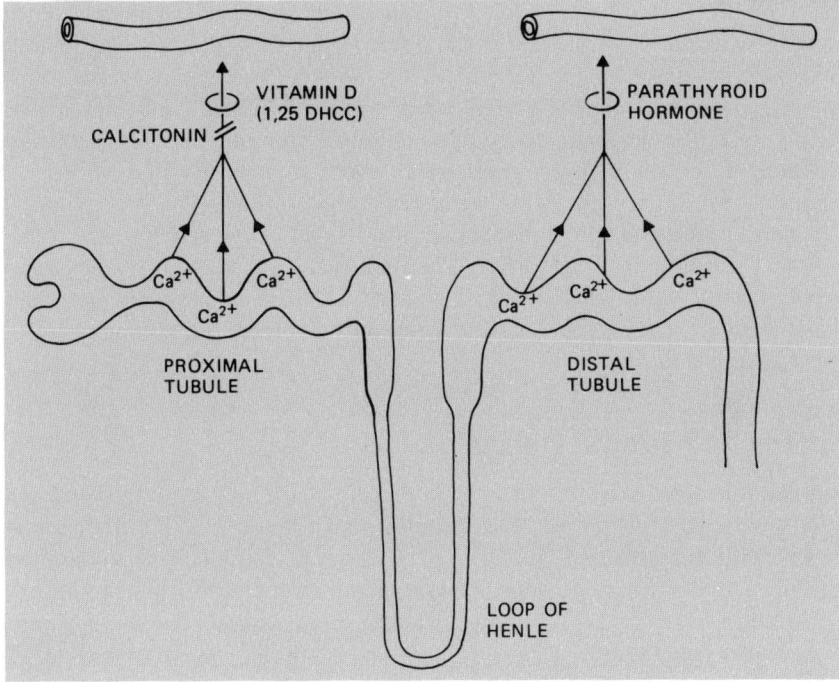

Fig. 20.2. Calcium homeostasis and the renal tubule.

Thus 1,25-DHCC enhances the absorption of calcium from the small intestine, and it also facilitates reabsorption of calcium ions from the proximal tubule (Fig. 20.2). Both 1,25-DHCC and parathyroid hormone mobilize calcium from bone.

Uses

Vitamin D is used to correct deficiency states (see below), and is available in three forms: cholecalciferol, ergocalciferol (vitamin D_2), and dihydrotachysterol. Dihydrotachysterol is more widely used because it bypasses renal regulation.

Unwanted effects

The main adverse effect associated with vitamin D preparations is hypervitaminosis D, characterized by hypercalcaemia, osteoporosis, soft tissue calcification, and renal calculi.

Deficiency

A deficiency of vitamin D, either from dietary sources or lack of sunlight, results in rickets or osteomalacia. Both conditions are characterized by a pathological defect in the mineralization of new bone. Rickets presents clinically during growth, whereas osteomalacia is the adult form of the disease. Oral manifestations of vitamin D deficiency depend upon the severity and age of onset. During growth, vitamin D deficiency will affect the mandibular condylar cartilage, causing retarded development of the mandibular ramus. There is often delayed eruption of the teeth and hypoplasia of tooth enamel. In both rickets and osteomalacia, the jaw bones are weak and prone to fracture.

Patients with chronic renal failure may suffer from renal rickets due to impaired synthesis of 1,25-DHCC. This will result in calcium malabsorption, hypocalcaemia, and a secondary rise in parathyroid hormone production. Hence, such patients will have the signs and symptoms of osteomalacia and (secondary) hyperparathyroidism.

Vitamin D-resistant rickets

This is a rare sex-linked familial disease characterized by a hypophosphataemia associated with a decreased renal tubular reabsorption of PO_4^{3-}. Patients will present with the signs and symptoms of rickets or osteomalacia depending upon their age. This form of rickets appears to respond to a metabolite of vitamin D—lα-hydroxycholecalciferol. This is an example of a disease due to a receptor abnormality (see Chapter 1).

PARATHYROID HORMONE (PTH)

The parathyroids are small, yellow glandular bodies, usually attached to the undersurface of the thyroid gland. They were first discovered in 1880, but their physiological function was not determined until the 1920s. The glands synthesize and secrete PTH.

Physiological functions

The PTH controls calcium metabolism and ensures that the extracellular fluid concentration of Ca^{2+} is kept constant. Hence it will regulate the absorption of Ca^{2+} from the gastro-intestinal tract, the deposition and mobilization of Ca^{2+} in bone, and the excretion of Ca^{2+} via the kidney.

The secretion of PTH is inversely related to the plasma concentration of calcium. When the concentration of Ca^{2+} is low there is an increased secretion of PTH; with normal or high concentrations of Ca^{2+}, secretion is reduced.

Parathyroid hormone increases bone resorption, especially from the older portion of mineralized bone, leading to an increase in the plasma concentration of Ca^{2+}. It acts directly on the osteolytic cells (osteoclasts and osteocytes), and increases the rate of mesenchymal cell differentiation to osteoblasts. Osteoclastic activity is evident some 20 minutes after an infusion of PTH.

The hormone has a dual action in the kidney: it increases tubular reabsorption of Ca^{2+}; and it inhibits tubular reabsorption of PO_4^{3-} (Fig. 20.2), which results in an increased renal excretion of inorganic phosphate. The overall effect of PTH on the kidney is to retain Ca^{2+} and maintain the plasma concentration.

Calcium and phosphate ions, as described earlier, are absorbed in the gastro-intestinal tract, and parathyroid hormone has an indirect effect on their absorption. The absorption of Ca^{2+} is dependent upon the active metabolite of vitamin D (1,25-DHCC); PTH enhances the renal hydroxylation of 25-HCC to 1,25-DHCC. The increase in the production of 1,25-DHCC increases Ca^{2+} absorption.

Disorders of parathyroid function

There are two such disorders, hypo- and hyperparathyroidism.

Hypoparathyroidism

This can result from either hypofunction of the parathyroid glands, surgical removal of the glands following thyroidectomy, or the rare genetic disorder of pseudohypoparathyroidism, in which target organs do not respond to PTH. This genetic disorder is yet another example of disease due to a receptor abnormality (see Chapter 1). In all varieties of hypoparathyroidism, the clinical symptoms are those of hypocalcemia, and include paraesthesia of the extremities, muscle twitching and, if severe, tetany. In chronic cases of hypoparathyroidism, there are various ectodermal changes including loss of hair, grooved and brittle fingernails, and enamel hypoplasia. Hypoparathyroidism is treated with vitamin D and, where necessary, calcium supplements.

Hyperparathyroidism

This is characterized by excessive production of parathyroid hormone. Three forms of the disease are recognized; primary, secondary, and tertiary. Primary hyperparathyroidism is associated with hyperplasia or neoplasia of the para-thyroid glands. In secondary hyperparathyroidism, the underlying cause is a hypocalcaemia associated with chronic renal failure. The hypocalcaemia stimulates excessive production of PTH. Patients with long-standing renal disease and secondary hyperparathyroidism may develop an apparent autonomous hypersecretion of PTH, and this is known as tertiary hyperparathyroidism.

Clinical features

Primary hyperparathyroidism has an incidence of $1:1000$ of the population, with females being more affected than males. Excessive PTH activity will cause a hypercalcaemia and hypophosphataemia. The presenting symptoms are those of hypercalcaemia, and include anorexia, thirst, polyuria, renal colic, and renal stones. Approximately one-third of patients show evidence of bone disease, including the bone disorder known as osteitis fibrosa cystica. This condition is characterized by foci of bone destruction leaving spaces filled with vascular and cellular connective tissue containing large numbers of osteoclastic giant cells. Such lesions often occur in the jaws, especially the mandible. Primary hyperparathyroidism is treated by surgical excision of the parathyroid glands. In secondary or tertiary hyperparathyroidism, the underlying renal disease must be corrected.

CALCITONIN

This was first described in 1964, and is a hormone secreted by the parafollicular cells of the thyroid gland. Like PTH, calcitonin secretion is controlled by plasma levels of calcium; it lowers plasma calcium and phosphate levels by an alteration in intracellular cyclic AMP. Calcitonin has two effects on calcium homeostasis. Firstly, it inhibits osteoclastic resorption, thus reducing the release of Ca^{2+} and PO_4^{3-} from the skeletal tissues. This inhibition is more pronounced when there is a high turnover of bone, as occurs in Paget's disease and thyrotoxicosis. Secondly, it has a minor effect on the kidneys, enhancing the excretion of phosphate, calcium, and sodium (Fig. 20.2).

Calcitonin (porcine or salmon varieties) is used to treat Paget's disease, and the hypercalcaemia secondary to malignancy or vitamin D excess. The hormone can only be given parenterally because it is destroyed by gastric secretions. Patients with Paget's disease usually show a response to calcitonin therapy within two months. Unwanted effects are pain at the site of injection, nausea, and flushing of the face. Because of the low doses of calcitonin used in Paget's disease, antibody formation leading to hypersensitivity is unlikely.

21

Unwanted effects of drugs, including immunopharmacology

UNWANTED EFFECTS DUE TO DRUGS

These appear to be fairly common in medical practice, although precise information about their incidence is not available. This is partly because unwanted effects may not be recognized as such either by the patient or by the doctor. Moreover, it will only be possible to calculate the incidence of such effects in relation to a particular drug when accurate information about the numbers of patients exhibiting adverse effects to that drug is available, together with accurate returns that indicate the total number of patients receiving it.

In dental practice, unwanted effects due to drugs would appear to be less common than in medical practice. They are likely to arise in two different ways. The dentist may be the first to observe an unwanted effect produced by a drug prescribed by the patient's medical practitioner; for example, ulceration in the mouth that accompanies agranulocytosis. On the other hand, as part of dental treatment, the dentist may prescribe a drug to which the patient reacts adversely. In order to obtain accurate information about the incidence of unwanted drug effects in dental practice, it is most important for all practitioners to report any suspected unwanted drug effect to the Medical Assessor (Adverse Reactions), Committee on Safety of Medicines, 33/37a Finsbury Square, London EC2B 2ZS. (Special yellow-coloured report cards with prepaid postage are available for this purpose from the Committee on Safety of Medicines).

Classification

It is difficult to classify unwanted effects satisfactorily because very often the mechanism is not clear. However, it is useful to have some form of classification for reference. One broad classification has divided unwanted effects into two classes, Type A Reactions and Type B Reactions (Rawlins and Thompson 1985).

Type A reactions
These are reactions that would be expected, or could be expected, from the known pharmacology of the drug or mixtures of drugs. Such reactions are relatively

common and usually not serious, although they may be unpleasant. An example of this sort of reaction arises from the use of antihistamines (H_1-blockers) to prevent histamine access to receptors involved in allergic responses. In addition to this blocking property the antihistamines have, in general, an intrinsic sedative effect, and this may be unwanted.

Type B reactions

These reactions cannot be predicted or explained by the known pharmacology of the drug. They are relatively uncommon and are often much more serious than the Type A Reaction. Allergic reactions to drugs generally come under this heading.

Another useful classification, a modified version of that proposed by Rosenheim and Moulton (1958), is given below. Both classifications fit well into each other.

(1) overdosage

(2) intolerance

(3) side-effects

(4) secondary effects

(5) idiosyncrasy

(6) teratogenic effects

(7) hypersensitivity

(8) drug interactions

These items are now considered in detail, except for drug interactions, which have been mentioned under individual drugs and will be discussed in Chapter 22.

Overdosage

Unwanted effects due to an excess of drug will be related to the amount of drug in the body. It is important to realize that all drugs are potentially poisonous, although some are relatively more poisonous than others. The safety of a drug will depend upon the size of the margin between the effective dose (ED) and the lethal dose (LD), as discussed in Chapter 1. This cannot be measured in man but can be determined in animals where, in order to allow for biological variation, a series of different doses are given to two groups of animals and two appropriate graphs of the results are drawn, one for effectiveness and one for lethality. From these graphs the amount of drug required to produce the desired effect in 50 per cent of animals (ED_{50}) can be read off, and also the amount required to kill 50 per cent of them (LD_{50}). The safety or, as it is termed, the Therapeutic Index can be obtained by determining the ratio LD_{50}/ED_{50} (see Fig. 1.13). The larger the value of this ratio, the safer is the drug, although it is important to relate the route of administration used in these determinations to that which may be used in man, and also to make allowance for species differences.

Absolute overdosage

This may be (i) immediate, due to the presence of too much drug given in error or taken deliberately with suicidal intent; on the other hand, it may be (ii) cumulative, which is brought about by slow excretion of the drug, with the result that there is a steady increase in the amount of drug in the body over a period of time. For example, digitalis and thyroxine take more than a week to be half-excreted; they therefore accumulate in the body unless steps are taken to reduce the initial dosage when an adequate therapeutic effect has been achieved. By contrast, penicillin is half excreted in less than an hour and is therefore not liable to accumulate.

Relative overdosage

This occurs when the mechanisms for metabolism and/or excretion of a drug are impaired. Under these circumstances, normal or even subnormal doses of the drug may cause signs of overdosage. In hepatic failure, drugs may be metabolized more slowly than normal, with the result that the amount of active drug in the body declines more slowly than usual, so leading to an increased and prolonged effect. For example, the duration of apnoea after a normal dose of the short-acting muscle relaxant, suxamethonium, may be greatly prolonged in patients with low plasma cholinesterase levels due to liver disease (Fig. 21.1). Similarly, renal

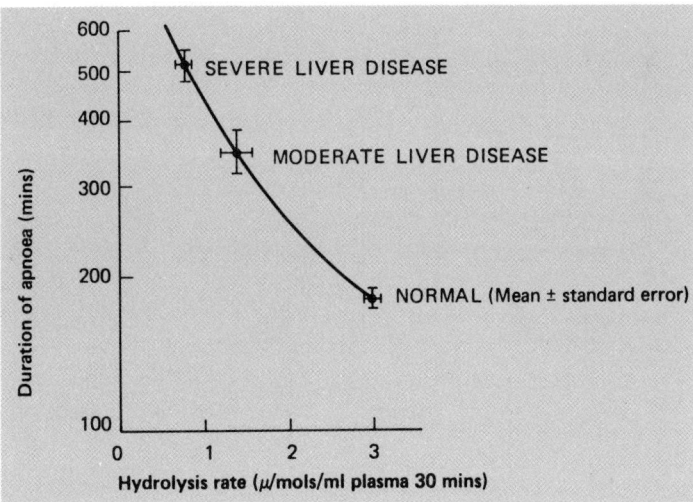

Fig. 21.1. The effect of liver disease on the rate of destruction (by hydrolysis) of the short-acting neuromuscular blocking drug suxamethonium. Plasma cholinesterase which is manufactured by the liver is responsible for the hydrolysis of suxamethonium. Since the presence of liver disease reduces the production of cholinesterase, it also affects the rate of breakdown of suxamethonium and hence the duration of neuromuscular block including apnoea after a dose of this drug. (Drawn from data of Foldes *et al.* 1956.)

failure will result in a diminished rate of excretion of a drug such as digoxin where this is the main route of excretion from the body.

Intolerance

This is said to occur when there is a lowered threshold to the normal pharmacological action of a drug; it is a phenomenon attributable to biological variation. Thus, whereas the normal therapeutic dose produces the desired effect in the majority of individuals, in a minority it may produce too large or too small an effect; the former is due to intolerance, the latter to tolerance. Put the other way round, the dose required to produce the desired effect in an intolerant patient is less than the normal dose, whilst the requisite dose for a tolerant patient is greater than the normal, as illustrated in Fig. 21.2. It follows that it is the intolerant patient who is liable to exhibit unwanted effects when the normal dose is used; the tolerant patient shows little or no effect.

Side-effects

These effects are therapeutically undesirable but pharmacologically unavoidable actions due to a drug. Side-effects can be subdivided into two main groups:

Extension of main action

Some side effects are due to an extension of the main action of the drug at sites additional to those required for therapeutic purposes. For example, atropine given

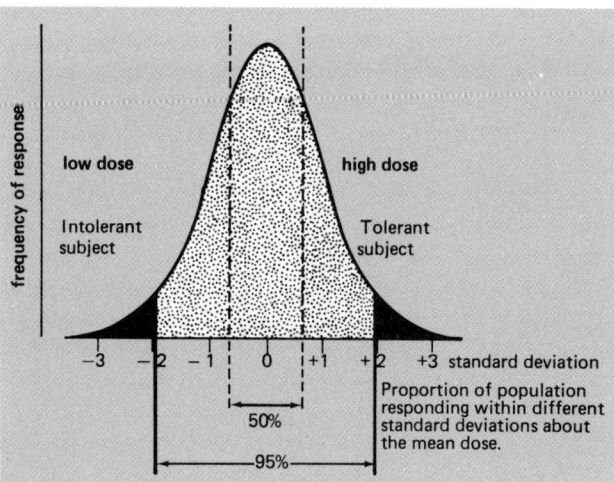

Fig. 21.2. Idealized frequency distribution curve for the responses of a population to a drug. The areas under the curve which represent 50 per cent and 95 per cent of the population are shown and subjects who are considered to be intolerant or tolerant have been arbitrarily shown as belonging to the remaining 5 per cent of the population (black areas). (Standard deviation is a measure of scatter; numerically the value will vary from drug to drug. Where the value is small, the range of doses required about the mean dose will be small, and vice versa.)

in order to produce a dry mouth may also interfere with the accommodation of the eye, and the normal functioning of the bladder and bowels. Although this drug produces widespread effects they are all due to a common mechanism, namely, that atropine competes with acetylcholine released from the postganglionic parasympathetic nerve endings for receptors situated on parasympathetic effector organs. On the other hand, a patient given atropine in order to relieve Parkinsonism may complain of a dry mouth, which under these circumstances becomes the side-effect.

Additional actions

Other side-effects are due to one or more additional actions that are inherent in the particular drug. For example, most antihistamines also possess hypnotic effects. In some circumstances, such as an itching urticarial rash that prevents sleep, these effects may be an added therapeutic benefit; in other situations, such as when used to treat hay fever in a bus driver, they may be highly undesirable. The occurrence of jaundice in patients taking certain of the monoamine oxidase inhibitors or some of the sex hormones is another example.

Secondary effects

These are not due to the direct pharmacological action of a drug but are the indirect consequences of it. For example, the prolonged use of broad-spectrum antibiotics may result in superinfection. Under these conditions, the normal bowel flora is altered by the antibiotic so that pathogenic organisms gain a hold. The result is that a new infection supervenes, and a patient who was originally being treated for a simple infection may contract and possibly die from a very serious one, for example staphylococcal enteritis. Another example is the prolonged use of a tetracycline mouthwash, which leads to a candidal infection of the mouth.

A number of patients treated with the antibiotic, clindamycin, have developed pseudomembranous colitis as a secondary effect; this can be a very dangerous syndrome (see Chapter 10).

Idiosyncrasy

This is a qualitatively abnormal reaction to a drug, which is due to some abnormality of the individual showing the response. For example, the prolonged apnoea that may occur after the administration of the neuromuscular blocking drug, suxamethonium, can be due to the presence of an abnormal cholinesterase, as shown in Fig. 21.3. It has been estimated that about 1 in 2800 persons possess this atypical esterase, which hydrolyses suxamethonium much more slowly than normal cholinesterase with the result that the duration of neuromuscular block is greatly prolonged. Another example is the precipitation of acute porphyria by the administration of barbiturates. This can only occur in patients who are qualitatively different in that they suffer from latent porphyria.

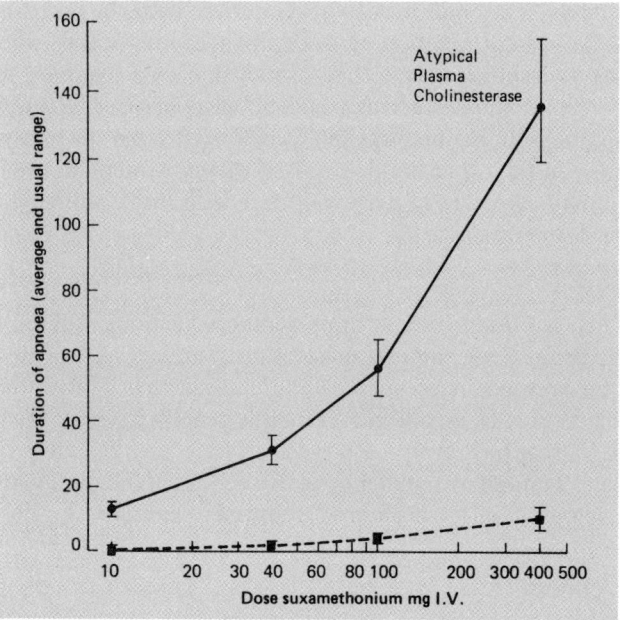

Fig. 21.3. The duration of apnoea after a single intravenous injection of different doses of suxamethonium in adult males with normal and atypical cholinesterase. The greatly reduced rate at which atypical cholinesterase hydrolyses suxamethonium is evident from the prolonged duration of apnoea (upper graph). (Drawn from data of Kalow and Gunn 1957. Reproduced by courtesy of Williams and Wilkins Co, Baltimore.)

Teratogenic effects

Drugs that damage the embryo, but which leave it compatible with prenatal life, and where the abnormalities are observable postnatally, are called teratogens. There are some drugs that have been positively identified as being teratogenic, thalidomide being the obvious example. Others include androgens, and tetracyclines—e.g. producing discoloured teeth. Yet other drugs are suspected as being potentially teratogenic, whilst others are possible teratogenic. For instance, the anticonvulsant, phenytoin, is suspected as a potential teratogen.

Hypersensitivity

Consideration of drug hypersensitivity (allergy) requires some understanding of the immune system; this is discussed now as a separate major section, which leads into the topic of drug allergy and its treatment.

The immune system

This is one of the body's significant defence mechanisms against infection; its functions include the recognition of foreign material (antigen) by various cellular components of the system (macrophages and lymphocytes). Recognition is followed by the production of specific neutralizing chemicals (immunoglobulins or antibodies) or cells (sensitized T-lymphocytes), and the formation of the antibody/antigen complexes. These complexes are finally phagocytosed by polymorphonuclear leucocytes.

The immune system has three important features: memory, specificity, and recognition of non-self. Certain diseases, such as measles, chicken-pox, and mumps, are usually suffered only once. The initial infection stimulates antibody production (primary response) and a memory facility, so that when the infection is encountered again antibodies are readily formed to the infecting agent (secondary response). This is the principle used in immunization. Antibodies raised against the mumps virus are specific for that virus and these antibodies will not render the patient immune to other viral infections. Finally, the immune system must also recognize what is foreign (non-self) and what is self. The failure to discriminate between self and non-self could lead to the synthesis of antibodies directed against tissues of the individual's own body. Such antibodies are referred to as auto-antibodies. The various components of the immune system are considered below.

Immunoglobulins

These are chains of peptides joined together by disulphide bridges. The chains of peptides can be further divided into heavy and light chains. In man, five classes of immunoglobulins can be identified, immunoglobulin G, M, A, D, and E, commonly abbreviated to IgG, IgM, IgA, IgD, and IgE.

Immunoglobulin G

This is the main immunoglobulin formed during the secondary response. It can cross the placenta and hence is essential for the early protection against infection in the new-born child. Immunoglobulin G is found in all cavities of the body where its main function is to neutralize bacterial toxins; such neutralization invariably activates the complement system (see later; and Chapter 4). The various activated complement products are chemotactic for white blood cells and cause an increase in capillary permeability.

Immunoglobulin A

This is referred to as the secretory immunoglobulin for it appears in all secretions produced by the body. Its function is the defence of exposed external body surfaces against infection from micro-organisms. The IgA is synthesized locally by plasma cells, and coats micro-organisms. This coating inhibits their adherence to the surfaces of mucosal cells, thereby preventing entry into the body.

Immunoglobulin M

This is a high molecular-weight immunoglobulin found on the surface of lymphocytes. It appears early in the response to infection and is very efficient at agglutinating bacteria. Hence high concentrations of IgM are associated with bacteraemias.

Immunoglobulin D

This is very susceptible to proteolytic degradation and hence has a short plasma half-life. Like IgM, IgD is found on the surface of lymphocytes and it would seem that both IgM and IgD function as mutually interactive antigen receptors controlling lymphocyte activation and suppression.

Immunoglobulin E

Only small amounts of this are found in serum as IgE is firmly fixed to the surface of mast cells. The combination between antigen and IgE on this surface results in mast cell degranulation, with the release of histamine and other potent chemicals. This is the underlying mechanism for hay fever, asthma, and anaphylaxis. Immunoglobulin E also protects the mucosal surfaces of the body by activating plasma factors and effector cells.

Cellular components of the immune response

Lymphocytes

There are two populations of lymphocytes found in man, thymus-dependent lymphocytes (T-lymphocytes), which are processed by the thymus gland, and bursa-dependent lymphocytes (B-lymphocytes), which are processed by lymphoid tissue equivalent to the structure known as the bursa of Fabricius found in birds. Both types of lymphocyte are derived from bone-marrow stem cells. B-lymphocytes, when stimulated by antigen, develop into plasma cells, which synthesize and release free antibody. T-lymphocytes, when challenged by an antigen, transform to lymphoblasts, which are responsible for cell-mediated immunity.

Macrophages

These are large mononuclear cells; their role in the immune response appears to be the processing and presenting of antigen to lymphocytes. Antigens are partly phagocytosed by macrophages and partly bind to their surface. The processed antigen, or that attached to the cell surface, is then presented to either a T- or B-lymphocyte. Macrophages also produce a chemical mediator, interleukin I, which stimulates T-helper cells (see below).

Cell-mediated response

T-lymphocytes are responsible for the cell-mediated immune response. The surface of the T-lymphocyte contains receptors that are triggered by antigens, which have either been processed by the macrophage or attached to the cell surface. Once the receptor is triggered, the T-lymphocyte undergoes blast transformation to several 'lymphocytes' with different functions. These include lymphokine producers, killer, memory, helper, and suppressor cells. Killer cells, or cytotoxic T-cells, will destroy any cells bearing the antigen that stimulated their formation. Killer cells are particularly involved in viral infections and graft rejection. Helper T-cells are necessary adjuncts to the initial proliferation and differentiation stages of the immune response. Suppressor cells limit the immune response to an antigen, and are important in modulating the immune system.

Lymphokines

These are a group of potent biological substances released from sensitized T-lymphocytes. Lymphokines have a variety of biological activities, as are listed below:

(1) macrophage chemotactic factor: attracts further macrophages to the site of antigen-mediated lymphokine production;

(2) migration inhibition factor: once attracted to the site, the macrophages and other white blood cells are inhibited from leaving;

(3) macrophage activating factor: macrophages are activated into phagocytosis;

(4) skin reactive factor: facilitates movement of macrophages from blood vessels and increases capillary permeability;

(5) interferon: inhibits viral replication;

(6) mitogenic factor and lymphocyte inhibitory factor: both affect the proliferation and suppression of T-lymphocytes;

(7) osteoclast activation factor: stimulates osteoclastic activity (and may be an important factor in bone loss associated with periodontal disease).

Humoral response

When B-lymphocytes are activated by an antigen they differentiate into memory cells and plasma cells. The plasma cells produce antibodies (immunoglobulins), which neutralize the antigen that caused their production. Such antigens are usually bacterial toxins and enzymes. Antibodies will also adhere to bacterial cell walls, often forming a coating on the cell surface. This coating effect enhances the phagocytosis of bacteria. Complement is often activated when antibody combines with an antigen attached to a cell surface (see Chapter 4).

Hypersensitivity (allergy)

Allergy, a term derived from two Greek words (*allos*, other; *ergon*, work or energy), means 'altered reactivity'; it was first introduced by von Pirquet and is concerned with a phenomenon that forms part of the subject of immunology. It is well-known that some unfortunate individuals are unable to eat certain foodstuffs, such as strawberries or lobster, because to do so makes them ill. Similarly, when the majority of people are enjoying summer weather, the pollen in the air causes others to suffer miserably from hay fever. These abnormal responses are examples of allergy and are attributable to an underlying antigen–antibody reaction of a particular type. Likewise, certain patients show abnormal responses to drugs, which are also due to an antigen–antibody reaction, and are examples of drug allergy.

Drug allergy

Incidence

Information about the incidence of drug hypersensitivity reactions is scanty, although it seems clear that whilst minor reactions are fairly frequent, serious or fatal reactions due to drugs are rare.

Antigen

An antigen is a substance that is able to evoke a specific immunological response, namely the production of antibodies. Antigens are substances of large molecular weight (MW), which are usually proteins but sometimes polysaccharides. Simple chemicals with MW of about 1000 or less cannot alone act as antigens. In food allergy, the affected individual reacts immunologically to some macromolecular constituents of the offending food.

Drugs as antigens

The majority of drugs consist of small molecules (MW less than 1000), which alone are unable to act as antigens. When an individual becomes hypersensitive to a drug, for example, acetylsalicylic acid or aspirin, it is believed that the aspirin reacts with a body protein. The aspirin–body protein conjugate is antigenic; substances that combine in this way with proteins and thereby form antigens are known as haptens (or pro-antigens). The hapten, in this case aspirin, confers specificity on the antigen (that is to say the production of antibodies that will react only with aspirin or some closely related chemical compound) whilst the protein confers antigenicity, as indicated below:

aspirin + body protein → aspirin–body protein conjugate.
(confers   (confers antigenicity)
specificity)

It appears that readily reversible drug/protein conjugation, which commonly takes place between drugs and plasma proteins, is much less likely to lead to sensitization than is the irreversible conjugation that occurs when covalent bonds link a drug to a protein.

Classification of hypersensitivity reactions

There are various types of hypersensitivity reactions, and these have been classified into types as now described.

Type I—Anaphylactic type reactions

We have seen that initial contact with an antigen causes activation of the various components of the immune system, and that secondary contact with the antigen leads to further boosting of the system (secondary response). However, in some individuals the secondary response may be excessive and lead to gross tissue damage. This excessive response (hypersensitivity) is well-exemplified by the Type I reaction. In Type I reactions, antigen combines with antibody (IgE) on the surface of mast cells, which degranulate bringing about the release of slow reacting substance (SRS), eosinophil chemotactic factor, serotonin, bradykinin, and prostaglandins, as well as histamine. This type of reaction causes systemic anaphylaxis, allergic asthma, rhinitis, and some forms of urticaria, as well as angio-oedema. Some of the chemical mediators of this reaction are now considered:

1. *Histamine* (see Chapter 4), an amine that is normally stored in an inactive form inside cells (in particular, mast cells), is one of the most important pharmacologically active substances released from immunologically damaged cells. It causes contraction of smooth muscle, dilatation and increased permeability of capillaries resulting in a sudden fall of blood pressure, weal formation, and stimulation of glandular secretions, especially those of the oxyntic cells of the stomach, which leads to an outpouring of gastric juice, rich in hydrochloric acid. There are other pharmacologically active substances released under these conditions that may contribute to the overall picture.

2. *Slow reacting substance* is released during anaphylactic shock and produces contractions of human bronchial muscle. It is now believed that this substance is identical to a mixture of the leukotrienes C_4 and D_4 (see Chapter 4).

3. *5-hydroxytryptamine* (5-HT, serotonin), another amine distributed in brain, intestine, and platelets, also stimulates a variety of smooth muscles and nerves.

4. *Bradykinin*, a nonapeptide, also causes a slow contraction of smooth muscle, vasodilatation with increased capillary permeability, and stimulates sensory nerve endings to produce pain.

It seems certain that other pharmacologically active agents are also involved in these reactions, e.g. prostaglandins (see Chapter 4).

The most dramatic and dangerous Type I hypersensitivity reaction is the anaphylactic reaction following the administration of a foreign protein or drug to which the subject has become sensitized. The clinical picture usually starts with flushing and itching of the skin, followed by severe difficulty in breathing due to laryngospasm and bronchospasm, and a severe fall in blood pressure. The pulse is rapid, weak, and may be almost imperceptible. The condition may be rapidly fatal unless immediate steps are taken to administer adrenaline. The earlier the onset of symptoms following administration of the drug allergen, the more severe and dangerous the reaction is likely to be; in fact, dangerous reactions are rare after the first 30 minutes. For this reason a counsel of perfection is to keep all patients who have received injections under observation for at least 30 minutes.

Penicillin is one of the drugs most likely to produce this dangerous reaction, and it has been estimated that in the USA the number of fatal reactions to penicillins may be as high as three hundred per year (Parker 1963). Although anaphylactic reactions are usually associated with injection of a drug or of a foreign protein (skin test, wasp or bee stings), aspirin taken by mouth has produced this reaction in a highly susceptible subject.

Not all reactions are so dramatic; the sort of acute, critical situation outlined above is unlikely to be encountered in ordinary clinical practice. Nevertheless, it must be anticipated and prepared for. What is more likely to occur is a paler version, appearing less dramatically and not causing such concern. The management of the acute and less dramatic event is somewhat different, although the same range of drugs is used, and these should always be available.

Treatment of anaphylactic shock

Treatment of a severe, acute anaphylactic reaction must be immediate, and the necessary drugs should always be at hand, e.g. adrenaline, corticosteroid, and antihistamine (H_1-blocker) (see Fig. 21.4). The patient should be placed horizontally either by appropriate adjustment of the dental chair or by placing them on the floor. If respiratory depression is present, oxygen should be administered or mouth to mouth respiration given.

Then 0.5 ml of 1:1000 (0.1 mg/ml) adrenaline solution should be injected intramuscularly (NEVER INTRAVENOUSLY). This should be followed by hydrocortisone sodium succinate, 100 mg intravenously. Further doses of adrenaline can be given as required at intervals of five minutes until the symptoms begin to subside. The maximum safe does is about 1.5 ml over a period of 15 minutes, a substantial dose that is not without its own risks (see later). Great care must be taken to see that adrenaline is not injected into a blood vessel because it may produce a fatal ventricular fibrillation if given intravenously.

The principal disturbances that occur in anaphylactic shock can be attributed to (a) damage to the endothelial lining of blood vessels with increased permeability and dilatation; and (b) spasm of smooth muscle in the bronchial tree. Adrenaline acts as a physiological antagonist to these effects by virtue of its vasoconstrictor and bronchodilator actions, and so opposes the potentially lethal actions that have been caused by histamine and other pharmacologically active agents explosively released during the anaphylactic reaction.

Although adrenaline is the first line of defence, the intravenous hydrocortisone 100 mg is also important. Glucocorticoids are anti-allergic agents and this dose should ensure that an adequate amount of hydrocortisone (which is normally required and released endogenously under a variety of 'stressful' conditions) is available. Hydrocortisone does not prevent the occurrence of the antigen–antibody reaction, but acts by protecting the cells from the outcome of this

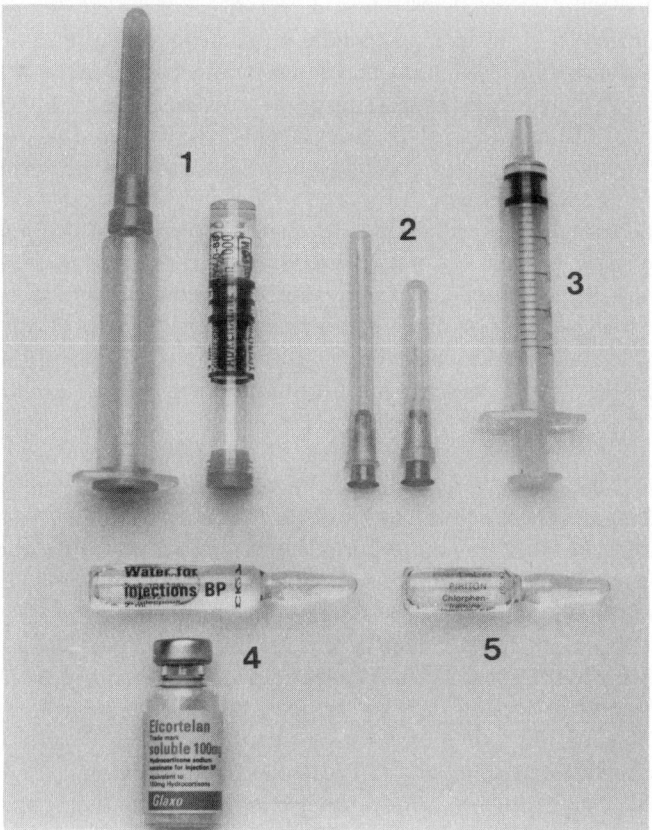

Fig. 21.4. Drugs, needles, and syringes which should always be immediately available for the treatment of drug hypersensitivity reactions.
1. Syringe and cartridge—1 ml, single dose of adrenaline hydrochloride 1:1000 (= 1 mg per ml).
2. Needles for IV, IM, and SC injections; IV = intravenous; IM = intramuscular; SC = subcutaneous.
3. 2 ml syring (removed from sterile wrapper for photograph).
4. Hydrocortisone sodium succinate 100 mg with 2 ml ampoule of water for injection in which it is dissolved.
5. Chlorpheniramine injection BP ('Piriton') 10 mg in 1 ml.

immunological reaction. The reversal of the vasodepressor response by adrenaline is dependent upon the presence of adequate hydrocortisone and if for any reason this is insufficient, for example, in a patient who has an impaired adrenocortical response following prolonged corticosteroid therapy, hydrocortisone is mandatory.

Antihistamines are usually *ineffective* in the treatment of acute anaphylactic shock for at least three reasons. Firstly, histamine is only one of the pharmacologically active agents released; the effects of the other mediators are not antagonized by H_1-blockers. Secondly, these drugs can at best only restore vasomotor tone to its original state and, at worst, may confound the situation due to their own vasodepressor action. Thirdly, in a reaction due to the liberation of histamine, antihistamines work by competing for the same receptor sites. If the receptor sites have already been occupied by histamine, then antihistamines are not likely to be that effective.

If the reaction to the introduction of the drug allergen is not so immediate and acute—the lesser version of what has so far been considered—another line of treatment may be used. In this instance it may suffice to administer hydrocortisone as the first line of defence, followed by an H_1-blocker. The antihistamine could be administered parenterally, e.g. chlorpheniramine 10 to 20 mg IM. Although H_1-blockers are very useful drugs as preventatives, e.g. in hay fever, we have seen that they are not likely to be effective in the very acute reactions where histamine is involved. Nevertheless, in a lesser reaction, antihistamine blockage of receptors may well be useful in preventing further access of histamine. An additional benefit is that antihistamines do have some sedative properties and this is useful as patients are likely to be apprehensive about their condition. Of course, adrenaline should always be available in this lesser situation in case the other remedies prove ineffective.

The question might be asked why adrenaline is not used routinely as it seems to be effective in all situations? The answer resides in the nature of adrenaline itself; it can be a dangerous substance and as such should be reserved for those life-endangering situations when other things won't do.

Other important examples of Type I reactions are asthma, rhinitis, (hay fever), angio-oedema, and urticaria. These are also known as the atopic states, which are usually less severe than acute anaphylaxis.

Asthma

Bronchial asthma has two components, increased tone of the smooth muscle within the bronchial walls (bronchoconstriction), and increased secretion of mucosal glands. In some asthmatic subjects, an attack of bronchoconstriction may be severe and prolonged, enough to cause an emergency almost as grave as that presented by anaphylactic shock. Asthma can be a very dangerous condition; many attacks are relatively mild, but it can kill.

The bronchospasm, as we have seen in Chapter 16, is due to the release of SRS and to a lesser extent, histamine, from sensitized mast cells in the bronchial mucosa. Typically the allergy is due to feathers, animal furs, and dusts. There is a form of asthma that occurs in later life, probably more common in women, where the cause is difficult to pinpoint. Drug-induced asthma is rare except as part of the picture of a systemic anaphylaxis.

Asthma is usually treated with sympathomimetic drugs, which stimulate β_2-receptors with relatively little action on cardiac receptors. Two such drugs are salbutamol and terbutaline; both of these can be used to abate an attack of acute asthma. Salbutamol, for instance, comes in various forms, i.e. as tablets, as a syrup, as an inhaler, as an injection, and as an infusion.

Provided that the airways are adequately open perhaps the best way of delivering the drug is by inhalation direct to the bronchioles. The therapeutic effect is rapid as the drug acts directly on the β_2-receptors of bronchioles and the action persists for four to six hours. Usually it does not adversely affect the cardiovascular system but constant usage can lead to tachycardia and arrhythmias.

Another drug that is useful in abating an acute attack of asthma is aminophylline, which is also a β_2-stimulant. It is a xanthine derivative, of which caffeine is another, and is often used by intravenous drip to terminate an acute attack of asthma that has proved resistant to the usual remedies. The place of drugs such as aminophylline in the treatment of asthma has varied from time to time, but there is no doubt that it is effective, although it does have an effect on the heart (e.g. tachycardia), thus providing a cautionary note.

A steroid, beclomethasone, used as an inhalant may be useful in certain situations. For instance, if the attack has not responded to a bronchodilator, a steroid may be required for a short period of treatment to re-establish the activity of the bronchodilator.

Sodium cromoglycate, a drug of relatively recent origin, stabilizes the mast cell and prevents degranulation. This at once implies that it will not terminate an attack of asthma, but may act as a preventative. Sodium cromoglycate is taken prophylactically several times a day and is effective in reducing the frequency and severity of attacks in many asthmatic subjects. It seems to be a very innocuous drug, free of unwanted effects by and large. It is usually prescribed in the form of an inhalant for maintenance therapy.

If an asthmatic attack occurs within the dental surgery, it is likely that the patient will have their remedy with them. It is unlikely that the dental surgeon will have either salbutamol or terbutaline available as part of an emergency kit, although there is no reason why not. However, adrenaline will certainly be part of that kit, and this should abate an attack. The asthma is likely to be relieved by a subcutaneous injection of adrenaline at the rate of about 0.5 ml per minute up to a total dose of 1.0 to 1.5 ml. If the attack is not relieved, an intramuscular injection of a corticosteroid (hydrocortisone 100 mg) should be given, oxygen administered, and medical aid sought. Antihistamines, as we have discussed, are likely to be totally ineffective as the principal mediator in the attack is not histamine.

Angio-oedema

This is a condition where leakage of fluid from vessels causes localized or more general swellings. It is commonly seen in the face, mouth, and upper respiratory tract, and is probably due to the release of histamine from sensitized mast cells. If the condition is very serious, the whole face may become swollen and there may be oedema of the pharynx and larynx to the degree that respiration is jeopardized.

The swelling occurs suddenly and dramatically, and is often preceded by the skin becoming very itchy. Immediate relief of the swelling, especially if the larynx is involved, can be obtained by the subcutaneous injection of adrenaline 1:1000 up to a total dose of 1.5 ml. The greatest danger in this condition is respiratory obstruction (more likely to occur in children) and, if the adrenaline fails to bring relief to the oedematous larynx, then it will be necessary to bypass the supralaryngeal airway. The recommended technique is that of laryngotomy, and this is performed by passing a fine-bore tube (cannula), or a large-gauge 'Venflor' between the thyroid and cricoid cartilages (i.e. through the cricothyroid membrane). Oxygen is then introduced through this tube and can be enough to maintain life. An emergency tracheostomy is not advocated; this is an extremely skilled procedure and, in an emergency situation, may prove a problem even to the experienced surgeon, never mind the dental surgeon unskilled in such techniques.

If the attack is less severe, an intramuscular injection of an antihistamine H_1-blocker, for instance chlorpheniramine, 10 to 20 mg, or promethazine, 25 to 50 mg, followed by an adequate oral dosage may suffice.

Rhinitis (hay fever)

This is a localized reaction due to the release of histamine by mast cells in the nasal and conjunctival mucosa. It usually occurs in people sensitized to pollens, and can more or less be regarded as a summer disease. Sneezing, itching and irritation of the nose, running nose, irritation of the eyes, and profuse lachrymation are all symptomatic. Some unfortunate individuals appear to be sensitive to materials of a non-seasonal nature and may show hay fever like symptoms at any time of the year. They are said to suffer from perennial paroxysmal rhinorrhea.

In rhinitis, antihistamines (H_1-blockers) may be the drugs of choice, bringing relief in about 80 per cent of cases. These drugs are effective preventatives rather than curatives. If given continuously to those suffering from hay fever, or at the appropriate season, then by blocking the histamine receptors they will prevent access of the histamine to receptors and may, therefore, prevent the occurrence of an attack.

Hay fever is more troublesome (and it may be very troublesome indeed) than life threatening, and so the problem can be tackled this way, by prevention rather than cure. However, cure can be considered by desensitizing the patient, and this is effective in some cases.

Urticaria

This is due to the release of histamine from sensitized mast cells in the skin. It is commonly known as 'nettle rash', not an inappropriate title, for the lesions are very like those of a nettle sting. In urticaria there is a widespread eruption of firm, pink or white weals, accompanied by intense itching. A very characteristic feature is its evanescent nature, the lesions appearing suddenly and disappearing within hours or even minutes. It is a common manifestation of allergic hypersensitivity to foods and drugs. In many ways, urticaria is an odd phenomenon: it sometimes occurs in people who are apparently not sensitive to any article of diet, but who are under some form of emotional stress; often no apparent cause can be found. The most common things in diet to produce urticaria are the proteins of shellfish, eggs, and milk, and some fruits—especially strawberries.

The best treatment of urticaria may be antihistamines acting as preventatives. Although the response is good, it is perhaps not quite as good as occurs in the subject who has rhinitis.

It will be appreciated that any of these atopic states can be a manifestation of allergy to a drug. All are Type I hypersensitivity reactions and are those most likely to be encountered by the dental practitioner.

Type II—Cytoxic reactions

These are mediated by IgG and IgM antibodies. The antibody combines with an antigen on the cell surface, the complement system is activated, and cell lysis occurs. The principal target cells are those in the circulatory system. An example of a Type II reaction is Rhesus incompatibility in the new-born child where antibodies are produced by a Rhesus negative mother against the Rhesus factor on the red cells of the fetus. The antibodies cross the placenta and cause haemolysis. Another example is sulphonamide-induced granulocytopenia.

Type III—Arthus reactions, serum sickness

These are primarily mediated by IgG; the combination between antigen and antibody forms complexes that subsequently activate complement. The rate of formation of antigen/antibody complexes depends upon the absolute amount of antigen and antibody present and their relative proportions to each other. In the presence of *antibody excess*, antigen/antibody complexes are readily precipitated and are localized at the site of antigen introduction. Complement factors are activated, and the responses occur at the site of antigen introduction. This reaction is known as the Arthus reaction and is characterized by local oedema and necrosis.

When there is *antigen excess*, soluble antigen/antibody complexes are formed that circulate and may become located in vascular endothelium producing a destructive inflammatory response called the serum-sickness syndrome. The clinical symptoms are fever, an urticarial rash, lymphadenopathy, and swelling of the joints (arthralgia). The condition usually lasts for about 6 to 12 days, and subsides on removal of the offending drug (antigen). Sulphonamides, penicillin, streptomycin, as well as other drugs, can cause this syndrome.

The treatment of serum sickness is by steroids; corticosteroids control all its manifestations and are drugs of first choice. Although urticarial and oedematous lesions respond well to H_1-blockers, these drugs often have no effect on the fever or arthralgia.

Type IV—Delayed hypersensitivity reactions

These are mediated by sensitized T-lymphocytes and macrophages, and are therefore cell-mediated ractions (see earlier). When sensitized T-lymphocytes come into contact with antigen, they undergo blast transformation and the resultant cells produce lymphokines (see The Immune System above). Type IV reactions take place one to four days after antigen exposure; examples include contact dermatitis and organ transplant rejection. Many reactions due to drugs, chemicals, and foods belong to this group; for example, contact dermatitis due to procaine, penicillin, or metals such as mercury and nickel. Cell-mediated hypersensitivity is also an important factor in periodontal disease.

These reactions do not respond to sympathomimetic agents or to H_1-blockers; indeed, the blockers, if applied topically, may themselves be responsible for producing delayed hypersensitivity. Corticosteroids are the most useful group of drugs in treatment of this type of reaction, but these cases should be referred to a dermatologist.

It is important for dental surgeons to remember that they themselves are particularly liable to become sensitized to drugs that they handle regularly, such as local anaesthetics and antibiotics, as is discussed in the appropriate Chapters.

Prevention of the unwanted effects due to drugs

A number of points should be noted. firstly, there is an increased incidence of adverse drug reactions in neonates and in the aged. For some unaccountable reason, it seems that women tend to suffer more from adverse drug reactions than do men. Patients with an allergic diathesis are also more prone to adverse reactions, and this may include reactions for which there seems to be no immunological explanation—the asthmatic's reaction to aspirin may be of this nature. Clearly, the presence of renal and hepatic disease can predispose to adverse effects; for example, the metabolism of a drug may be seriously impaired. Certain drugs appear to be especially liable to produce unwanted effects, e.g. anticoagulants, antihypertensive drugs, non-steroidal anti-inflammatory drugs, antimicrobials (penicillin being particularly prone—perhaps because of its extensive usage).

In order to reduce the incidence of adverse reactions, the following points should be considered:

1. Medical history taking must include a drug history; any previous untoward experiences with drugs should be noted and the drug withheld if there is a history of allergy.
2. If a patient is sensitized to one drug, he or she is likely to be sensitized to all drugs in the same group and possibly also to related drugs, e.g. penicillin and the cephalosporins.

3. Has the patient any underlying medical conditions that might predispose to a build-up of the drug and toxicity, e.g. renal failure?
4. Is the drug really necessary at all—is the medical condition self-limiting?
5. Is the safest drug possible being used for the treatment?
6. Is there a possibility of a drug interaction?

In spite of taking into account all factors, no doubt therapeutic misadventures will still occur. However, a proper consideration of all of these factors will minimize the problem.

Oral reactions to drugs

These are relatively rare considering the extent of consumption of drugs. This is a wide subject, and is dealt with fully in specialized textbooks, e.g. *Textbook of Adverse Drug Reactions* (see Further reading). Table 21.1 gives some examples of the sort of reaction that can occur in the mouth, but it makes no pretence to be exhaustive. In general, the mechanisms behind these oral reactions are ill-understood, although in some instances there is an immunlogical basis.

IMMUNOSUPPRESSANTS

When foreign tissue or cells are introduced into the body, the immune system is activated and the foreign material eliminated. Despite the essential protective role of the immune response, the system may need to be suppressed. Immunosuppression is required in organ transplants and in the treatment of certain autoimmune diseases. Cytotoxic drugs and corticosteroids suppress the immune system and these are discussed elsewhere (see Chapters 17 and 18). The main immunosuppressants used clinically are cyclosporin and azathioprine.

Cyclosporin

Cyclosporin is a relatively new immunosuppressant obtained from the fermentation of two fungi, *Trichoderma polysporum* and *Clindrocarpon lucidum*. Although first developed as an antifungal, and then as an antibiotic, both of these actions proved unsatisfactory. However, it was soon realized that cyclosporin induced a selective type of immunosuppression and the drug is now widely used to prevent the rejection of organ transplants.

Pharmacological properties

Cyclosporin can be administered orally or parenterally. When given orally, the drug is rapidly absorbed from the gastro-intestinal tract and has a half-life of approximately four hours. Cyclosporin is metabolized in the liver, and the metabolites excreted in the bile and elminated in the faeces.

Table 21.1. Unwanted effects of drugs in the orofacial region

Disorder	Drug(s) involved
Xerostomia	Ganglion blockers; atropine and atropine-like antispasmodics, e.g. propantheline bromide; antidepressants—tricyclic and tetracyclic; antiparkinsonian drugs, e.g. benzhexol, biperiden, benztropine, and orphenadrine; antihistamine drugs, H_1-blockers; phenothiazines; clonidine
Disturbances of taste:	
(i) partial or total loss of taste	Penicillamine; clofibrate; carbimazole; lithium carbonate; lincomycin; phenindione; prothionamide; griseofulvin.
(ii) metallic taste	Metronidazole; biguanide antidiabetic drugs, e.g. metformin
Halitosis	Isorbide dinitrate (sublingually); disulfiram
Pain and swelling of the salivary glands	Phenylbutazone and oxyphenbutazone; iodides; bretylium; guanethidine; bethanidine; methyldopa; clonidine; nitrofurantoin; chlorhexidine
Cervical lymphadenopathy	Phenytoin and primidone
Erythema multiforme	Barbiturates; carbamazepine; chlorpropamide; clindamycin; ethambutol; meprobamate; minoxidil;penicillin; phenylbutazone; phenytoin; sulphonamides (long-acting); sulindac; salicylates; rifampicin
Lupus erythematosus (systemic)—SLE	A wide variety of drugs has been implicated in the production of SLE. The oral mucosa is involved in about 25 per cent of patients. Drugs involved range from antihypertensives to anti-infective agents, e.g. penicillin, tetracycline.
Lichenoid eruptions	Chlorpropamide; indomethacin; methyldopa; a-adrenoceptor blocking drugs, e.g. labetalol; chloroquine; mepacrine; gold salts; quinine; quinidine; streptomycin; sodium aminosalicylate
Gingival hyperplasia and hypertrophy	Phenytoin; cyclosporin; oral contraceptives; nifedipine
Discolouration of the oral mucosa and teeth	
(i) mucosal tissues	Lead poisoning; chloroquine; phenothiazines; oral contraceptives; chlorhexidine
(ii) teeth	Tetracyclines; stannous fluoride toothpastes; chlorhexidine
Oral ulcerations	
(i) a number of chemicals can cause 'burns' of the oral mucosa if injudiciously applied	e.g. trichloracetic acid in the treatment of pericoronitis
(ii) Drugs used for other purposes may cause local irritation of the mouth	Aspirin; potassium; isoprenaline (used as sublingual tablets); pancreatin powder or tablets; emepromium bromide; gentian violet; cocaine
(iii) Oral ulceration, either primary or secondary to leucopenia	Antineoplastic agents, such as methotrexate, fluorouracil, actinomycin D, doxorubicin and bleomycin
(iv) Oral ulceration with neutropenia	Naproxen
Oral infections induced or aggravated by drugs	Corticosteroids: given in non-physiological amounts over a long period, these carry an increased risk of bacterial, fungal, or viral infections.

Table 21.1. Unwanted effects of drugs in the orofacial region

Disorder	Drug(s) involved
	Antibiotics: particularly broad-spectrum types, can alter the normal bacterial flora of the mouth, throat and gut, so that resistant organisms may proliferate; overgrowth of *C. albicans* may result, causing oral candidiasis.
	Antimetabolites: topical fluorouracil therapy has been associated with the activation of herpes labialis (and the development of telangiectasia).
	Immunosuppressive drugs: (e.g. azathioprine and prednisone in renal transplants)—bacterial or fungal infections; severe herpes simplex infection has been observed.
	Oral contraceptives: their use has been associated with 'dry socket' after tooth extraction.
Extrapyramidal syndromes	
(i) acute dyskinesia (involuntary movements of the tongue, trismus, and grimacing—together with spontaneous dislocations of the TMJ)	Phenothiazines; butyrophenones; metoclopramide; tricyclic antidepressants; phenytoin; carbamazepine; lithium
(ii) tardive dyskinesia	As above

Pharmacodynamics

An important component of the immune response is the interaction between macrophages and lymphocytes. As a result of this interaction, macrophages produce a chemical mediator called interleukin I, which stimulates T-helper cells. Once stimulated, the T-helper cell produces interleukin II, another chemical transmitter, which activates other uncommitted T-lymphocytes to differentiate into helper, suppressor or killer cells.

Cyclosporin is a selective immunosuppressant, affecting the T-cell or cell-mediated response with little or no effect on the B-cell or humoral response. The action on the cell-mediated system is as follows. Cyclosporin inhibits the priming or 'activation' of macrophages and therefore interferes with the synthesis of interleukin I. Following this action on the macrophage, cyclosporin acts on the T-helper cell by preventing the production of interleukin II. Finally, the drug inhibits the formation of interleukin II receptors on undifferentiated T-cells, which blocks the production of more helper, suppressor, and killer T-cells. It also appears that cyclosporin affects helper cells more than suppressor cells, resulting in a net imbalance in favour of suppressor action.

Unwanted effects

These include nephrotoxicity, hepatotoxicity, mild anaemia, tremors, transient paraesthesia, and excessive hair growth (hirsutism). Of particular interest to the dental surgeon is the action of the drug on the oral structures, causing gingival hyperplasia and transient perioral hyperaesthesia.

Gingival hyperplasia occurs in approximately one-third of those taking cyclosporin. It is more frequent in children than adults, and begins in the interdental papilla. The labial gingiva of the anterior teeth are more commonly affected than the posterior teeth. Local irritants, such as plaque, calculus, faulty restorations, prosthetic and orthodontic appliances, may increase the severity of the hyperplasia.

Many patients experience a perioral tingling sensation when they first start cyclosporin therapy. The sensation usually disappears within a few days; it may be dose-related.

Uses

Cyclosporin is mainly used to prevent rejection of organ transplants, such as kidney, heart, and liver. It has also been used in the treatment of insulin-dependent diabetes, cirrhosis, psoriasis, and rheumatoid arthritis.

Azathioprine

This is a purine derivative with selective immunosuppressant activity against the cell-mediated system. The drug appears to increase T-cell suppressor activity and reduce T-cell helper activity. Azathioprine can be given orally or parenterally.

Unwanted effects

There are many of these, and because of these risks the use of this drug should be balanced against the severity of the patient's condition and the expected clinical effect. The most serious unwanted effect of azathioprine therapy is depression of bone marrow function causing a leucopenia and thrombocytopenia. Routine haematological screening is required for all patients taking azathioprine. Other unwanted effects include gastro-intestinal intolerance, allergic reaction, and skin rashes.

Uses

Azathioprine is mainly used to prevent rejection of organ transplants. The drug is also used as an alternative to corticosteroids in pemphigus, systemic lupus erythematosis, severe rheumatoid arthritis, and thrombocytopenic purpura.

REFERENCES

Foldes, F. F., Swerdlow, M., Lipschitz, E., VanHees, G. R., and Shanor, S. P. (1956). Comparison of the respiratory effects of suxamethonium and suxamethonium in man. *Anaesthesiology*, **17**, 559–68.

Kalow, W., and Gunn, D. R. (1957). The relation between dose of succinylcholine and duration of apnoea in man. *Journal of Pharmacology and Experimental Therapeutics*, **120**, 203–14.

Parker, C. W. (1963). Penicillin allergy. (Editorial). *American Journal of Medicine*, **34**, 747–51.

Rawlins, M. D. and Thompson, J. W. (1985). Mechanisms of adverse drug reactions. In *Textbook of adverse drug reactions*, (3 edn), (ed. D. M. Davies). Oxford University Press.

Rosenheim, M. L. and Moulton, R. L. (ed) (1958). *Sensitivity reactions to drugs*. Blackwell, Oxford.

FURTHER READING

Daley, T. D. and Wysocki, G. P. (1984). Cyclosporin therapy: its significance to the periodontist. *Journal of Periodontology*, **55**, 701–11.

Roitt, I. M. and Lehner, T. (1983). Immunology and oral disease, (2nd edn,). Blackwell, Oxford.

Walton, J. G. and Seymour, R. A. (1985). Dental disorders. In *Textbook of adverse drug reactions*. (3rd edn), (ed. D. M. Davies). Oxford University Press.

22

Drug interactions

INTRODUCTION

It is sometimes necessary to give more than one drug at the same time, and when this is so their effects may be exerted independently or they may interact. It must be made clear at the outset that not all drug interactions are therapeutically undesirable. Thus some interactions may be deliberately planned in order to produce some useful effect that cannot be achieved by means of a single drug; for example, the antimicrobial combination co-trimoxazole (trimethoprim + sulpha-methoxazole), or the combined oral contraceptive (oestrogen + progestogen). On the other hand, the interaction may be undesirable and potentially dangerous (Macgregor 1965; British National Formulary, 1987); one of the earliest and best known examples is that between ethyl alcohol and barbiturates, which can produce a profound depression of the CNS. Other examples are aspirin + warfarin, or a monoamine oxidase inhibitor (MAOI) + cheese (Blackwell *et al.* 1967). The result of the interaction may be the potentiation or antagonism of one drug by another (Type A in the classification of Unwanted effects; Chapter 21), or it may be the production of some different effect that is not readily predictable (Type B in the same classification). Whatever the mechanism, all drug interactions should be reported to the Committee on Safety in Medicines using the special yellow pre-paid postcards that are made available for the report of adverse drug reactions. Clearly the dental surgeon may, in the absence of sufficient knowledge about drug interactions, prescribe a drug to a patient who is already taking another one for some medical condition, and thereby unwittingly precipitate a drug interaction.

INCIDENCE AND IMPORTANCE OF DRUG INTERACTIONS

In theory, many such interactions are possible but in practice only a relatively small number are of clinical importance. An accurate estimate of their incidence amongst out-patients is not available but, for hospital in-patients, it has been estimated to be in the range 0.5–2 per cent. This suggests that adverse drug interactions represent a minor contribution to adverse drug reactions as a whole, and there is little doubt that in the past the potential incidence of drug interactions has been exaggerated. However, for certain drugs the potential for reaction is much higher than it is for others and it is these that must be avoided. For example, in a study of 277 patients taking oral anticoagulants of whom 94 were receiving other drugs with which the anticoagulants might have interacted (33.9 per cent of the total), clinically significant interactions were considered to have developed in 6 patients. This represents an incidence of 6.4 per cent in those taking drug combinations (2.2 per cent in all patients; Williams *et al.* 1976).

Drug interactions of clinical importance

These are likely to be due to two main reasons:

1. *The drug has a steep dose–response curve.* Under these conditions a relatively small quantitative change in the concentration of drug at the target site (receptor, enzyme), or in the tissue, leads to substantial changes in the therapeutic or adverse effect—for example; digoxin, lithium.

2. *The drug has a major effect on a vital process.* Drugs that alter such vital processes as blood pressure, blood coagulation, or control of breathing fall into this category. It will be appreciated that a drug that interacts with another given in a dose carefully determined to produce a particular effect, could produce potentially lethal effects.

In practice, the chief sources of serious clinical interactions are drawn from a short list of drugs that fall into the following classes (Dollery and Brodie, 1980):

(1) oral anticoagulants (coumarins);

(2) oral contraceptives (oestrogen and progestogen);

(3) oral hypoglycaemics (tolbutamide, chlorpropamide, glibenclamide);

(4) cardiovascular: (a) cardiac glycosides, (b) anti-arrhythmics, (c) antihypertensive (hypotensive);

(5) anticonvulsants (phenytoin, phenobarbitone, primidone, carbamazepine);

(6) CNS drugs;

(7) aminoglycoside antibiotics (amikacin, gentamicin, kanamycin, neomycin, netilmicin, streptomycin, and tobramycin);

(8) cytotoxics and immunosuppressants.

CLASSIFICATION OF DRUG INTERACTIONS

Such interactions may be classified into three groups, namely pharmaceutical, pharmacokinetic, and pharmacodynamic.

Pharmaceutical interactions

These are due to the formulation or mixing of chemically incompatible substances. Thus pharmaceutical interactions are most likely to occur when drugs interact in the same infusion solution, e.g. ampicillin with glucose; or when one drug interacts with the solution (e.g. amphotericin is unstable in dextrose–saline solution). Details about the addition of medication to infusion fluids are included in the *British National Formulary* (BNF; see Appendix 2, 1988). This form of interaction is unlikely to occur in dental practice because of the nature of the drugs and the routes of administration normally used. Nevertheless, the dental practitioner should be aware of and alert to this form of interaction.

Pharmacokinetic interactions

These are due to altered absorption, distribution (protein binding), metabolism, or excretion of one drug by another.

Suitable examples will now be given under these headings; Table 22.1 (below) lists other interactions.

Absorption

An example of adverse interactions related to increased absorption are those between MAOIs and sympathomimetic amines (see Chapter 14). Here the drug restricts the action of an intestinal enzyme (monoamine oxidase), allowing the absorption of abnormal quantities of amines, which may have serious effects.

By contrast, an important and useful way in which one drug may decrease the absorption of another is the addition of a vasoconstrictor, usually adrenaline, to solutions of local anaesthetics. This serves a dual purpose: by delaying absorption, it prolongs the duration of anaesthesia; and simultaneously it reduces the rate of increase of the plasma concentration of local anaesthetic and thereby lessens the likelihood of systemic effects.

The absorption of tetracyclines may be reduced as a consequence of interacting chemically with antacids that contain divalent and trivalent cations (e.g. Ca, Al, Mg), dairy products (e.g. milk), oral iron preparations, sucralfate, and zinc sulphate. These combinations of drugs should therefore be avoided otherwise the therapeutic effect of tetracyclines will be reduced.

Distribution

In the context of drug interactions, the factor most likely to affect the distribution of a drug in the body is an alteration in the extent to which it is bound to protein (Brodie, 1964). Thus the displacement of drug X from some of its binding sites on plasma protein by drug Y (which has a stronger affinity) leads to an elevation of the plasma concentration of drug X; and if drug Y is withdrawn the reverse will occur. However, it is important to realize that for a *significant* alteration of the free

Table 22.1. Some drug interactions with which the dental practitioner may be concerned

1st Agent Prescribed as part of MEDICAL treatment		2nd Agent, which might be prescribed as part of DENTAL (or other) treatment	Clinical result of interaction between 1st and 2nd agent	Course of action and comments	Possible mechanism of interaction
Group	**Drug**				
1. Gastro-intestinal	Metoclopramide	Antimuscarinic (anticholinergic) e.g. atropine; Opioid (opiate) e.g. morphine	Antagonism—reduced effect of both drugs	Avoid combination	Physiological antagonism
	Antacids containing salts of calcium (Ca), magnesium (Mg), aluminium (Al) Oral iron (Fe)	Tetracyclines	Therapeutic failure (tetracyclines used for treating rapid forms of periodontal destruction see Chapter 11)	Stop antacids that contain Ca, Mg, Al, and oral Fe during therapy with tetracyclines	Chelation
2. Cardiovascular: β-adrenoceptor blocking drugs	Acebutalol Atenolol Metoprolol Nadolol Oxprenolol Penbutolol Pindolol Propranolol Sotalol Timolol	Sympathomimetic amines, e.g. adrenaline phenylephrine (amphetamines), including cold remedies	Severe hypertension, particularly with non-selective β-blockers. Rarely, severe hypertension	Hypertensive crisis should be treated with an α-adrenergic receptor blocking drug (Elis et al. 1967) e.g. phentolamine (Rogitine) 5 mg IV or im, repeated if necessary.	In the presence of β-blockers, the α-agonist actions of the sympathomimetic are exerted unopposed, especially with vasopressor effect.
Antihypertensive drugs	Vasodilators e.g. hydralazine Centrally acting, e.g. methyldopa Adrenergic neurone blockers e.g. bethanidine α-adrenoceptor blockers, e.g. prazosin. Angiotensin-converting enzyme inhibitors e.g. captopril	Hypnotics, sedatives e.g. benzodiazepines, H₁-blockers with sedative property	Potentiates antihypertensive effect	Use combination with care	Hypnotics and sedatives depress vasomotor centre
Anticoagulants	Heparin	Aspirin Compound analgesics containing aspirin	Potentiation of anticoagulant	Avoid combination	Reduced aggregation of platelets. Reduced prothrombin production (chronic use)

Table 22.1. Some drug interactions with which the dental practitioner may be concerned

1st Agent Prescribed as part of MEDICAL treatment		2nd Agent, which might be prescribed as part of DENTAL (or other) treatment	Clinical result of interaction between 1st and 2nd agent	Course of action and comments	Possible mechanism of interaction
Group	Drug				
Anticoagulants	Warfarin	Aspirin (D and I) Possibly some other NSAIDs (but ibuprofen and naproxen usually safe) Co-trimoxazole (I) Erythromycin (I) Ketoconazole (I) Metronidazole (I) Paracetamol (regular treatment or high doses)	Potentiation of anticoagulant	Avoid combination; if not possible adjust dose of warfarin appropriately	D = displacement from binding sites, but not clinically significant I = inhibition of warfarin metabolism
3. CNS hypnotics and sedatives	Benzodiazepines: alprazolam chlordiazepoxide clobazam diazepam nitrazepam triazolam	Alcohol Antihistamines (H_1-blockers) Narcotic analgesics	Potentiation of hypnotic/sedative effect of benzodiazepine	Avoid combination or adjust dose of 1st or 2nd agent	Synergism of two drugs with central depressant actions
Antidepressants monoamine oxidase inhibitors (MAOIs)	Phenelzine Iproniazid Isocarboxazid Tranylcypromine Pargyline (antihypertensive only)	Indirectly (or mixed) acting sympathomimetic amines: ephedrine phenylephrine Amine-containing foods: cheese pickled herrings Marmite yoghourt Bovril broad beans strong wines and beers	Acute hypertensive crisis with stimulation of CNS Hypertension with headache. Risk of cerebral haemorrhage	Hypertensive crisis should be treated with an α-adrenergic receptor blocking agent, e.g. phentolamine 5 mg IV or IM repeated if necessary. Patients on MAOI must be WARNED not to take these foods	Inhibition of MAO by MAOIs interferes with the biotransformation of those amines which are normally substrates for this enzyme. MAOIs *also* inhibit other enzyme systems e.g. pethidine demethylase, and this may be responsible for the serious interaction which can occur when a narcotic analgesic such as pethidine is given to a patient taking an MAOI. Many of the other interactions between MAOIs and other drugs reported may be due to similar mechanisms.

	Drug	Interacting drug	Effect	Action	Mechanism
	Narcotic analgesics: pethidine morphine codeine barbiturates general anaesthetics		Coma with hypotension/hypertension, CNS stimulation.	Treat with hydrocortisone hemisuccinate 100 mg IV or IM repeated as necessary; symptomatic treatment including the use of α-adrenergic receptor blockers for hypertension where necessary; medical aid should be sought immediately. IMPORTANT: These combinations of drugs should not be used. Patients who are receiving MAOIs should *wear a locket* indicating that they are taking these drugs, as well as carrying written evidence from the doctor who prescribed the drug, warning against these dangers. In the event of one of these emergencies hospital treatment should be sought immediately.	
Tricyclic and related compounds	Amitriptyline Butriptyline Clomipramine Desipramine Dothiepin Iprindole Maprotiline Mianserin Nortriptyline Protriptyline Trazodone Trimipramine Viloxazine	Adrenaline noradrenaline (alone or with local anaesthetics)	Hypertension; but it is important to note that the small amount of adrenaline added to a solution of local anaesthetic is usually safe for administration to a patient taking tricyclic antidepressant.	If a hypertensive attack occurs it should be treated with an α-adrenergic receptor blocking agent, e.g. phentolamine 5 mg IV or IM repeated if necessary.	Tricyclic compounds interfere with uptake of adrenaline and noradrenaline (both directly acting sympathomimetic amines) into adrenergic nerve endings.
Anti-epileptics	Phenytoin	Barbiturates (also alcohol, carbamazepine)	Reduced phenytoin effect	Avoid combination or adjust dosage appropriately.	Increased metabolism of phenytoin due to induction of DMES (see text).
Anaesthesia	General anaesthetics	Adrenaline	Arrhythmias with halothane, cyclopropane, trichlorethylene	Avoid combination	Some general anaesthetics sensitize the myocardium to the arrhythmogenic action of adrenaline
4. Infections	Griseofulvin	Barbiturates	Reduced therapeutic effect of griseofulvin	Adjust dose of either drug appropriately	Accelerated inactivation of griseofulvin

Table 22.1. Some drug interactions with which the dental practitioner may be concerned

1st Agent Prescribed as part of MEDICAL treatment		2nd Agent, which might be prescribed as part of DENTAL (or other) treatment	Clinical result of interaction between 1st and 2nd agent	Course of action and comments	Possible mechanism of interaction
Group	Drug				
5. Miscellaneous	Ethyl alcohol (ethanol) (most likely to be taken for social reasons)	Barbiturates Benzodiazepines Phenothiazines Antihistamines (H_1-blockers)	Enhanced depression of CNS	Patient must be warned of the risk of these interactions	Additive or synergistic effects due to combination of actions of two centrally depressant drugs
		Metronidazole	May produce unpleasant disulfiram-like effects e.g. flushing, nausea and epigastric discomfort	Advise patient to avoid use of alcohol during treatment with metronidazole.	Inhibits hepatic metabolism of ethanol causing disulfiram-like ('Antabuse') effects
	Oestrogen and progestogen	Rifampicin, possibly other broad-spectrum antibiotics	Failure of contraception.	Where there may be special concern, alternative methods of contraception should be instituted.	Although there are anecdotal reports of this interaction, convincing evidence is lacking; patient compliance failure is a more likely explanation.

plasma concentration to take place, two conditions must obtain. First, the drug to be displaced (drug X) must be highly bound to plasma protein, e.g. 99 per cent, so that a small change in binding, for example 1 per cent, will result in a doubling of its free plasma concentration (from 1 per cent to 2 per cent of the total). Second, the major part of the total dose of drug X must be distributed in plasma; if the converse is true, then extensive displacement from the plasma binding sites would produce little clinical effect. Three groups of drugs that fulfil these criteria are (i) oral anticoagulants, e.g. warfarin (bound 99 per cent volume of distribution (Vd 9 l)); (ii) oral hypoglycaemics e.g. tolbutamide (bound 96 per cent, Vd 10 l); and (iii) the antiepileptic, phenytoin (bound 90 per cent, Vd 35 l); (Aronson and Grahame-Smith 1981).

The clinical dangers of drug interactions due to displacement from protein-binding sites have turned out to be much less than originally anticipated. This is because for those drugs likely to be involved, the total clearance rate is proportional to the fraction of unbound drug in the plasma. As a consequence, the increase in plasma concentration that follows from binding displacement is offset by a compensatory increase in clearance, so that the plasma *concentration* remains virtually unchanged once the new steady-state has been reached. Nevertheless, until such time as this state has been reached, there will be an increase in the amount of free (i.e. pharmacologically active) drug in the plasma, and this will produce an effect that may result in a potentially adverse reaction; for example, haemorrhage due to excessive anticoagulation (coumarins). In practice this mechanism occurs rarely and other mechanisms are involved, usually inhibition of drug metabolizing enzymes (DMEs; see below and Chapter 1).

Metabolism (biotransformation)

The intensity and duration of effect of many drugs depend largely upon their rate of biotransformation, chiefly in the liver, to less active or inactive metabolites (Gillette, 1967). Therefore, if the rate of metabolism of one drug is altered by another drug, this will substantially modify the effect of the first drug.

Stimulation (induction) of drug-metabolizing enzymes (DMEs)

Certain drugs such as phenobarbitone, phenytoin, primidone, carbamazepine, rifampicin, griseofulvin, and ethanol (ethyl alcohol)—chronic use, as well as cigarette smoking, are powerful inducers of DMEs with the result that the half-life $(T_{0.5})$ of some drugs may be reduced substantially. The enzyme induction develops over several weeks and takes about the same time to disappear after the inducing agent has been withdrawn. Drugs with a metabolism likely to be altered by enzyme inducers are anticoagulants and oral contraceptives. Thus the metabolism of warfarin may be increased, so leading to a diminished anticoagulant effect and the need for an increased dosage. If the inducer is then withdrawn, the subsequent reduced metabolism will lead to an increased effect with possible haemorrhagic complications.

A potentially important interaction belonging to this group is that between oral contraceptive steroids and antibiotics (Dossetor, 1975). Over the past decade there have been sporadic reports of women who have become pregnant whilst taking an antibiotic at the same time as an oral contraceptive steroid. As a consequence, the impression has gained ground that oral contraceptive steroids may fail in the presence of antibiotics. This suggestion received support from the results of animal studies, where there is clear evidence of an entero-hepatic circulation of steroids that can be modulated by broad-spectrum antibiotics. Antibiotics suppress the gut microflora, which normally deconjugate (and therefore reactivate) steroids previously inactivated by conjugation in the liver. However, human studies suggest that in most women entero-hepatic recirculation of contraceptive steroids plays only a minor metabolic role and is therefore most unlikely to account for contraceptive failure in the presence of broad-spectrum antibiotics (Orme and Back 1986). A much more likely explanation is failure of compliance. When there is special concern about the possible effect of an antibiotic on a particular patient already taking contraceptive steroids, then she should be given either co-trimoxazole (because this appears least likely to cause an interaction problem), or she should be advised to use an alternative method of contraception.

Inhibition of drug-metabolizing enzymes (DMEs)

A number of drugs may inhibit DMEs; these include metronidazole, chloramphenicol, phenylbutazone, cimetidine, ethanol (acute intoxication), isoniazid, and MAOIs. The commonest drugs to be affected through this inhibition are phenytoin and anticoagulants; thus the effects of phenytoin are increased in the presence of isoniazid (in slow acetylators) or chloramphenicol.

Unfortunately, despite their name, MAOIs are very unspecific and may also decrease the rate of biotransformation of barbiturates, phenothiazines, and alcohol. It has also been shown in animals that the metabolism of pethidine (and other opioids) is slowed by MAOIs due to inhibition of pethidine demethylase (Clark 1967), the enzyme that demethylates pethidine to norpethidine. The potentially lethal interaction between pethidine and MAOIs that may occur in man could be due to a similar mechanism (Clark and Thompson 1972).

General anaesthetic agents should not be given to any patient receiving an MAOI. If, for the purposes of dental treatment, a general anaesthetic is necessary, the MAOI should be withdrawn, but only after consultation with the patient's medical adviser, and the anaesthetic should not be given until a period of three weeks has elapsed. If it is absolutely essential to give the general anaesthetic in the presence of an MAOI, then the patient must be admitted to hospital and the psychiatrist responsible must, for that patient, vouch that the risk of stopping the MAOI is greater than the risk of a possible interaction.

Excretion

The rate of excretion of drugs that are weak electrolytes can be modified by altering the pH of the urine (see Chapter 1). Thus, the rate of excretion of weak acids, such as salicylates, can be expedited by making the urine alkaline. This increases the proportion of salicylate molecules present in the ionized form; these are more water-soluble (less fat-soluble) than the corresponding un-ionized molecules, which would be reabsorbed by the tubules. This effect is exploited in the treatment of aspirin poisoning, when it is necessary to remove the drug from the body as quickly as possible. Conversely, the excretion of a weak base, such as pethidine, can be hastened by making the urine acid so that once again the drug will be present in the urine predominantly in the ionized and water-soluble form.

The diuretics, frusemide and ethacrynic acid, decrease excretion of gentamicin thus enhancing its potential for ototoxicity and nephrotoxicity. Phenylbutazone reduces the renal clearance of chlorpropamide so increasing the risk of hypoglycaemia. The anti-arrhythmic agent, quinidine, reduces the excretion of digoxin by the kidney and, as it may double the plasma concentration (see Chapter 1), it can precipitate digoxin toxicity.

An alternative form of interaction occurs when two drugs compete for the same transport system in the kidney. It is by this mechanism that probenecid reduces the rate of excretion of the penicillins.

Pharmacodynamic interactions

This type of drug interaction takes place either directly or indirectly at the site of the action of the drug, in other words, in the vicinity of the receptor.

The most common *direct* ones are those that act either on the central or autonomic nervous systems. Thus, many drugs that depress the CNS will produce synergistic effects when given together. A well-known, although not always heeded example, is the danger of drinking ethyl alcohol (ethanol) in the presence of benzodiazepines or antipsychotic drugs. Similarly, antihypertensive drugs may interact in either a useful way (hydralazine and propranolol), or in a potentially harmful way (verapamil and propranolol). There are many other examples; here are some that may have relevance to the dental practitioner:

Potentially hazardous combination	Effect
Frusemide (ethacrynic acid) with gentamicin	Ototoxicity
Competitive neuromuscular with aminoglycoside blockers or antibiotic or quinidine	Increased muscle relaxation
warfarin with tetracyclines	Increased anticoagulant effect

N.B. The interaction warfarin–tetracycline may be due to altered affinity of Vitamin K for clotting factor receptors. Except when there is a dietary deficiency of Vitamin K, antibiotics of the penicillin, cephalosporin, and aminoglycoside groups are safe to use in a patient already taking warfarin (Aronson and Grahame-Smith 1981).

Indirect pharmacodynamic interactions are of two types. In the first, the normal action of a drug is altered as a result of change in fluid or electrolyte balance induced by the interacting drug. An important example (although one unlikely to be of relevance to the dental practitioner) is the potentiation of effect of cardiac glycosides or the antagonism of the anti-arrhythmic drugs, quinidine or lignocaine, as a result of hypokalaemia induced by diuretics.

The second type is of much greater relevance to the dental practitioner. This is the interaction between oral anticoagulants and drugs that either cause gastro-intestinal erosion or ulceration (aspirin and other NSAIDs; corticosteroids), or decrease the aggregation of platelets (aspirin, indomethacin, phenylbutazone). Under these circumstances the tendency to bleed will be increased and, if it occurs, haemostasis may be impaired.

PREDICTION OF DRUG INTERACTIONS

When drugs are being prescribed together, or when an additional drug is prescribed to those already being taken, there are several pointers that should help the prescriber be on the alert to the possibility of a drug interaction (Dollery and Brodie 1980). These are as follows:

1. Does the drug belong to the short list (see p. 433) of those more likely to be involved in drug interactions?
2. Is the drug metabolized in the liver? It is not possible to predict with accuracy the way in which the body will metabolize a particular drug. However, there is a high correlation between the lipid solubility of a drug and its ability to (i) cross the blood–brain barrier and hence have CNS actions, and (ii) enter the hepatocytes and so be metabolized by the liver. The corollary of this is that drugs which gain access to the CNS will be metabolized in the liver, an example being chlorpromazine.
3. Is it highly protein bound? Warfarin is 98 to 99 per cent bound (see Chapter 1) and so can be displaced from its binding site on the plasma proteins by another drug that binds to protein more avidly, for example aspirin.
4. Is it an enzyme inducer? The barbiturates and cimetidine are enzyme inducers; they induce DME systems (see earlier) and hence reduce the half-life of a drug so affected, with potentially serious results.
5. Is it an enzyme inhibitor? The MAOIs are powerful inhibitors of other enzyme systems, including DMEs, and may as a result potentiate the effects of many other drugs (see Chapter 1).
6. Is it excreted unchanged in the urine? Digoxin is excreted unchanged in the urine, so that any drug with the capacity to alter the renal clearance of digoxin can produce potentially dangerous effects.

CONCLUSIONS

It can be seen that drug interactions form a large, heterogeneous, and potentially hazardous group of problems, and it is most important for the dental practitioner to be aware of their existence. Through ignorance of this subject, a dental practitioner may prescribe a drug which interacts with one already being taken by the patient. The list of interactions is growing steadily, and dental practitioners must be prepared to keep themselves informed of them. Table 22.1 has been prepared as a guide to these, and includes those interactions that the dental practitioner is most likely to meet, although it must be pointed out that this Table is not exhaustive. The Table indicates the clinical outcome, the course of action and, wherever possible, the probable mechanism of action for each example.

REFERENCES

Aronson, J. K. and Grahame-Smith, D. G. (1981). Clinical pharmacology: adverse drug interactions. *British Medical Journal,* **282,** 288–91.

Blackwell, B., Marley, E., Price, J., and Taylor, D. (1967). Hypertensive interactions between monoamine oxidase inhibitors and foodstuffs. *British Journal of Psychiatry,* **113,** 349–65.

British National Formulary No. 15 (1988). British Medical Association and The Pharmaceutical Society of Great Britain.

Brodie, B. B. (1964). *Physico-chemical factors in drug absorption* In *absorption and distribution of drugs,* (ed. T. B. Binns). Livingstone, Edinburgh.

Clark, B. (1967). The *in vitro* inhibition of the N-demethylation of pethidine by phenelzine (phenylhydrazine). *Biochemical Pharmacology,* **16,** 2369.

Clark, B. and Thompson, J. W. (1972). Analysis of the inhibition of pethidine N-demethylation by monoamine oxidase inhibitors and some other drugs with special reference to drug interactions in man. *British Journal of Pharmacology,* **44,** 89–99.

Dollery, C. T. and Brodie, M. J. (1980). Drug interactions. *Journal of the Royal College of Physicians, London,* 14, 190–6.

Dossetor, J. (1975). Drug interactions with oral contraceptives. *British Medical Journal,* 467–8.

Elis, J., Laurence, D. R., Mattie, H., and Prichard, B. N. (1967). Modification by monoamine oxidase inhibitors of the effect of some sympathomimetics on blood pressure. *British Medical Journal,* **2,** 75.

Gillette, J. R. (1967). Individually different responses to drugs according to age, sex and functional or pathological state. In *Drug responses in man* (ed. G. Wolstenholme and R. Porter). Churchill, London.

MacGregor, A. G. (1965). Clinical effects of interaction between drugs. Review of points at which drugs can interact. *Proceedings of the Royal Society of Medicine,* **58,** 943–6.

Orme, M. L'E. and Back, D. J. (1986). Drug interactions between oral contraceptive steroids and antibiotics. *British Dental Journal,* **160,** 169–70.

Williams, J. R. B., Griffin, J. P., and Parkins, A. (1976). Effect of concomitantly administered drugs on the control of long term anticoagulant therapy. *Quarterly Journal of Medicine,* **45,** 63–73.

23

Non-medical use of drugs: alcohol and alcoholism

INTRODUCTION

The dental surgeon is most unlikely to be called upon to treat drug dependence or to prescribe drugs in such quantities as would result in dependence. However, the incidence of drug abuse is likely to increase, and dental practitioners are going to encounter this problem amongst their patients. It is therefore important that they be familiar with the problems of common drug abuse. Drug abusers may suffer hallucinations from LSD or withdrawal symptoms from opioids; both problems can occur when abusers attend the dental surgery, and it is thus important that the dental surgeon should recognize their signs and symptoms.

This Chapter defines the non-medical use of drugs (including alcohol), and gives a brief outline of the widely abused drugs and the clinical picture of abuse.

DEFINITIONS

Drug abusage

This is defined as:

the consumption of a drug where there is is no medical indication, or;

the consumption of a drug in therapeutically excessive amounts without medical supervision.

Consequences of drug abusage

1. The effects on the individual, i.e. the action of the drug on the physiological and psychological state of the individual.
2. The effects on society, i.e. the interplay between environmental, sociological, and economic conditions in relation to drugs of dependence.

Drug dependence

Drug dependence is a state of psychic or physical dependence, or both, on a drug, arising in a person following administration of that drug on a periodic of continuous basis. (WHO Expert Committee of Addiction-producing Drugs 1964)

Psychic dependence

In this situation, there is a feeling of satisfaction and a psychic drive that require periodic or continuous administration of the drug to produce pleasure or to avoid discomfort. (WHO 1965)

Physical dependence

Physical dependence is an adaptive state that manifests itself by intensive physical disturbances when the administration of the drug is suspended or when its action is affected by the administration of a specific antagonist. (WHO 1965).

Forces that come into play in drug dependence (Paton 1968)

(1) production of a primary pleasurable reward;

(2) social and environmental factors;

(3) withdrawal or abstinence effects;

(4) drug tolerance.

Motives (WHO 1973)

(1) to satisfy curiosity about drug effects;

(2) to achieve a sense of belonging, to be accepted by others;

(3) to express independence and sometimes hostility;

(4) to have pleasurable, new, thrilling or dangerous experiences;

(5) to gain an improved 'understanding' or 'creativity';

(6) to foster a sense of ease of relaxation;

(7) to escape from something.

ALCOHOL AND ALCOHOLISM

Alcohol (ethanol, ethyl alcohol) is derived from the fermentation of sugars and refined carbohydrates. The compound has little therapeutic usage, but its social significance is enormous.

Pharmacokinetics

Alcohol is rapidly absorbed from the upper part of the gastro-intestinal tract, partly from the stomach, but mainly from the small intestine. Absorption is delayed by food, especially dairy products and fatty foods. Another factor that affects absorption is the concentration of the solution, with strong solutions inhibiting gastric peristalsis. Alcohol is also more rapidly absorbed in habitual drinkers. After absorption, it rapidly diffuses throughout the body fluids and tissues.

Ninety per cent of absorbed alcohol is metabolized (oxidation) by the enzyme system in the liver (alcohol dehydrogenase). The first stage of this metabolism is the formation of acetaldehyde, then acetate, and finally carbon dioxide and water. The remaining 10 per cent is excreted unchanged in the urine, sweat, and breath. The rate of alcohol metabolism varies, but is generally thought to be quicker in heavy drinkers. Alcohol is unusual in that it follows zero-order kinetics (see Chapter 1).

Pharmacological properties

Alcohol has anaesthetic properties and causes depression of the central nervous system (CNS). Hyperactivity, when it occurs, is due to removal of inhibitions. In normal doses, alcohol acts on the brain-stem reticular formation but, with high doses, direct cortical depression occurs. The effect of alcohol on the CNS in relation to consumption is shown in Table 23.1. Alcohol induces peripheral vasodilation by depressing the vasomotor centre; this accounts for the feeling of warmth that people notice after drinking. As a result of the vasodilation there is a loss of body heat, and therefore it is unwise to take alcohol before going out into the cold. There is no firm evidence to suggest that alcohol usefully dilates the coronary arteries, although it does relieve the pain of angina by reducing peripheral resistance through vasodilatation.

In moderate concentrations, alcohol increases the secretion of gastric acid but, at high concentrations, it reduces such secretion. Thus, it is unwise to drink where there is a history of peptic ulceration. The diuretic properties of alcohol are familiar to all drinkers; this property is due to alcohol inhibiting the secretion of antidiuretic hormone (ADH).

Table 23.1. The effect of alcohol on the CNS relationsup to alcohol consumption. NB, 1 unit of alcohol is equivalent to 1 measure of spirits, or $\frac{1}{2}$ pint of beer/lager, or 1 glass of wine

Number of units	Effect
1–2	Normal
3–4	Warmth, friendliness, digestive discomfort, lengthening of reaction to visual field
6	Diminished sense of depth, impaired driving
8	Loss of inhibition, euphoria, aggressive behaviour, visual disturbances
10	Deterioration of motor reaction and loss of precision
12	Uncertain movements, reduced ability for adaptation
14	Accommodation disturbances, loss of balance
16	Obvious drunkenness, muscular inco-ordination
18	Irritability, depression, nausea, loss of sphincter control
24–8	Stupor
30–6	Coma
40–60	Paralysis of respiratory centre, death

Alcohol has a dual effect on blood glucose: initially it increases blood glucose due to reduced glucose uptake by the tissues; but this leads to increased insulin output, which will cause hypoglycaemia, an event that is likely to occur if alcohol is taken after severe exercise.

Tolerance develops to alcohol: the more frequently an individual drinks, the more they require to obtain the same effect.

Alcoholism

This can be defined as a chronic disease manifested by repeated drinking so as to cause injury to the drinker's health or to their social and economic functioning. An alcoholic can be defined as an individual who is unable, consistently, to choose whether he/she shall drink or not, and who, if he/she drinks, is unable consistently to choose whether he/she shall stop or not.

Alcoholism has been classified into five types:

(1) alpha: in which the individual drinks as a relief from mental pain, thus using alcohol as a drug;

(2) beta: in which the individual drinks because their position or environment demands it;

(3) epsilon: in which the individual drinks to excess, but only periodically;

(4) gamma: in which the individual cannot control their intake once they have taken their first drink;

(5) delta: in which the individual drinks intermittently without necessarily getting drunk.

The alpha, beta, and epsilon forms of alcoholism demonstrate psychological dependence that can lead into physical dependence. The gamma and delta types demonstrate both psychological and physical dependence.

Thus, alcohol can produce different effects according to the way it is used. It is a drug that can cause psychological dependence when used for the relief of anxiety. It can lead to a strong physical dependence with serious consequences in the physical, psychological, moral, and social senses. In view of this, it is worth noting that whereas we often see drinking, sometimes to excess, and drunkenness, we seldom see alcoholism. This is for two reasons:

Firstly, drinking and drunkenness are physical states and can, therefore, be seen. However, alcoholism is a state of mind, which exists even when it is not showing any symptoms.

Secondly, the drunkard usually gets drunk in public and does not care who sees. The alcoholic is often protected by friends and family, who cover up for deficiencies and do everything possible to prevent the condition from being discovered.

It is necessary to make this distinction between drinking, drunkenness, and alcoholism, not only because of the immediate effects on the drinker, but also because of the long-term ones that influence the drinker and those who come into contact with him or her. This distinction is very much in evidence in the attitudes of society, as well as in the measures taken to deal with the condition. Thus, drunkenness, especially if only occasionally, is often regarded as a temporary lapse that, even if not completely condoned, is looked upon with a certain tolerance. On some occasions, drunkenness is even encouraged and viewed with a certain amount of amusement. This is hardly justifiable in view of the high incidence of alcohol-related driving accidents. The regular drunkard does not enjoy much sympathy from either society or the law. They are usually avoided as an embarrassment by friends and are easily picked up by the police because they are a nuisance. They may run into serious financial difficulties and their family invariably suffers. With help and self-control, the drunkard may be able to overcome their drinking problem.

The picture with alcoholics is very different: they are dependent upon alcohol for their everyday functioning, and all efforts are directed at obtaining drink. They need alcohol to get started in the morning, to keep them going throughout the day, and even more alcohol in the evening before retiring to bed. Alcoholics have to keep themselves continuously topped-up. They may be able to function in society for a time, but eventually their work deteriorates until they are unable to work at all. Their interests become more restricted until they become centred on the one thing that matters—alcohol. Their family and friends desert them, hence alcoholism is often known as the lonely disease.

Stages of alcoholism

It is now recognized that anyone who regularly consumes more than 20 units of alcohol a week is seriously at risk from becoming an alcoholic. (One unit of alcohol is defined as either one glass of wine, one measure of spirits, or half a pint of beer or lager). Four stages of alcoholism can be recognized; these are as follows:

1. *The pre-alcoholic symptomatic phase.*   The individual starts drinking socially, but soon realizes that alcohol provides relief from psychological difficulties. At the start he or she seeks relief only occasionally, but soon their tolerance for tension decreases and they resort to alcohol more frequently. Drinking is heavier in the evening and soon becomes noticeable to family and friends.

2. *The prodromal phase.*   At this stage, the drinker may consume a considerable quantity of alcohol and still carry on with normal activities, but does not remember anything about them the following morning. The onset of these amnesic episodes (black-outs) may be followed by a change in drinking behaviour, which indicates that alcoholic drinks have ceased to be social pleasure and have become 'drugs of necessity'. The subject may become unduly preoccupied with alcohol, start drinking surreptitiously, and develop guilty

feelings about drinking. The prodromal phase may last anything from six months to five years.

3. *The crucial phase.* The main feature of this phase is loss of control, which means that as soon as a small quantity of alcohol is taken, then a demand for more alcohol is set up. This is felt as a physical demand by the drinker and lasts until they are too intoxicated or too sick to ingest any more alcohol. At about this time, they begin to rationalize their drinking behaviour by inventive excuses for drinking. Drinking now becomes conspicuous and, as a result, the drinker develops markedly aggressive behaviour and suffers persistent remorse. Both add to his or her tension and provide a further reason for drinking. During the crucial phase, there may be periods of total abstinence or attempts to change the pattern of drinking. The drinker invariably loses his or her job, and family and friends desert them, which leads to the development of unreasonable resentment. They often neglect their food and start drinking at any hour of the day. Progressively, this disease process undermines the morals and physical resistance of the drinker.

4. *The chronic phase.* At this stage, drinkers begin to find themselves intoxicated during the daytime and continues in this state for several days. Marked ethical deterioration and impairment of thinking occur, and sometimes true alcoholic psychoses. By some strange phenomenon, the drinker becomes less tolerant to alcohol, and undefinable fears and tremors develop.

Table 23.2 lists both the physical and psychological signs and symptoms of the early, the probable, and the certain alcoholic.

Treatment

This can be by aversion therapy, the use of sensitizing drugs, or psychological therapy. Aversion therapy is aimed at creating a conditioned reflex so that the alcoholic feels sick and vomits when they see, smell, or taste alcohol. Drugs used for aversion therapy are emetine and apomorphine. Sensitizing drugs, such as disulfiram, block the metabolism of alcohol by inhibiting the conversion of acetaldehyde to acetate. Thus disulfiram produces a fall in blood pressure, headaches, chest pain, nausea, and vomiting. Psychological therapy, as provided by groups such as Alcoholics Anonymous, has proved to be of tremendous value in the treatment of alcoholism.

VOLATILE SUBSTANCE ABUSE (SOLVENT ABUSE)

The first case of solvent abuse was reported in the UK in 1969. Since that time, there has been a steady increase in the number of fatalities and the age of the abusers has fallen; the range of ages involved is now from 8 to 23 years. It appears that curiosity or peer-group pressure is responsible for the transient indulgence of many teenagers in this activity. Nevertheless, chronic volatile substance abuse does occur, and may lead to hepatic and renal damage, encephalopathy, and

Table 23.2. Physical and psychological signs and symptoms of the early, probable, and certain alcoholic

---

Early alcoholic—physical signs and symptoms
    Chronic gastritis
    Anaemia
    Dimness of vision (amblyopia)
    Vitamin deficiencies (especially vit. C)
    Cardiac irregularities (tachycardias and arrhythmias)
    Flushed face
    Nocturnal sweating
    Bruising on body and limbs
    Cigarette burns
    Increased tolerance to alcohol

Early alcoholic—psychological signs and symptoms
    Gulping drinks
    Person looks for easy employment that offers facilities for drinking
    Frequent car accidents
    Behavioral problems in the family and inexplicable behaviour within it
    Frequent changes of residences
    Changes in social and business relationships
    Major disruption: loss of job
    Feelings of aggression, resentment, and jealousy
    Paranoid attitudes
    Depression and isolation

Probable alcoholic—physical signs and symptoms
    Black-outs
    Increased infections
    Pancreatitis, peripheral neuropathy, alcoholic myopathy, cardiomyopathy
    Constant odour of alcohol on the breath
    Vascular enlargement—characteristic facial appearance

Probable alcoholic—psychological signs and symptoms
    Subjective loss of control
    Surreptitious drinking—morning drinking
    Repeated conscious attempts at abstinence
    Frequent absences from work
    Changing drinks
    Loss of interest
    Outburst of rage and threats of suicide
    Frequent references to alcohol
    Drinking for the relief of anger, insomnia, fatigue, depression, and social discomfort

Certain alcoholic–physical and psychological signs and symptoms
    Withdrawal symptoms when drinking is stopped, i.e. drowsiness, hallucinations, fits, and
        delirium tremens.
    Tolerance—high blood alcohol levels without intoxication
    High consumption of alcohol
    Liver cirrhosis and alcoholic cerebral degeneration
    Blatant indiscriminate use of alcohol
    Drinking continues despite strong medical and social contra-indications

---

peripheral neuropathy, as well as psychological and social problems (Volans and Byatt 1986).

Solvent abuse, now renamed volatile substance abuse (because other substances in addition to glues and solvents are abused), takes the form of deep inhalation from a cloth soaked in the agent or from a plastic bag into which it has been poured.

The clinical picture of solvent abuse is similar to that which follows intoxication with alcohol or volatile anaesthetics. Thus, there is initial stimulation of the CNS followed by depression, but the time-course is different. The onset is rapid, the effects last for minutes and not hours, and the occurrence of disorientation and hallucinations is much more frequent than with alcohol or volatile anaesthetics. The breath smells of the particular solvent used, and there may be evidence of it on the hands and face, including a rash over the muzzle area. It is well-known that solvents can sensitize the heart to catecholamines and hypoxia, so that cardiac arrhythmias may occur during the exposure. There may also be a metabolic acidosis with coma in which the reflexes are exaggerated. Solvent abuse has also precipitated status epilepticus (Allister et al. 1981).

Treatment of volatile substance abuse can be difficult and should be left to those experienced in these problems. The treatment includes psychotherapy (listening and talking to the victim; discussing his or her problems), behaviour therapy (retraining to prevent this behaviour when the urge or opportunity arises), and relaxation therapy, including hypnotic techniques (O'Connor 1981).

DENTAL PROBLEMS OF DRUG ABUSERS

All drug abusers will show signs of dental neglect; their oral hygiene will be poor and they often only attend for emergency treatment. Thus, routine dental care is difficult to achieve for such patients. The specific dental problems of the different types of drug abusers are discussed below.

Intravenous drug abusers

Opioids are the common group of drugs taken intravenously. There is a risk of hepatitis B and AIDS amongst intravenous drug abusers, and the dental surgeon should take every precaution to avoid both infection and cross-infection (see Chapter 9). Patients taking opioids may also suffer withdrawal symptoms whilst undergoing dental treatment, and the dental surgeon should be able to recognize this problem. Pentazocine, which is a mixed agonist/antagonist, should not be given to such patients as it may induce withdrawal symptoms.

Alcohol abuse

The chronic alcoholic may suffer from vitamin deficiencies, which will cause oral symptoms such as stomatitis, glossitis, and angular cheilitis. Liver damage following alcohol abuse may result in impaired blood clotting and poor wound healing. General anaesthetics and sedation techniques should be avoided where possible in the alcoholic as they show resistance to the agents used. Other drugs to avoid in alcoholics are aspirin, because of its effect on haemostasis and the gastric mucosa, and metronidazole, which inhibits the metabolism of alcohol.

Smoking

Smoking tobacco results in brown or black stains on the teeth, but does not normally lead to conspicuous changes in the gingiva. In heavy smokers there may be a greyish-white gingival discolouration and, in pipe smokers, the palatal mucosa may be characterized by 'cobblestone' surface, the so-called 'smokers palate', in which the orifices of accessory palatal salivary glands become inflamed and undergo hyperkeratotic change. The degree of bleeding elicited on blunt probing of the gingival crevice may be reduced in smokers with periodontitis (Preber and Bergstrom 1985).

Acute ulcerative gingivitis occurs more frequently in smokers (Kowolik and Nisbet, 1983), and some reports suggest that smoking is associated with an increased prevalence of chronic periodontal disease. Smokers have more dental plaque than non-smokers, but smoking does not appear to increase the rate of plaque formation (Macgregor et al. 1985); the major reason for the increased plaque accumulation in smokers is probably inadequate oral hygiene. It has long been known that smoking causes an increase in salivary flow, and this may partly explain the increased amounts of salivary calculus found in smokers.

Evidence that smoking increases the incidence of 'dry socket' (Sweet and Butler 1978) has not subsequently been confirmed. However, it has been shown that smoking impairs post-extraction socket filling with blood (Rogers et al. 1986); this may impair the healing of tooth sockets.

The generalized keratosis of the normally unkeratinized oral mucosa sometimes seen in heavy smokers appears to be benign, but there is evidence that smoking is a causative factor in leukoplakia (Pindborg 1980), which may be a premalignant lesion. Curiously, smoking seems to have a therapeutic effect on oral aphthous ulceration (Chellemi et al. 1970). Smoking is an important cause of carcinoma of the mouth (Pindborg 1980); the main prospective studies have found that carcinoma of the mouth, pharynx, and oesophagus are all associated with smoking. The risk of developing oral carcinomas has been estimated to be six times greater in smokers than in non-smokers.

Smokeless tobacco

This term is used to describe alternative forms of taking tobacco, which include snuffing, sneezing, dipping, and chewing. Smokeless tobacco consumption is on the increase, especially in school-age children (Schaefer et al. 1985). There is increasing evidence that this form of tobacco consumption is associated with alterations in the oral mucosa and dental tissues. These include gingival recession, periodontal bone loss, leukoplakia, and tooth abrasion. Products from smokeless tobacco have been shown to have the potential for causing carcinoma of the oral mucosa, pharynx, larynx, and oesophagus (Christen 1980). Some smokeless tobacco products have recently been banned in the UK.

REFERENCES

Allister, C., Lush, M., Oliver, J. S., and Watson, J. M. (1981). Status epilepticus caused by solvent abuse. *British Medical Journal,* **283,** 1156.

Chellemi, S. J., Olson, D. L., and Shapiro, S. (1970). The association between smoking and aphthous ulcers. *Oral Surgery,* **29,** 832–6.

Christen, A. G. (1980). The case against smokeless tobacco: five facts for the health professional to consider. *Journal of the American Dental Association,* **101,** 464–9.

Eddy, N. B., Halbach, H., Isbell, H., and Seevers, M. H. (1965). Drug dependence: its significance and characteristics. *Bulletin of World Health Organization,* **32,** 721–33.

Kowolik, M. J. and Nisbet, T. (1983). Smoking and acute ulcerative gingivitis. *British Dental Journal,* **154,** 241–2.

Macgregor, I. D. M., Edgar, W. M., and Greenwood, A. R. (1985). Effects of cigarette smoking on the rate of plaque formation. *Journal of Clinical Periodontology,* **12,** 335–41.

O'Connor, D. J. (1981). Glue sniffing and solvent abuse problems: causes and treatments. *The Police Surgeon, Journal of the Association of Police Surgeons in Great Britain,* **19,** 48–57.

Paton, W. D. M. (1968). Drug dependence—a socio-pharmacological assessment. *Advancement of Science,* **25,** 200–12.

Pindborg, J. J. (1980). *Oral cancer and precancer.* John Wright & Sons, Bristol.

Preber, H. and Bergstrom, J. (1985). Occurrence of gingival bleeding in smokers and non-smoker patients. *Acta Odontologica Scandinavica,* **43,** 315–20.

Rogers, S. N., Meechan, J. G., Macgregor, I. D. M., and Hobson, R. S. (1986). The effect of smoking on immediate post-extraction socket filling with blood and on the incidence of dry socket. *Journal of Dental Research,* **65,** 489.

Schaefer, S. D., Henderson, A. H., Glover, F. D., and Christen, A. G. (1985). Patterns of use and incidence of smokeless tobacco consumption in school-age children. *Archives of Otolaryngology,* **111,** 639–42.

Sweet, J. B. and Butler, D. P. (1978). Predisposing and operative factors. Effect on the incidence of localised osteitis in mandibular third molar surgery. *Oral Surgery,* **46,** 206–15.

Volans, G. N. and Byatt, C. M. (1986). Poisoning from domestic products. *Prescribers' Journal,* **26** (no. 4), 87–97.

WHO Expert Committee on Addiction-producing drugs, Thirteenth Report. (1964). World Health Organization Technical Report Series No. 273.

WHO Technical Report Series. (1973). Youth and drugs. No. 516. Geneva.

24

Emergencies in dental practice

MOST of the emergencies to be considered here are likely to be very rare in dental practice. However, the practitioner must be familiar with methods of dealing with the immediate crisis. The treatment given by the dental practitioner must be as simple as possible, and the emergency kit of drugs (described at the end of the Chapter) as limited as is compatible with need. Too many drugs included in an emergency kit will mean that the practitioner is likely to be familiar with the use of none.

The emergencies will be considered under the following headings:

(1) fainting;

(2) angina or myocardial infarction;

(3) cardiac arrest;

(4) acute allergic reactions;

(5) epilepsy;

(6) hypoglycaemia;

(7) adrenal crisis.

General anaesthetic problems and those associated with bleeding have been dealt with in the appropriate Chapters.

FAINTING

Fainting is likely to be the most common cause of loss of consciousness in the dental surgery. It is due to a transient lack of blood supply to the brain. Very often a fainting attack can be anticipated, and therefore prevented, by careful observation of the patient, particularly at the time of administration of a local anaesthetic. A patient who is pale, sweating, and feels sick and dizzy, is one providing a warning. Such a patient may go quickly into unconsciousness. The pulse is weak at first, slow, and then becomes fuller and bounding.

Fainting in the dental surgery is less common today than in the past, and this is because patients are now treated in the supine position. The sort of patient who is likely to faint is one who is unduly anxious, and the one who has decided not to eat before any dental treatment. If food has not been taken prior to dental treatment, then a glucose drink should be provided.

The treatment for fainting is to lie the patient flat with the head in a dependent position to allow the cerebral blood flow to be maintained.

ANGINA PECTORIS AND MYOCARDIAL INFARCTION

Angina is a symptom of ischaemic heart disease; an attack is characterized by a sudden, very severe substernal pain that often radiates to the left shoulder and arm. Very occasionally the pain may radiate to the left mandible and teeth. The typical anginal attack is often brought on by exercise and by emotion, such as anxiety. Because of the anxiety association, such an attack is a possibility in the dental surgery. The patient may have had anginal attacks for a long time and so will recognize the symptoms; they will be carrying their usual remedy, e.g. glyceryl trinitrate tablets (see Chapter 15). If an attack occurs they should place one tablet under the tongue. If a patient with recurrent angina pectoris happens to develop an acute myocardial infarction, he or she may take several tablets in quick succession in an attempt to relieve the intractable pain. All this will do is to produce a further reduction in myocardial blood flow, and this will clearly have a further adverse effect. Patients should be advised that in the event of very prolonged attacks of pain, when two tablets have not proved helpful, then to take any more will not be effective, but could be harmful.

If the patient has a myocardial infarct, the pain will be similar to that experienced in an attack of angina, the difference being that it will be more severe and persistent. The patient is often breathless and vomiting is common. The pulse will be weak and the blood pressure falls. They may become unconscious for a time, and may suffer cardiac arrest and die.

Once a myocardial infarct has been diagnosed the following steps should be taken:

1. An ambulance must be called for by an assistant.

2. Pain and anxiety must be relieved.

The nature of the pain experienced will provoke acute anxiety. This, in itself, will cause the outpouring of endogenous adrenaline with possible precipitation of cardiac ventricular fibrillation. Fibrillation is a cause of sudden death and should, as far as possible, be prevented by dealing effectively with the pain and anxiety. For this purpose, morphine has been the drug of choice for a long time. Although it is a drug that can be held by dental surgeons, and can be administered by them, it is a controlled drug (see Chapter 3) and is unlikely to be stored in the dental surgery by many practitioners. On the other hand, pentazocine, although also a controlled drug, is more familiar to dental surgeons. It is listed in the *Dental Practitioners' Formulary 1986–88*, and is used in some dental sedative techniques. However, it is *not* recommended for use in the case of myocardial infarction. Even parenterally it is not as good an analgesic as morphine, and unfortunately it cannot be guaranteed to relieve anxiety. Indeed, the reverse may be the case; it may produce anxiety and, in certain instances, hallucinations. When a patient has experienced a myocardial infarction, it is important to maintain their haemodynamic status. Morphine is much more likely to do this than is pentazocine. High doses of pentazocine, unlike morphine, increase the blood pressure and heart rate, and this in itself could put an extra strain on the already overtaxed heart.

The best treatment for myocardial infarction in this context is the use of Entonox, a premixture of gases—50/50 mixture of nitrous oxide and oxygen (see Chapter 8). This gaseous mixture provides more rapid pain relief than morphine. If Entonox is not available, nitrous oxide may be administered with oxygen, but the concentration of nitrous oxide must not exceed 70 per cent, as above this concentration anaesthesia and hypoxia may occur. Nitrous oxide is a weak anaesthetic agent but possesses excellent analgesic properties. In addition it has an euphoriant effect. What is being done should be explained to the patient as the anaesthetic mask may well cause them to feel more anxious.

The patient should be placed in the position that feels most comfortable to them. Pulmonary oedema is a possible consequence of infarction due to left ventricular failure and this causes dyspnoea. To lie the patient flat in these circumstances could cause the lungs to fill with fluid and make breathing virtually impossible. All tight clothing around the neck should be loosened.

CARDIAC ARREST

There are many causes of cardiac arrest, e.g. myocardial infarction, anaesthetic agents, acute anaphylactic reactions, adrenal crisis. Apart from the obvious fact that the patient will be unconscious, there are some signs to look for, namely:

(1) colour of the skin;
(2) absence of arterial pulse.

Pallor indicates under-perfusion of the skin with blood. If the colour is white, then this may indicate a circulatory problem and could be the result of a mild cardiac infarct. If the colour is grey, this would indicate that the remaining oxygen tension in the peripheral vessels has been further reduced. A whitish grey skin suggests circulatory collapse of some duration. Indications of such circulatory collapse would also include lack of pulse. Time is of the essence, and only the radial and carotid pulses should be felt. A stethoscope to listen for heart sounds is worse than useless. Sometimes heart sounds may be difficult to ascertain in this way even in the normal patient; they may be very difficult to find if the patient is obese.

There may also be lack of bleeding from a surgical wound, and the pupils will be dilated. However, eye signs should not be considered an essential feature of early diagnosis because they occur later on in the catastrophe. Do not waste time looking for eye signs!

Cardiopulmonary resuscitation

The brain is the organ most sensitive to oxygen deprivation. If its oxygen supply is cut off for three minutes, then brain death will occur. This presupposes that the patient was in a reasonable condition beforehand. If they were in an agitated state, for example, where the oxygen demand would be raised, then the brain would suffer even more rapidly following cardiac arrest. Such a possibility may arise in the dental chair. So the emergency techniques must be well-known and rehearsed, for no time can be spent reading them up in a book once the emergency has begun. Although a single operator can provide both cardiac and respiratory resuscitation, this is difficult and extremely exhausting.

Procedures

1. *Aid the venous return.* Place the patient on the floor or onto a firm flat surface. Get their feet up to help the flow of blood back to the heart.

2. *Thump the patient's chest mid-sternum.* One or two blows with the side of the closed fist may restart the heart. The sole purpose of this is to shock the heart into electrical activity and if two blows produce no response, further ones will be a waste of time for this will not restart the heart.

3. *Start external cardiac massage.* The operator kneels by the side of the patient and the sternum is depressed 1–1.5 inches. One hand is placed over the other on the lower sternum and a forceful compression started. A rate of 60 to 70 should suffice for an adult. This is a risky business and, in older patients with less elasticity of the rib cage, as many as 50 per cent may suffer fracture of the ribs. In very small children, the compression rate is about 100 and only the thumbs are used to press on the chest.

4. *Artificial ventilation.* This must be given during the period of cardiac massage. The neck should be extended and the lower jaw held forward in order to keep the airway clear. The ventilation can be accomplished by mouth to mouth respiration or by some sort of face mask and oxygen. The lungs should be inflated after every fifth compression of the chest. During artificial respiration the patient's nose should be closed.

Resuscitation is a very exhausting procedure and where possible one person should attend to the cardiac massage, and another to the respiratory ventilation. If only one person is available, then five compressions to one ventilation is suggested.

Medical help should be sought by an assistant, and the cardiopulmonary resuscitation maintained until there is a return to a good pulse or alternatively until the arrival of expert help. A patient who recovers will be admitted to hospital. It is no part of the dentist's job to try using drugs such as lignocaine to deal with any arrhythmias that may occur.

ACUTE ALLERGIC REACTIONS

See Chapter 21 and the Table at end of this Chapter.

EPILEPSY

Major epilepsy is a convulsive disorder with attacks that are characterized by an aura (a disorder of sensation), a tonic and a clonic phase (see Chapter 14). In the tonic phase the patient is rigid and may stop breathing; in the clonic phase convulsions occur; in either phase the patient may bite their tongue.

If the patient has an attack in the dental surgery, they must be prevented from injuring themselves during the seizure. All appliances should be removed from the mouth as quickly as possible. Recovery is fairly rapid, a matter of a few minutes. Whether or not dental treatment is continued can only be decided by the operator, taking into account the circumstances prevailing at the time. As some patients feel a little drowsy after recovery from a seizure, it is sensible to see they are accompanied home by a responsible adult.

If a patient is known to be an epileptic it is important for them to continue medication before attending for dental treatment.

If the patient does not recover in a matter of minutes, and seizures occur in rapid succession (status epilepticus), then an anticonvulsant drug must be given. The drug of choice is the benzodiazepine, diazepam. The ultrashort-acting barbiturate, thiopentone, will also cut short an attack, but it should be remembered that the ultrashort-acting barbiturate normally used in dental practice, methohexitone, has convulsant properties *and should never be used*. Status epilepticus is a dangerous condition and the patient should be taken into hospital as soon as possible.

HYPOGLYCAEMIA

The diabetic patient's regime can become unbalanced and they may then suffer from too much insulin or too little. Too much will lead to hypoglycaemia, a condition brought about if the diabetic taking insulin has their dietary regime disrupted; too little insulin can produce a state of diabetic ketosis. It is important to distinguish between hypoglycaemia and diabetic ketosis; both can cause the patient to become unconscious. However, it is extemely unlikely that diabetic ketosis would present with unconsciousness in the dental surgery as it takes several days to develop. The differential signs and symptoms are:

Ketosis (lack of insulin)	Hypoglycaemia (excess of insulin)
Weakness	Weakness
Excessive thirst	Hunger
Dehydration (dry skin and mucous membrane)	Sweating
	Blood pressure normal or elevated
Decreased blood pressure	Pulse—full and rapid
Sweet breath—said to be acetone	Patient anxious (adrenaline release)
Deep laboured respirations	Later: coma
Later: coma (unlikely to be seen in dental surgery)	

One characteristic feature of hypoglycaemia is that the patient may become difficult to manage and even aggressive.

Patients experienced in the management of their condition may well be able to distinguish between the onset of a hypoglycaemic attack and ketosis. If there is any doubt about the diagnosis, a few lumps of sugar or sugar sweets will normally rectify the hypoglycaemia fairly rapidly. A hypoglycaemic attack requires urgent treatment and, if the patient is unable to swallow, intravenous dextrose should be administered. If a vein cannot be found, then glucagon should be administered intramuscularly. Glucagon is a hormone secreted by the α-cells of the islets of Langerhans of the pancrease, the β-cells producing insulin. Glucagon raises plasma glucose concentration by mobilizing glycogen stored in the liver (see Chapter 18). Hypoglycaemia must be treated promptly: a prolonged hypoglycaemic coma is likely to lead to irreversible brain damage.

When there is doubt about the diagnosis of whether the coma is hypoglycaemic or hyperglycaemic in origin, insulin must not be administered by the dental surgeon as it can be very dangerous in hypoglycaemic coma. The likelihood is that a coma occurring in the dental surgery in a diabetic patient will be caused by hypoglycaemia.

ADRENAL CRISIS

If the adrenal glands are unable to provide sufficient cortisol to meet the needs of 'stress', an adrenal crisis may occur. This is a state of profound shock, and a warning of such an occurrence would be weakness, vomiting, pallor, perspiration, tachycardia, weak pulse, and hypotension. If surgery is to be carried out on a patient when there is this risk of an inadequate response to 'stress', special precautions should be taken. Adrenocortical function is likely to be depressed if (a) the patient is taking corticosteroids as a prolonged course (month or over), or (b) if the patient has been taking corticosteroids regularly for a month or more during the last year. There is no general agreement on the time taken to restore normal adrenocortical function after prolonged steroid therapy has been discontinued. The approach to prophylactic steroid replacement is shown in Table 24.1.

Table 24.1. Prophylactic steroid replacement for dental procedures

Procedure	Patients currently on a prolonged course of steroid therapy	Patients who have had a prolonged course of steroid therapy during the previous year
Minimal procedures, e.g. an extraction under local anaesthesia	Give 200 mg hydrocortisone orally 2 hours pre-operatively; this is followed by the patient's usual steroid regimen	Give 200 mg hydrocortisone orally 2 hours pre-operatively
Minor oral surgery, e.g. impacted third molar removal and minor procedures under a general anaesthetic	Give 100 mg hydrocortisone intravenously pre-operatively followed by the same dose intramuscularly every 6 hours for a period of 24 hours; this is followed by the patient's usual steroid regimen	Give 100 mg hydrycortisone intravenously pre-operatively followed by the same dose intramuscularly every 6 hours for a period of 24 hours
Major oral surgery	Give 100 mg hydrocortisone intravenously pre-operatively followed by the same dose every 6 hours for a period of 72 hours; this is followed by the patient's usual steroid regimen	Give 100 mg hydrocortisone intravenously pre-operatively followed by the same dose intramuscularly for a period of 72 hours
Routine restorative procedures (other than surgical)	No prophylactic cover required; steroids should be available in case of collapse	No prophylactic cover required; steroids should be available in case of collapse

If, in spite of all the precautions itemized in Table 24.1, the patient shows signs of collapse, hydrocortisone (500 mg) should be given intravenously and immediately. This is a very serious situation and the patient should be admitted to hospital as soon as possible, if not already an in-patient.

Patients who are considered to be vulnerable should have their blood pressure monitored; this may provide a reasonable guide to their general condition. For just how long this should be done, and at what intervals, is not established with any certainty. It is recommended that the blood pressure should be measured in such patients at half-hourly intervals over a period of two hours. If, after this time, the blood pressure is still significantly low, the patient should be referred to hospital.

THE EMERGENCY KIT

Table 24.2 shows the basic emergency drug kit for dental practices, together with recommended dosages for various emergencies.

Table 24.2. The emergency drug kit for dental practice and the dosages for various emergencies

Drug	Dosage	Emergency
Hydrocortisone sodium succinate	100 mg IV or IM (powder in vial plus 2 ml of water for injection)	Anaphylactic shock; adrenal crisis; acute asthma: repeat as required
Adrenaline (1 1000 solution)	0.5 ml IM (MUST NEVER BE GIVEN INTRAVENOUSLY)	Anaphylactic shock
Chlorpheniramine	10–20 mg IV or IM	Allergic reactions
Dextrose (10 ml ampoules containing 50% solution)	5–20 ml IV	Hypoglycaemic coma
Glucagon injection	0.5–1 unit IV, IM, or SC	Acute hypoglycaemic reactions
Nitrous oxide and oxygen ideally Entonox 50:50, alternatively a mixture of gases with NOT more than 70% N_2O	inhalation	Myocardial infarction
Morphine sulphate injection BP	8–20 mg IM	Myocardial infarction
Diazepam	by slow intravenous injection: 2.5 mg increments until condition is controlled, up to 20 mg. (2.5 mg increments per 30 s.)	Status epilepticus

25

Therapeutic measures for common dental conditions

LISTED below are some of the common dental conditions that often require treatment. The possible methods of treatment are outlined as being either operative, that is treatment carried out by the dental surgeon, or non-operative, that is the use of medication. In some conditions both types of treatment are necessary. The list of non-operative measures is by no means exhaustive and only serves as a guideline; many of the conditions have been also discussed under various drug treatments. It is beyond the scope of this Chapter to discuss the differential diagnoses of these conditions. For these, the reader is referred to standard texts on oral surgery and medicine for details.

Dentine hypersensitivity

Operative treatment: for cases that do not respond to desensitizing agents, then root canal therapy may have to be carried out.
Non-operative treatment: application of either Lukomasky's paste, stannous fluoride, or Tresiolan to the area of exposed dentine may be of some short-term benefit. Toothpastes containing either strontium chloride or formaldehyde should be used as the regular dentifrice (see Chapter 11).

Pulpal hyperaemia

Operative treatment: remove the cause, either a 'high spot' on a new filling, caries, lack of a lining under a restoration, or a leaky amalgam. The cavity should then be dressed with either a calcium hydroxide base and zinc oxide–eugenol, or just zinc oxide–eugenol.

Acute pulpitis

Operative treatment: remove the pulp or extract the tooth.
Non-operative treatment: Ledermix may be applied to the cavity floor if there is pulpal inflammation causing inadequate anaesthesia. Analgesics are of little value in this common dental condition (see Chapters 5 and 6).

Periapical abscess

Operative treatment: establish drainage via the root canal or extract the tooth.
Non-operative treatment: if the infection is not localized, or treatment has been delayed, antibiotics should be prescribed. Both phenoxymethyl penicillin (250 mg every six hours for five days) and metronidazole (200 mg every eight hours for five days) have been shown to be effective for this condition. For severe infections, the patient should be treated with intramuscular benzylpenicillin (600 mg), followed by oral penicillin. If the patient is allergic to penicillin, a higher dose of metronidazole (400 mg every 12 hours) should be used.

Cellulitis

Operative treatment: if suppuration is present then drainage should be established. The cellulitis may be due to a carious tooth and this should also be removed.
Non-operative treatment: early treatment with antibiotics is essential. If the patient is not allergic to penicillin, then they should be given benzylpenicillin IM, 600 mg every 6 hours for at least 24 hours. If allergic to penicillin they should be treated with intramuscular linocmycin, 600 mg every 12 hours for 24 hours. Any pus obtained during drainage must be sent for culture and antibiotic sensitivity. After the initial course of intramuscular drugs, the patient can usually receive antibiotics orally; the dose regime for oral phenoxymethyl penicillin is 250 mg every six hours for five to seven days, and for clindamycin, 250 mg every six hours, also for five to seven days. Antibiotic therapy may need to be changed depending upon the results of culture and sensitivity.

Osteomyelitis

Operative treatment: if possible, remove the sequestra and any remaining portions of necrotic bone.
Non-operative treatment: initial treatment with intramuscular benzylpenicillin, 600 mg six-hourly, followed by phenoxymethyl penicillin, 250 mg six-hourly. Lincomycin and clindamycin may be useful alternatives to penicillin in this condition. Antibiotic treatment should be continued for 5 to 10 days depending on the severity of the osteomyelitis. Any pus obtained from the wound should be sent for culture and sensitivity, and antibiotic therapy will depend upon these findings.

Pericoronitis

Operative treatment: extract the opposing upper third molar, or reduce the cusps if they are traumatizing the swollen gingival tissue around the erupting lower third molar. Once the pericoronitis has resolved, the lower third molar should be removed.

Non-operative treatment: hot salt-water mouth washes (one teaspoon of salt in a cup of hot water) may be of benefit in pericoronitis. Such mouthwashes should be used every two hours until the inflammation resolves. Trichloroacetic acid can be placed under the gingival tissues and then immediately neutralized with glycerine. The efficacy of this treatment is not established and great care should be taken when the caustic is applied. Moderate cases of pericoronitis should be treated with oral antibiotics, either metronidazole, 200 mg every eight hours for five days, or phenoxymethyl penicillin, 250 mg every six hours for five days. Severe cases with trismus, marked buccal swelling, pyrexia, and lymphadeno-pathy should be treated with intramuscular penicillin, 600 mg, or penicillin triple injection, which contains benethamine penicillin 475 mg, procaine penicillin 250 mg, and benzylpenicillin sodium 300 mg.

Acute ulcerative gingivitis

Operative treatment: local debridement of the gingival tissues and removal of a supra-gingival calculus if possible.

Non-operative treatment: If the condition is mild then oxygen-releasing agents, such as hydrogen peroxide or sodium peroxyborate, may be of some benefit. For the moderate to severe cases, oral metronidazole is the treatment of choice (200–400 mg every eight hours for three to five days depending on severity).

Periodontal abscess

Operative treatment: curettage of the pocket to establish drainage and irrigation with 0.2 per cent chlorhexidine.

Non-operative treatment: hot salt-water mouth baths should be prescribed to encourage drainage. Severe cases should be treated with oral antibiotics; penicillin or metronidazole are both efficacious. Where possible, the patient should be instructed to irrigate the periodontal pocket with 0.2 per cent chlorhexidine solution.

Acute herpetic gingivostomatitis

Non-operative treatment: reduce the pyrexia with either aspirin or paracetamol (Aspirin cannot be given to children under 12 years of age because of the risk of Reyes syndrome). The patient should be kept well-hydrated. Idoxuridine 0.1 per cent solution should be painted on the lesions, but this may prove difficult in children. Chlorhexidine 0.2 per cent mouthwash should be used six-hourly to reduce the incidence of secondary infection. Severe or generalized cases may need to be treated with oral acyclovir, 200 mg five times daily for five days.

Teething

Operative treatment: massage the gums over the erupting tooth or allow the baby to chew on something hard.

Non-operative treatment: choline salicylate (Bonjela) rubbed into the gums may be of some benefit. Paracetamol elixir (5–10 ml) should be prescribed to reduce the pyrexia that often accompanies 'teething'.

Herpes labialis

Operative treatment: if patient is prone to herpes labialis, avoid trauma to the lips during dental procedures, and keep the lips coated with vaseline.

Non-operative treatment: idoxuridine 5 per cent in dimethyl sulphoxide should be applied at the earliest opportunity every two hours. Alternatively, acyclovir cream can be used.

Postoperative dental pain

Non-operative treatment: pain after a dental surgical procedure is usually of short duration and responds to aspirin or any of the other NSAIDs. Dosages should be taken every four to six hours. If pain persists after 48 hours, then secondary infection may have occurred and this should be treated with antibiotics. Analgesics recommended are aspirin 1 g, paracetamol 1 g, ibuprofen 400 mg, and diflunisal 500 mg.

Postoperative swelling and trismus

Non-operative treatment: cold compresses applied buccally and hot salt-water mouth baths may be appropriate local measures to reduce swelling. Aspirin or one of the other NSAIDs will help to reduce postoperative swelling and trismus. The pre-operative administration of corticosteroids has been shown to be of some benefit in reducing the incidence and magnitude of swelling after dental surgical procedures (see Chapter 4). Steroids used for this purpose include intramuscular dexamethasone 20 mg, methylprednisolone 80 mg, and hydrocortisone 100 mg. Steroids are administered one to two hours before surgery, and may be repeated six hours after surgery.

Dry socket (alveolar osteitis)

Operative treatment: the socket should be irrigated with warm saline to remove any remains of blood clot.

Non-operative treatment: a sedative dressing should be placed in the socket; examples include ribbon gauze soaked in Whiteheads varnish or bismuth iodoform paste (BIPP). Alternatively, cotton wool impregnated with zinc oxide and eugenol may help to reduce the pain commonly associated with this condition. Such socket dressings are not without problems and may cause necrosis of bone. Inert cores impregnated with a variety of antibiotics have been tested for reducing the incidence of 'dry socket' after tooth extraction. Of those evaluated, tetracycline appears to be the most efficacious. Patients should be prescribed analgesics, either aspirin or other NSAIDs, to help reduce pain. Prophylactic systemic antibiotics should be considered in patients prone to dry sockets; phenoxymethyl penicillin is the antibiotic of choice.

Sinusitis

Operative treatment: ensure that the antrum is free of foreign bodies, such as root fragments, and that there is no oro-antral fistula present. Recurrent cases should be treated by antral washout.
Non-operative treatment: inhalations with either menthol and benzion 2 per cent, or menthol and eucalyptus dissolved in hot water. Ephedrine nose drops, 0.5 per cent will produce vasoconstriction of the nasal mucosa and facilitate drainage. Acute cases should be treated with antibiotics; doxycycline 200 mg as an initial dose, followed by 100 mg daily, is particularly effective. Alternatively, any of the broad-spectrum penicillins can be used.

Candidal infections
Thrush

Non-operative treatment: a two-week course of nystatin lozenges, 500 000 units, four times a day; alternatively, amphotericin B lozenges 10 mg, four times a day for two weeks, or miconazole gel, 5–10 ml, four times daily. All preparations are held in the mouth for as long as possible then finally swallowed.

Angular cheilitis

Operative treatment: in edentulous patients, check the vertical height of their dentures. Investigate blood for deficiencies of iron, folate, and vitamin B_{12}.
Non-operative treatment: Sore areas should be treated with a topical antifungal agent, such as nystatin cream, amphotericin cream, or miconazole cream; creams should be applied four times a day.

Denture stomatitis

Operative treatment: leave out dentures as much as possible and keep them in a cleansing agent such as sodium hypochlorite. Dentures should be replaced when the condition resolves. Full haematological investigation should be carried out.
Non-operative treatment: the dentures should be left out, and the patient given

nystatin pastilles or amphotericin B lozenges to suck four times a day. However, patients will be reluctant to leave their dentures out for any length of time. When inserted, the denture fitting surface should be coated with miconazole cream.

Candidal leukoplakia

Operative treatment: biopsy or, if small, surgical excision and graft.
Non-operative treatment: miconazole appears to be the antifungal of choice for this condition; treatment may have to be continued for several months.

Minor aphthous ulceration

Operative treatment: remove local causes of irritation, such as sharp edges of teeth and restorations; check that the clasps of appliances or dentures are not traumatizing the oral mucosa. Investigate blood for deficiencies of iron, vitamin B_{12}, and folate.
Non-operative treatment: chlorhexidine mouthwash 0.2 per cent or a tetracycline mouthwash (DPF) may reduce the incidence of secondary infection associated with aphthous ulceration. Carmellose gelatine paste DPF may provide a mechanical protection of the oral mucosa. Hydrocortisone pellets (2.5 mg) are useful if the patient gets a prodromal symptom, i.e. a tingling sensation in the oral mucosa prior to the ulcers breaking out; the pellets should be applied to the area every six hours and allowed to dissolve. Once ulcers have occurred, triamcinolone acetonide dental paste or betamethasone aerosal spray applied six-hourly may help.

Major aphthous ulceration

Operative treatment: check for haematological deficiencies.
Non-operative treatment: as above for minor aphthous ulceration, but the condition usually requires treatment with systemic corticosteroids. Prednisolone is the treatment of choice, and the dose regime will depend upon the severity of the condition. Very severe cases may need treatment with azathioprine.

Xerostomia

Operative treatment: investigate salivary glands for mechanical obstruction, i.e. calculi.
Non-operative treatment: repeated application of fluoride is necessary to prevent caries, which has a high incidence in dry mouths. Artificial saliva may be of some help. Sugar-free fruit pastilles and chewing gum may promote any residual salivary flow.

Index